Third Edition

A Practical Approach to
PEDIATRIC ENDOCRINOLOGY

Third Edition

A Practical Approach to
PEDIATRIC ENDOCRINOLOGY

George E. Bacon, M.D.
Professor and Chairman
Department of Pediatrics
Texas Tech University
Chief, Pediatric Service
Lubbock General Hospital
Lubbock, Texas

Martha L. Spencer, M.D.
Chairman, Department of Pediatrics
Park Nicollet Medical Center
Vice President of Youth
International Diabetes Center
St. Louis Park, Minnesota

Nancy J. Hopwood, M.D.
Professor, Department of Pediatrics
Section of Pediatric Endocrinology
University of Michigan
Ann Arbor, Michigan

Robert P. Kelch, M.D.
Professor and Chairman
Department of Pediatrics
University of Michigan
Physician-in-Chief
C.S. Mott Children's Hospital
Ann Arbor, Michigan

YEAR BOOK MEDICAL PUBLISHERS, INC.
CHICAGO • LONDON • BOCA RATON • LITTLETON, MASS.

1 2 3 4 5 6 7 8 9 0 M R 94 93 92 91 90

Library of Congress Cataloging-in-Publication Data
A practical approach to pediatric endocrinology / George E. Bacon . . .
[et al]. — 3rd ed.
    p.   cm.
    Includes bibliographical references.
    ISBN 0-8151-0405-7
    1. Pediatric endocrinology.   I. Bacon, George E., 1932-
    [DNLM: 1. Endocrine Diseases—in infancy & childhood.   WS 330
P895]
RJ418.P7   1990   89-22484
618.92'4—dc20   CIP
DNLM/DLC
for Library of Congress

Sponsoring Editor: Bethany L. Caldwell
Assistant Managing Editor, Text and Reference Books: Jan Gardner
Production Project Coordinator: Diane K. Purcell
Proofroom Supervisor: Barbara M. Kelly

Preface

Like the first two editions, this book is designed as a practical guide for the medical student, pediatric house officer, and practicing pediatrician. It may also be of value as a preliminary text for beginning fellows in pediatric endocrinology, but is not intended to be as detailed as the more exhaustive works currently available. In general, the chapters deal with disease entities rather than organ systems, and greater attention is given to those disorders that occur most frequently. Many of the special studies commonly utilized in pediatric endocrinology are described in the appendices, and extensive references are provided at the end of each chapter for further study.

In this third edition, additional endocrine physiology appropriate to the ensuing subject matter has been provided at the beginning of most chapters, and we have endeavored to make the substantial revisions necessary to encompass the new or changing information that has accumulated since the previous edition. For example, education and management of children with newly diagnosed diabetes on an outpatient basis is emphasized, newer concepts of the interpretation of growth hormone data and the treatment of short stature are reviewed, and our expanding knowledge and understanding of the broad spectrum of congenital adrenal hyperplasia is discussed. Thyroid screening programs, barely under way when the first edition was published nearly 15 years ago, have subsequently proved to be a major factor in the diagnosis and successful treatment of congenital hypothyroidism, and data derived from these programs are presented.

Finally, in most cases we have not attempted to define precisely what could be accomplished in a private office setting and what should be referred for evaluation and management by a pediatric endocrinologist; rather we have chosen to present a practical plan for diagnosis and treatment, and allow the reader to determine at which point his or her comfort level dictates that referral is appropriate.

George E. Bacon, M.D.
Martha L. Spencer, M.D.
Nancy J. Hopwood, M.D.
Robert P. Kelch, M.D.

Acknowledgment

Once more, we express our gratitude to Frances Rupp (University of Michigan), who provided the sole secretarial support for the first two editions and vowed never to do it again—but did anyway. For this third edition, the assistance of Mary Lou Smith (Texas Tech University) is likewise greatly appreciated. Our sincere thanks to both for their vital contributions to the preparation of this book.

George E. Bacon, M.D.
Martha L. Spencer, M.D.
Nancy J. Hopwood, M.D.
Robert P. Kelch, M.D.

Contents

Diabetes Mellitus

DIAGNOSIS AND TREATMENT

Diabetes mellitus is a common metabolic abnormality in children. In the United States it affects about 1.6 per 1,000 school-age children.[1,2] The impact of diabetes on the quality of life and on mortality and morbidity through the development of complications is enormous. Health care providers have a responsibility to help the child maintain as normal a metabolic state as possible while facilitating child and family adjustment to this chronic disease. Each child and its family react differently to the physical and emotional stresses of diabetes and must be treated on an individual basis.

Classification

Diabetes is a group of disorders with glucose intolerance in common. It is associated with abnormalities in carbohydrate, fat, and protein metabolism and with the development of abnormalities of small blood vessels, large blood vessels, and nerves. These disorders have been classified into three clinically and pathologically different types: type I, insulin-dependent diabetes mellitus (IDDM); type II, non-insulin-dependent diabetes (NIDDM); and other types resulting from or associated with specific conditions or syndromes[3] (Table 1–1). Modifications of this classification will probably be made as disorders are better defined.

TABLE 1-1.
Classification of Glucose Intolerance*

Diabetes mellitus
Type I: Insulin-dependent
Type II: Non-insulin-dependent
Nonobese
Obese
Other types (drugs, pancreatitis,
syndromes)
Impaired glucose tolerance
Gestational diabetes
Previous abnormality of glucose tolerance
Potential abnormality of glucose tolerance

* Adapted from the National Diabetes Data Group. *Diabetes* 1979; 28:1039.

Etiology

Type I diabetes occurs primarily in children. They are insulinopenic and ketosis develops easily. Ninety-five percent of persons with type I diabetes have either DR3 or DR4 histocompatibility leukocyte antigen. Inheritance of one of these antigens increases the risk of developing IDDM threefold to fivefold over that of the general population; when both are present, the risk increases tenfold to 20-fold.[4]

Genetic factors alone are inadequate to explain the onset of type I diabetes. Environmental factors such as viruses and drugs have been proposed to initiate an autoimmune process in beta cell destruction in susceptible persons. This process may take months to years. Islet cell antibodies and insulin antibodies are evidence that the destruction is ongoing. The earliest detectable abnormality in insulin secretion is a progressive reduction of first-phase plasma insulin response to intravenous glucose stimulation. Overt glucose intolerance can be demonstrated when insulin secretory reserves are less than 20% of normal.[5, 6]

In an attempt to link these observations, it has been suggested that a virus (or other environmental factors) may be an inciting factor for the development of diabetes, in persons with the appropriate genetic predisposition, by way of an autoimmune mechanism.

Accurate genetic counseling is difficult, and statistics on the relative risk of developing clinical diabetes are approximations. The observed risk to individuals with one first-degree relative with IDDM is less than 5%. Concordance rates in identical twins are less than 50%.[6] More specific counseling should be possible as the group of disorders that result in diabetes is better defined.

In contrast, type II diabetes more often develops in persons over 40 years of age who are obese. Insulin levels may be low, normal, or high. The presentation is insidious, with minimal or no symptoms. Ketosis is usually not present except with stress. A subgroup of type II diabetes, maturity-onset diabetes of youth, has been described that is autosomal dominant. Children in these families frequently have abnormal blood glucose levels with infection.[7]

In a few patients diabetes is difficult to categorize as either type I or type II. There is no reliable test that differentiates between the two types. The clinical course may be the distinguishing feature. For example, some black youths with typical signs and symptoms of type I diabetes tolerate being without insulin therapy for prolonged periods. Studies show that they have more endogenous insulin secretion than most persons with type I diabetes but less than that in persons with type II. It seems to be dominantly inherited and nonautoimmune.[8]

Children in high-risk minority groups (Hispanic, Native American, black) may have type II diabetes. Diagnosis and intervention with diet and exercise early, as well as preventive health maintenance are important.

Diabetes mellitus and glucose intolerance are also associated with other diseases, drugs, and syndromes. The incidence of diabetes in children with cystic fibrosis is reported to be about 7.6% and is associated with progressive clinical deterioration.[9]

Diagnosis of Insulin-Dependent Diabetes Mellitus

Most children experience an abrupt onset of IDDM, with polydipsia, polyuria, enuresis, and weight loss. Frequently, a urinary tract infection is suspected. When a family is aware of these symptoms, recognition is rarely delayed more than 2 weeks, and weight loss is minimal. Occasionally children are seen with a protracted course of intermittent glucosuria and poor weight gain (Table 1–2). An oral glucose tolerance test (OGTT) is not necessary once a child has

TABLE 1–2.
Presenting Characteristics of Diabetes Mellitus in 250 Children (University of Michigan)

Presence of one or more of the following symptoms:	89%
Polydipsia Polyuria	
Enuresis Fatigue	
Weight loss Abdominal pain	
Sticky urine Infection	
Patients asymptomatic; glucosuria detected on routine examination	11%
Duration of symptoms	
<1 month	63%
1–2 months	27%
>2 months	10%
Age at diagnosis	
<1 year	2%
1–5 years	37%
6–10 years	41%
11–15 years	20%*

* This figure may be biased since it includes only adolescents treated in the Pediatric Endocrine Clinic.

exhibited glucosuria, elevated random plasma glucose (greater than 200 mg/dL), preferably on at least two occasions, and symptoms.

The peak age of onset of symptoms in our experience is 9 years, with only 2% of patients diagnosed before the age of 1 year.

If appropriate ambulatory facilities are available, hospitalization of children with IDDM is usually not necessary unless they have diabetic ketoacidosis or there are complicating medical or psychosocial factors. Occasionally children are stabilized with intravenous fluids as either hospitalized patients or outpatients and then followed up in an ambulatory setting. The advantages of such an approach in addition to reduced cost are the continuity of medical care; the immediate assumption of diabetes care by the family and child; and more realistic nutrition, activity, and insulin adjustment in the home setting.[10]

The initial education of the family involves three appointments of 2 to 3 hours each with the health care team, which consists of a physician, nurse educator, nutritionist, and a family counselor. There is a follow-up visit in 1 to 2 weeks, with frequent phone contact in the interim.

The physician conducts a medical history and physical examination, supervises insulin adjustment, and is available on 24-hour call. The diabetes nurse educator and dietitian focus on providing the patient with the basic (survival) knowledge and skills to manage diabetes. A more extensive educational program is recommended in 3 to 6 months.

Much of the initial anxiety centers around the first blood test and insulin injection. This is done immediately by the child who is old enough (usually age 7 years and older) or by a member of the family. All family members are encouraged to give themselves an injection of saline solution.

Once this is accomplished, a simplified explanation of the pathophysiology of diabetes can be given so the child and family will understand the rationale for the treatment plan. Acute complications such as hyperglycemia and hypoglycemia are discussed, as are brief illnesses. Each session begins with a review of blood glucose and urine ketone test records. Blood glucose self-testing is taught using visually read strips so that children can test in any place and at any time.

The nutritionist obtains a history of usual food intake and food preferences. The importance of consistency in timing of meals and the amount of food consumed is stressed. A simplified meal plan is given. At the next appointment an individualized meal plan using the exchange system is introduced. The average daily caloric needs may be calculated as 1,000 kcal plus 100 kcal per year of age until the child is 12 years old. During adolescence boys often need 3,000 to 4,000 kcal, and girls need to decrease their intake depending on activity level. Lifestyle issues such as work, school, dating, and sports are discussed during the last session (see Appendix 1-E).

The counselor is introduced as part of the health care team and emphasizes the interrelationship between emotions and blood glucose levels. The family's coping strategies and psychosocial concerns are identified. Counseling may be suggested when indicated.

The initial insulin dose consists of a mixture of short-acting (regular insulin,

insulin injection) and intermediate-acting (insulin zinc suspension, lente; iso-phane insulin suspension, NPH) human insulin. A child with moderate to large urine ketone bodies may need 0.3 to 0.4 U/kg given in a ratio of 2:3 regular-intermediate insulin. Subsequent insulin doses range from 0.7 to 1 U/kg/24 hr, with approximately two thirds given before breakfast and one third given before supper.

The ratio of regular-intermediate insulin is usually between 1:3 and 1:1. Children without urine ketones may be more sensitive to insulin. Therefore, the initial dose is 0.2 U/kg, with subsequent needs of 0.4 to 0.5 U/kg/24hr.

Insulin doses are modified according to blood glucose responses. The blood glucose goals initially are 120 to 240 mg/dL. These are modified quickly to 70 to 180 mg/dL after the first few days (Appendix 1–A).

Children have constantly changing insulin requirements, associated not only with insulin reserve but also with growth, activity, and stress. Each child needs an individualized insulin regimen. The average preadolescent requires a daily amount of insulin equivalent to about three times age in years, or 0.5 to 1 U/kg. Insulin requirements tend to increase rapidly during adolescence, and then decrease somewhat when adulthood is reached (Fig 1–1).

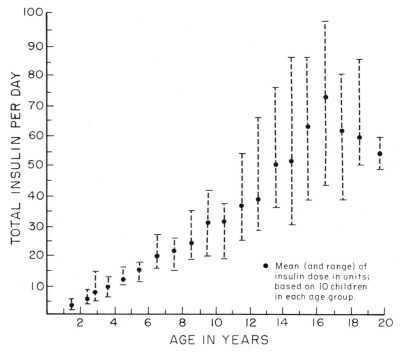

FIG 1–1.
Mean daily insulin requirement in relation to age (University of Michigan).

About 60% to 70% of children with diabetes experience an early remission phase ("honeymoon" period) during which little or no insulin is required. This phenomenon, which is probably due to transient recovery of beta cell function,[6] usually occurs within a few weeks after treatment is initiated and may persist for weeks or even months. We generally recommend that a child continue to take 1 or 2 U of insulin daily even if none is necessary. This practice tends to reduce the psychologic trauma related to reinstitution of insulin shots.

Knowledge of insulin timing and action (Appendix 1–B) as well as the results of blood glucose self-testing is necessary to determine an appropriate insulin regimen. In most instances, children are started on the twice-a-day mixed regular-intermediate insulin regimen described. Table 1–3 shows other regular-intermediate regimens.

Changes in insulin dose are based on blood glucose patterns (Appendix 1–C). Food intake, activity, stress, and insulin all affect blood glucose test results. In children it is rare for any of these to be consistent or predictable; therefore, it is important to *prevent* high or low blood glucose levels rather than *react* to them. Usually only one insulin is adjusted, 0.5 to 2 U at a time. Regular insulin may be diluted (e.g., 1:1, 1:4) to allow more accuracy to insulin adjustments for children receiving small doses.

Supplements (adding or subtracting regular insulin) may be used when blood glucose control is not stable or there is a planned increase in food or activity. These are temporary insulin adjustments and should be recorded separately.

It is extremely important to test after using a supplement to see whether it was successful and to use this information for future adjustments. When supplements are consistently needed at a particular time of day, the basic insulin dosage should be adjusted.

Monitoring the success of the health care plan involves daily blood glucose testing by the child or family. Children are usually asked to test their blood before each meal and at bedtime. Additional tests may be needed at 2:00 or 3:00 AM, before and after exercise, when ill, or when a low blood glucose level is

TABLE 1–3.
Intermediate (NPH) and Regular (R)
Mixtures*

AM	Noon	Supper	Bedtime
NPH	—	NPH	—
R		R	
NPH	—	NPH	—
R	R	R	—
NPH	—	—	NPH
R	—	R	—
NPH	—	NPH	—
R	R	R	R
R	R	R	NPH

* See Appendix 1-B for explanation.

suspected. This is the best way for a person with diabetes to learn about diabetes and how the body reacts to different situations. Usually new patients start testing with visually read strips. Use of meters is taught after 3 to 6 months if desired. Many meters are available; all are accurate if the test is done carefully and the meter is maintained. Problems that arise are usually the result of poor technique, poor timing, and inaccurate recording. Memory meters are helpful, but the family still needs to observe blood glucose patterns to adjust the insulin dose.

The blood glucose records should be reviewed quarterly by the health care team, and a hemoglobin A_1 (glycosylated hemoglobin) level obtained. The hemoglobin A_1 or A_{1c} assay provides an objective measure of the average blood glucose levels for the previous 4 to 6 weeks.[11]

The child's blood pressure, height, and weight are plotted; clinical thyroid status and injection sites should also be assessed every 3 to 4 months. Urinary protein should be monitored annually, preferably by a microalbumin test.[12] Evaluation of the retinas by direct ophthalmoscopic examination is particularly important after puberty. Fasting lipid profiles are assessed every 2 years.

Treatment of Ketoacidosis and Hyperosmolar Diabetic Coma

Correction of ketoacidosis and hyperglycemia is dependent on reversal of the pathophysiologic derangement. Insulin deficiency results in decreased glucose utilization and increased gluconeogenesis, lipolysis, ketogenesis, and proteolysis. Triglycerides and cholesterol levels are elevated. The result is hyperglycemia that exceeds the renal threshold for glucose reabsorption, causing osmotic diuresis with water loss greater than that of electrolytes. Extracellular hyperglycemia also causes intracellular dehydration and depletion of intracellular potassium. Thus treatment consists of:

1. Insulin.
2. Replacement of water and electrolytes.
3. Correction of acidosis.
4. Replacement of caloric deficiencies.

Ketoacidosis is suspected with the onset of polydipsia, polyuria, weight loss (which can be profound over a short time), abdominal pain, and vomiting. If diabetes has been previously diagnosed, alert parents and children can reverse early symptoms (polydipsia and polyuria) with extra insulin as needed, based on frequent monitoring of blood glucose and ketones. Once a child is vomiting secondary to ketoacidosis, the progression to serious acidosis is rapid, and intravenous (IV) fluids become necessary. In severe acidosis (CO_2 <10 mEq/L), the characteristic Kussmaul breathing is obvious. Children generally are mentally alert; if not, other causes for change of sensorium should be sought.

Initial laboratory studies should include serum electrolytes, glucose, urea nitrogen, ketones, and complete urinalysis. A milky plasma indicates hyperlipemia, which may be marked in some patients. Serum ketones may be measured, but this is not necessary. Once treatment is instituted, a careful search is made for any infection that could be a precipitating factor. A detailed flow sheet is maintained to record vital signs, laboratory data, urine test results, urine volume, IV fluids, and insulin dose. Catheterization of the bladder is not necessary, nor is gastric aspiration, unless the patient is comatose.

The details of therapy vary greatly among physicians, but are based on the same principles. Individualization and close monitoring are essential. Traditionally, large doses of insulin were used because of "insulin resistance." However, it is now well established that small doses of insulin are effective, given as a continuous IV infusion, intramuscularly (IM), or subcutaneously (SC). Complications with hypokalemia and hypoglycemia are less frequent.[13–16]

Continuous IV infusion is a simple physiologic method of administering insulin and allows greater flexibility in blood glucose regulation. A "priming" dose of insulin is not necessary.[17] Twenty units of regular insulin are added to 100 mL of normal saline solution. Some of this mixture is run through the IV tubing and discarded, "saturating" the insulin binding sites in the tubing. An infusion pump controls the rate of infusion, which is calculated initially to provide 0.1 U/kg/hr of insulin. This rate is adjusted to provide a decrease in blood glucose of approximately 100 mg/dL/hr. When the blood glucose level approaches 250 mg/dL, 5% glucose is added to the electrolyte solution. The use of IV insulin should be continued until the acidosis is largely corrected (pH >7.3, bicarbonate >15 mEq/L). Because this may follow the fall in blood glucose by several hours, the insulin infusion rate may need to be decreased to maintain blood glucose concentration between 100 and 150 mg/dL. One-half hour before discontinuing the infusion, SC regular insulin, 0.25 to 0.5 U/kg, or the patient's usual insulin dose, should be given.

The initial IM dose of regular insulin in the treatment of ketoacidosis is 0.25 U/kg, followed by hourly doses of 0.1 U/kg IM.[16]

Subcutaneous administration of insulin usually requires a "priming" dose of 0.5 U/kg regular insulin, half of which is given IV and the remainder SC. Additional SC doses of 0.25 to 0.5 U/kg regular insulin are given every 3 to 4 hours.

Maintenance requirements of fluid and electrolytes in children consist of 80 mL of water per kilogram body weight for infants, decreasing to 30 to 40 mL/kg for adolescents and adults, and 2 to 3 mEq of both sodium and potassium/kg.[18]

Fluid deficits in children with diabetes average about 100 mL/kg (10% dehydration).[19] Calculation of fluid replacement is based on a correction of losses over 24 hours, with half given in the first 8 hours and the remainder over the next 16 hours.

Body potassium stores are depleted as a consequence of acidosis, diuresis, and vomiting.[20] Generally, initial serum potassium levels are normal or increased because of the shift from intracellular to extracellular fluid accompanying an increase in hydrogen ion concentration. With correction of acidosis, serum potassium concentration rapidly declines and hypokalemia is a frequent complication.

Replacement therapy consists of 40 mEq of potassium chloride or phosphate per liter of fluid. (The latter has been less commonly used but probably is preferable because phosphate stores are depleted in ketoacidosis.)[21] Large amounts of phosphate potentiate hypocalcemia; thus we advise using an equal mixture of potassium chloride and neutral potassium phosphate salts.[22, 23] Larger amounts of potassium salts (e.g., 80 mEq/L of fluid) may be given if necessary, with careful monitoring of T waves by electrocardiography. Traditionally, potassium has been withheld until urinary flow has been established; however, this policy probably is unnecessarily conservative and may contribute to hypokalemia in some patients. Close attention to serum potassium concentration is essential.

Initially, normal saline solution, 20 mL/kg, may be given over 1 hour to expand extracellular volume, improve circulation, and enhance renal function. Thereafter, a more hypotonic solution of 0.33% to 0.45% saline is appropriate.

Serum sodium concentration is falsely low in the presence of hyperglycemia, secondary to the extracellular shift of intracellular water to compensate for hyperosmolality. Serum sodium is thereby decreased 1.6 mEq/L for every 100 mg/dL rise in serum glucose above 100 mg/dL.[24] Hyperlipemia also causes spuriously low laboratory measurements of electrolytes. Underestimation of serum sodium probably is not significant unless hypertonic sodium solutions are administered.

There is no consensus on the use of alkali. After initial respiratory stimulation, severe acidosis (plasma pH less than 7.1) may depress respiration by a direct effect on the respiratory center as well as impairing cardiovascular function.[25] However, rapid IV administration of sodium bicarbonate may cause a paradoxical cerebrospinal fluid acidosis while plasma pH is normalized,[26] and rapid correction of plasma pH with alkali shifts the oxygen dissociation curve to the left, causing decreased oxygen supply to the tissues and potentiating the development of lactic acidosis.[27, 28] The significance of this latter finding is disputed by Munk et al.[29] Treatment with hydration and insulin *alone* usually corrects the metabolic acidosis by interrupting ketogenesis and permitting endogenous bicarbonate production.[14]

Our present recommendation is to use sodium bicarbonate, 2 mEq/kg, infused over one-half hour when the plasma pH is less than 7.1. This may be repeated in 1 hour if there has been no improvement.

Summary of Therapy for Diabetic Ketoacidosis

1. *Regular insulin*:
   SC: 0.5 U/kg (half IV, half SC) followed by 0.25 U/kg SC every 2 to 4 hours, or
   IM: 0.25 U/kg followed by 0.1 U/kg IM hourly, or
   IV: 0.1 U/kg/hr infusion. (This is the most popular program. Also, an initial bolus of 0.1 U/kg IV can be given if blood glucose level is very high or usual daily insulin dose has not been administered, although this is controversial and not proved to be necessary.[17])
2. *Fluids*:
   Maintenance: (dependent on age) 30 to 80 mL/kg/24 hr.

Deficit: usually 100 mL/kg (10% dehydration).
3. *Sodium*: Normal (0.9%) saline solution, initially 20 mL/kg over 1 hour, then 0.33% to 0.45% solution. Monitor with serum sodium determinations.
4. *Potassium*: Give 40 mEq potassium salts (phosphate and chloride) per liter of fluid; 60 to 80 mEq/L may be given *with caution* if necessary. Monitor with serum potassium determinations and electrocardiogram. (Note that serum potassium level may be normal in the presence of total body depletion.)
5. *Bicarbonate*: If serum bicarbonate is <10 mEq/L or venous pH <7.1, calculate dose of sodium bicarbonate based on 2 mEq/kg; infuse over one-half hour.
6. *Glucose*: Add 5% solution when blood glucose is <250 mg/dL.

Hazards of treatment are (1) hypokalemia, (2) hypernatremia; (3) water intoxication and cerebral edema, and (4) late hypoglycemia.

Hyperosmolar diabetic coma is characterized by severe hyperglycemia, dehydration, and elevated serum osmolality. Metabolic acidosis is a feature of the syndrome in children (although not in adults), but ketonuria is minimal or absent. The typical clinical history is that of rather acute onset of fever, anorexia, vomiting, and progressive stupor, usually developing within 48 hours. Frequently there is little or no previous evidence of diabetes mellitus, although a strong family history may be obtained. There is a high incidence of preexisting neurologic disorders.[30, 31]

Chemically, blood glucose concentration often is 750 to 1,500 mg/dL. Total cation (sodium and potassium) usually exceeds the anion (chloride and bicarbonate) by more than 25 mEq/L. The unidentified anion may be largely lactate (lactic acidosis) or other organic acids.

Serum osmolality (mOsm/L) may be estimated by the formula:

$$\frac{2 \times \text{Serum sodium (mEq/L)} + \text{Blood glucose (mg/dL)}}{18} + \frac{\text{Blood urea nitrogen (mg/dL)}}{2.8}$$

Levels well in excess of 300 mOsm/L are observed, compared with the normal of approximately 290 mOsm/L.

The essence of treatment of hyperosmolar nonketotic coma is *slow* correction of the fluid deficit to reduce the risk of cerebral edema. Isotonic solution (0.9% saline) is recommended if this diagnosis is suspected. Blood glucose concentration should be determined frequently, because extreme insulin resistance has been reported.[31] Thrombotic episodes may occur,[30] and the mortality rate is about 50%.

Cerebral Edema

Cerebral edema develops suddenly several hours after treatment has begun.

The onset is marked by an abrupt change in the level of consciousness. Respiratory arrest may occur in association with herniation of the brain stem. The mortality of cerebral edema complicating ketoacidosis is very high.[32]

Brain swelling has been described to occur in asymptomatic patients with diabetic ketoacidosis.[33] It is thought that an osmotic dysequilibrium may occur between the central nervous system and extracellular fluid during treatment of diabetic ketoacidosis, with water moving into the brain.[34] Insulin, bicarbonate, and excessive or hypotonic fluid have also been implicated. Cerebral edema is treated with intubation, hyperventilation, and other methods to reduce intracranial pressure (e.g., mannitol).

Therapeutic Goals

Each physician has criteria for good diabetes management and methods for achieving it. The American Diabetes Association has endorsed the policy of urging physicians to strive for as normal a metabolic state as possible in their patients, while acknowledging the difficulties encountered in trying to achieve this in children.[35] Some children do not adhere to their diet, change their insulin dose appropriately, or test their blood frequently, and yet they are in good control by some criteria. On the other hand, some show a course of instability even though they adhere strictly to the regimen. In our clinics, important therapeutic goals are:

1. To achieve as normal a metabolic state as possible.
2. To encourage a realistic attitude toward diabetes.
3. To promote emotional well-being of the child and family.
4. To provide the child and family with knowledge of diabetes to enable them to assume a primary role in daily diabetes management.
5. To encourage the family to share the responsibility for management of the diabetes appropriately with health care providers.

Criteria to assess attainment of these goals are detailed in Appendix 1-A.

The universal goal is prevention of vascular complications. Unfortunately, until complete normalization of blood glucose levels is feasible, the controversy about the degree to which vascular changes of diabetes are secondary to the biochemical abnormalities will remain unresolved.[36–40] (See the section on Summary of Current Research.) Continuous blood glucose monitoring affirms the within-day and day-to-day variability that emphasizes the lack of normal blood glucose homeostasis even in "stable" diabetes. In the meantime, the best biochemical control *practicable* with the methods available, taking into consideration the child's comfort and ability to live a happy and rewarding life, is the objective of treatment.

COMMON MANAGEMENT PROBLEMS

Growth and Development

Growth rate is one parameter used to assess metabolic control in children with diabetes. A syndrome of poorly controlled juvenile diabetes, short stature, truncal obesity, and hepatomegaly was first described by Mauriac in 1930.[41] Abnormalities of Mauriac's syndrome tend to resolve with better control of diabetes. A study involving monozygotic twins, one of whom developed diabetes before the onset of puberty, reported that the affected twin was significantly shorter (mean of 2 inches) in 11 of 12 pairs, even though diabetes control was judged adequate.[42] However, other studies indicate that children with diabetes are of average height.[43] Data from the University of Michigan Pediatric Endocrine Clinic support this observation (Fig 1–2). Jackson et al. reported that only children in lesser degrees of control by their criteria (poor compliance, glycosuria, elevated hemoglobin A_1 or A_{1c}) have delayed growth and maturation.[44] Growth in poorly controlled diabetes may be related to abnormalities in net somatomedin activity.[45]

Hepatomegaly

Hepatomegaly in poorly controlled diabetes may occur without the associated features of Mauriac's syndrome. Liver function studies usually are normal, but serum lipids may be elevated. Liver biopsy reveals fat and glycogen deposits.[46]

Infections

Evidence has related altered immunologic defense mechanisms with ketoacidosis. However, these changes seem reversible with normalization of the metabolic state.[47, 48] Increased risk of infection may be associated with hyperglycemia, ketoacidosis, peripheral vascular insufficiency, and neuropathy. Candidiasis is a typical complication in children with persistent hyperglycemia. Staphylococcal infections are not more frequent in diabetics, but may be more severe. In summary, increased susceptibility to infection generally is not expected in the diabetic child whose blood glucose control is satisfactory and who is free of vascular and neurologic complications.

Hypoglycemia

Insulin reactions may occur with insulin overdose, with inadequate intake of food, or in association with excessive physical activity. Early symptoms of low blood glucose often consist of headache, hunger, fatigue, or inability to concentrate. Parents note irritability and personality changes in their children.

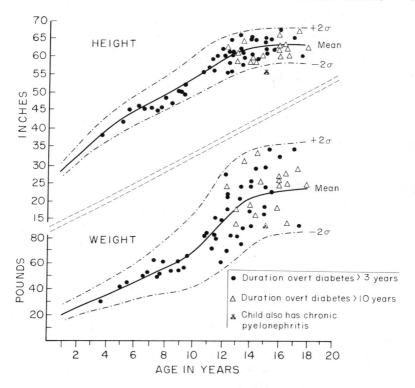

FIG 1–2.
Growth in height and weight of girls with prepubertal onset of diabetes (University of Michigan).

In severe hypoglycemia, coma can occur with or without convulsions.

Permanent neurologic sequelae may result from hypoglycemia.[49] The young child in particular seems to be at risk.[50] Repeated episodes appear to be a predictor for subsequent hypoglycemia. Many episodes can be prevented.[51] Hypoglycemia without warning (hypoglycemia unawareness) occurs more frequently in persons with diabetes of long duration or receiving an intensive insulin regimen.[52]

Treatment with 15 to 20 gm of carbohydrate in the form of sugar cubes or juice usually is successful. Injectable glucagon (available as a 1-mg kit with powder and diluting fluid) may be used when a child is unconscious and unable to accept glucose orally. Recovery occurs in 5 to 15 minutes if the patient has been treated promptly. It is important that parents be instructed in the use of this preparation, which should be available in the home at all times. Episodes of vomiting may occur as a result of glucagon administration or the hypoglycemia itself. When the child awakens, carbohydrate should be given orally to prevent relapse.

Ideally, potential periods of low blood glucose should be anticipated and prevented. More food may be necessary prior to increased physical activity, and simple sugars should be available at these times. If insulin reactions recur at similar times during the day, appropriate adjustment of insulin dose or diet can be made. Often the problem may be traced to insufficient calories or lack of protein with meals or snacks. Younger children, particularly, are prone to insulin reactions during the night because of their earlier bedtime and longer periods of sleep. An adequate evening snack is essential in such cases. It is also important that children with a history of early morning hypoglycemia not be allowed to sleep beyond the usual time.

Posthypoglycemic Hyperglycemia (Somogyi Effect)

Children are unpredictable in their eating habits, activity patterns, and emotional behavior. In addition, most children with diabetes have only minimal pancreatic function and may be unable to compensate for relatively small errors in insulin dosage. These conditions contribute to the wide, rapid fluctuations in blood glucose sometimes encountered. In an effort to reduce intermittent hyperglycemia, there is a natural tendency to administer excessive amounts of insulin. A possible consequence is the Somogyi effect: hypoglycemia followed by marked hyperglycemia, glucosuria, and ketonuria.[53, 54] Hypoglycemia often is asymptomatic and may not be reflected in routine tests. Hyperglycemia presumably results from release of endogenous glucose via secretion of cortisol, growth hormone, and catecholamines. Hyperglycemic phases lasting several days following a single episode of hypoglycemia have been reported.[55]

Posthypoglycemic hyperglycemia may be suspected in the following circumstances:

1. Rapid fluctuations of blood glucose tests.
2. Symptoms of hypoglycemia (hunger, headache, dizziness) despite marked hyperglycemia.
3. Random blood glucose determinations, particularly in the late evening or early morning, revealing hypoglycemia.
4. Sudden appearance of urine ketone bodies, particularly in the early morning.
5. Persistence of marked hyperglycemia despite increasing insulin dose.

If any of these conditions is present, a trial of gradual reduction of insulin dosage is justified and may be both diagnostic and therapeutic. A decrease in blood glucose level confirms that the problem was secondary to the Somogyi effect.

In some children diabetes is more difficult to manage and further documentation of the pattern of blood glucose fluctuations is required before appropriate changes in insulin dosage can be made. Twenty-four hour blood glucose profiles and daily diaries indicating time, quality, and quantity of food intake and exercise will help to clarify each child's individual daily routine at home (Appendix 1-C).

Fasting hyperglycemia and ketonuria can be an indication that more insulin is needed or a sign of too much insulin. Increased insulin requirements have been noted between 6:00 and 9:00 AM (dawn phenomenon).[56-58] However, note that the clinical significance of nocturnal hypoglycemia has recently been questioned.[58]

Insulin Resistance and Allergy

True insulin resistance (total dose exceeding 200 U/day in adults or more than 2 U/kg/day in children in the absence of ketoacidosis) is rare.[59] A few patients have been reported in whom insulin resistance to SC insulin resulted from increased insulin degradation. These patients responded to continuous intravenous infusions.[60]

Antibody formation may cause local allergic reactions to insulin consisting of erythema and induration at the injection site. Usually this resolves despite continued use of insulin. If serious hypersensitivity occurs, a change of insulin type may be beneficial. The antibodies causing these reactions may be related to species (beef, pork), to impurities present, or to zinc. Human insulins have alleviated the need to desensitize in most cases.

Lipodystrophy

Localized atrophy of subcutaneous fat is rare; however, hypertrophy may occur following repeated injections of insulin into the same site. Rotation of sites is essential.

Psychological Aspects

Emotional stress has been related to the onset of symptoms of IDDM.[61] While this may be one of many factors involved in the cause of IDDM, more convincing evidence supports the significant role of emotional stress on diabetes management. The ability of the family to incorporate the diabetes health care plan into their lifestyle depends on their adjustment to the diagnosis of diabetes and their ability to cope with its ramifications. This in turn affects the child's reaction to the diagnosis and his future psychological development. In addition, the child's adjustment probably has a significant effect on the family's response. Studies have related poorly controlled diabetes to chaotic family situations, unresolved conflicts, and inadequate coping mechanisms.[62, 63] Self-esteem of the child may be affected along with ego development, although the relationship of metabolic control to these factors is not clear.[64, 65] Longitudinal psychological studies of the child and family in relation to metabolic control are needed.

Emotional stress has been shown to precipitate ketoacidosis by means of "stress" hormones.[66, 67] This seems to occur more frequently with adolescents, but it is evident, and the stress more easily identified, in younger children.

Finally, the blood glucose level is directly related to a child's behavior; both hyperglycemia and, more frequently, hypoglycemia may be manifested by irritability, irrational behavior, and confusion. Thus diabetes management requires an understanding and appreciation of the psychological status of the child and family and its influence on metabolic control. Baseline psychosocial data need to be obtained on all children at the time of diagnosis so that problems in adjustment may be anticipated and counseling provided. Continued assessment of family interactions and providing time for discussions of developmental issues, such as peer relationships, school problems, and feelings of isolation and being "different," are the responsibility of the members of the health care team. Support groups consisting of parents of children with diabetes are valuable for resolving parenting concerns and for lessening parental feelings of isolation.

Diabetes and the Adolescent

Adolescence is a period of marked emotional as well as physical change. Teenagers with diabetes tend to react to stressful situations with emotional responses that are excessive and may precipitate episodes of hyperglycemia and ketonuria. Diabetes in the teenager complicates the process of establishing independence from the parents. Teenagers perceive diabetes as a flaw that impairs their self-image. Fear of the impact of diabetes on future vocational and marital plans is immense.[68] Unfortunately, these fears often distort teenagers' knowledge of their disease.[69]

Denial, projection, and regression are frequent mechanisms used by adolescents to cope with their diabetes. Denial is exemplified by poor adherence to diet, omission of insulin doses, and failure to test the urine. This behavior is reinforced by the secondary gain resulting from increased attention of parents and physician as they attempt to force compliance.

A study at the University of Michigan Pediatric Diabetes Research and Training Center revealed a marked decrease in the number of hospitalizations of adolescents with IDDM for recurrent episodes of ketoacidosis when the hospital ceased to be a haven from the stresses of home and school.[67] Projection of a patient's anger to the parents who "caused" the diabetes is common. Temporary regression also occurs. Parents must be understanding, but cannot allow their own guilt feelings to encourage these defense mechanisms. Threats and accusations are not appropriate.

Adolescents need to participate with their parents and other members of the diabetes team in developing their health care plan. The rationale for the plan is discussed as well as the consequences of deviating from the program. Peer pressures, particularly in respect to diet adherence, are recognized and discussed. Poor dietary habits are common in teenagers; a frequent pattern consists of periods of relative starvation followed by excessive eating. This cycle readily lends itself to improper insulin dosage. If ketoacidosis develops, it should be treated vigorously and the adolescent discharged promptly. The use of drugs and alcohol also is discussed openly. The possibility of severe hypoglycemic reactions following moderate alcohol ingestion is emphasized.[70, 71] All adolescents should be seen alone and their confidence respected except in circumstances where the adolescent might be harmful to self or others. However, communication with the family must be maintained. Although independence is encouraged, the family needs to provide the structure to enable easier adherence to the health care plan. Preparing meals, reviewing the blood glucose records, and setting limits are all part of being parents.

Diabetes and Pregnancy; Infant of a Diabetic Mother

Although pregnancy is not generally in the realm of the pediatrician or pediatric endocrinologist, the incidence of pregnancy in teenagers with diabetes suggests that some capability in this area is necessary, particularly pertaining to counseling. Furthermore, care of the infant is the responsibility of the pediatrician.

Despite increasing knowledge and a steady improvement in perinatal survival, diabetic pregnancies are still considered in the high-risk category. The infant perimortality rate is less than 10% in most centers; however, congenital anomalies have replaced respiratory distress syndrome as the major cause of neonatal death. The risk of major congenital malformations is increased threefold. Abnormalities most commonly involve the cardiac, skeletal, or central nervous system.[72] Evidence links these abnormalities with poor diabetes control during embryogenesis (gestational weeks 3 through 7). All women of childbearing age should be made aware of these risks, and if pregnancy is considered, glycemic control optimized.

Good metabolic control during pregnancy also appears to be important in improving infant survival. In one study the infant perimortality rate was 23.6% when mean maternal blood glucose level was greater than 150 mg/dL, but only 3.8% when average concentration of blood glucose was below 100 mg/dL; there also was a corresponding decrease in morbidity.[73] Churchill et al.[74] reported a positive correlation between neurologic defects and ketonuria but not hypoglycemia. Self glucose monitoring is especially useful during pregnancy as an aid in achieving such blood glucose regulation (fasting blood glucose [FBG] less than 90 mg/dL and postprandial blood glucose less than 120 mg/dL).[75] Normal FBG values during pregnancy average 65 mg/dL, with nonfasting blood glucose mean values of 80 to 87 ± 8 to 11 mg/dL.[76]

Advances in obstetric management have also contributed to the steady improvement in perinatal survival. Ultrasonography, maternal serum alphafetoprotein, fetal biophysical profile, non-stress test, contraction stress test, amniotic fluid phospholipid assays (lecithin-sphingomyelin ratio), and antepartum fetal heart rate monitoring are procedures commonly used to estimate the maturation and well-being of the fetus.[77] These factors largely determine the time of delivery.

Even with good prenatal care and delivery at the optimal time, intensive pediatric supervision of the infant is important during the neonatal period. Maternal hyperglycemia causes hyperinsulinism in the fetus, which persists for several days after birth. Increased insulin levels in the cord blood of the infant of a diabetic mother (IDM) have been documented by C peptide immunoreactivity.[78] (This method of determining insulin concentration is not influenced by antibody formation.) Hypertrophy and hyperplasia of the islets of Langerhans have also been demonstrated. The lipogenic action of insulin is responsible for increased body fat and enlargement of the heart and liver.

Table 1–4 is a list of the clinical problems observed in the IDM. With careful medical and obstetric management, these complications should occur rarely. Respiratory distress syndrome due to hyaline membrane disease is no longer the leading cause of death in these infants. A major factor in reducing the incidence of respiratory distress syndrome is delivery of the infant after 37 weeks' gestation.[77]

Transient tachypnea ("wet lung" syndrome) is secondary to retention of extravascular fluid in the lung, the cause of which is not clear.[79] Symptoms usually subside after 24 hours. A chest roentgenogram is helpful in differentiating this syndrome from hyaline membrane disease. It should be noted that tachypnea also may be a symptom of hypoglycemia, polycythemia, or cardiac failure.

In addition to hyperinsulinism, decreased epinephrine response may contribute to hypoglycemia in the IDM.[80, 81] In general, the higher the cord glucose level, the lower the infant's blood glucose concentrations will fall. The peak incidence of hypoglycemia occurs at about 2 hours of age, and recovery is often complete by 24 hours.

In contrast to the large infants seen in most hyperglycemic mothers with IDDM, infants of diabetic mothers with vascular disease have low birth weight and are small for gestational age. Such infants have a greater incidence of both perinatal and postnatal mortality.

All IDM should be fed within the first 6 hours of life. Early feedings also may reduce the incidence of hyperbilirubinemia. Diagnosis and therapy of hypoglycemia in the neonate are outlined in Chapter 2. In the IDM, it may be prudent to initiate treatment with 10% dextrose IV shortly after birth rather than waiting for documentation of hypoglycemia by obvious symptoms or periodic blood glucose determinations. It is important to taper IV glucose gradually, as abrupt cessation often results in hypoglycemia.

Hypocalcemia, a frequent complication in the IDM during the first 2 days of life, may be secondary to elevated maternal serum calcium levels suppressing the fetal parathyroids[82]; however, immaturity is an important factor, because the

TABLE 1–4.
Clinical Problems of the Infant of a
Diabetic Mother

Respiratory distress syndrome
Hyaline membrane disease
Transient tachypnea
Hypoglycemia
Hypocalcemia
Hyperbilirubinemia
Polycythemia

incidence is markedly decreased in infants delivered after 37 weeks' gestation.[77] Symptomatic infants should be treated initially with 10% calcium gluconate (5 to 10 mL) IV, injected slowly until symptoms disappear. Maintenance consists of oral supplementation of calcium and a formula with a high ratio of calcium to phosphorus (at least 2:1).

Later growth and development in IDMs are usually normal,[83] except when there are obvious birth defects or other serious complications in the prenatal or neonatal periods. An adverse effect on intellectual development of IDMs whose mothers had acetonuria during pregnancy has been found by several investigators.[74, 84] Transient hypoglycemia in these infants seems to be well tolerated.

Management of gestational diabetes and the fetus is similar, with the emphasis directed to close control of blood glucose and high-risk pregnancy surveillance.

Other Types of Diabetes

In asymptomatic and aglycosuric children, routine glucose tolerance testing is not indicated. When there are clear indications, an OGTT should be performed under carefully standardized conditions[86] (Appendix 1–D). Results are difficult to interpret in acutely or chronically ill children or in those receiving such medications as steroids, thiazides, or phenytoin. Adequate carbohydrate intake (greater than 50% of the calories or at least 150 gm) is important for 3 days prior to the test. Quiet activity is permitted and emotional stress minimized. The recommended amount of glucose given to children is 1.75 g/kg ideal body weight up to a maximum of 75 g.[3]

Diabetes is diagnosed only when the fasting blood glucose (FBG) level is greater than 140 mg/dL, the 2-hour value is equal to or greater than 200 mg/dl, *and* one additional value between 0 and 2 hours is also equal to or greater than 200 mg/dL.[3] (Plasma and serum glucose concentrations are approximately 15% higher than blood glucose.)[86]

Children who have venous FPG less than 140 mg/dL and a 2-hour postprandial glucose level greater than 140 mg/dL are considered to have impaired glucose tolerance[3] (Appendix 1–D).

Insulin levels may be elevated or depressed in NIDDM,[87, 88] and a delayed response may be observed.

The clinical course of a child with NIDDM is unpredictable. In the few studies involving children, some patients with an abnormal OGTT progressed to insulin dependence, others remained asymptomatic, and in a few the OGTT became normal. Low insulin responses to glucose are thought to be associated with a higher incidence of deterioration of glucose tolerance.[7] Additional controlled data on the natural history of these children are obviously needed.

At present, the treatment for children with NIDDM includes a diabetic diet (Appendix 1–E), which tends to reduce hyperglycemia, eliminate reactive hypoglycemia, and prevent excessive weight gain. In the event that insulin treatment becomes necessary, the transition will be easier since the child already will be accustomed to the modified diet. There is no convincing evidence that dietary programs delay the onset of overt diabetes.

Oral hypoglycemic agents do not appear to be of significant value in children,[89-91] although evaluation has been difficult because of the lack of a uniform definition of NIDDM and the variable natural history. These drugs carry the risk of symptomatic hypoglycemia and are probably of little additional benefit in the child who is adhering to a diet plan.

As a general rule, children with NIDDM should test their blood postprandially about once a day for glucose. Increasing hyperglycemia, polyuria, polydipsia, and growth failure are indications for reevaluation. Otherwise, fasting and 2-hour postprandial blood glucose determinations and a glycosylated hemoglobin level should be assessed at 6-month intervals. Unless overt diabetes intervenes, repeat OGTTs should probably be performed every 2 or 3 years. Fasting hyperglycemia is an indication for the use of exogenous insulin.

"Potential abnormality of glucose tolerance" is a statistical risk class that includes children who have never exhibited glucose intolerance but are at increased risk for development of diabetes for a variety of reasons. This classification should be used primarily for identifying groups of individuals who could participate in prospective research studies.

Those who have an increased risk to develop IDDM include[4]:

1. Individuals who have islet cell antibodies.
2. Monozygotic twin of a patient with IDDM.
3. Sibling of a patient with IDDM.
4. Offspring of a patient with IDDM.[3]
5. Individuals with certain HLA types (e.g., DR3, DR4).

Transient neonatal hyperglycemia (transient diabetes of the newborn) usually occurs during the first week of life in infants who are small for gestational age. The condition may persist for less than 24 hours, but average duration is several months. It is characterized by dehydration, glucosuria, and hyperglycemia in the absence of ketonemia. Insulinopenia has been documented in some patients.[92-94] Infants with milder cases require nothing more than close observation. If dehydration occurs, treatment with insulin often is required.[95] The initial insulin dose should not exceed 0.25 to 0.5 U of regular insulin. Occasionally, the diabetes may be permanent, but this can be determined only by the clinical course.[96] Pancreatic agenesis is rare and typically accompanied by evidence of intestinal malabsorption.

CHRONIC COMPLICATIONS OF DIABETES

Dermopathies

Erythematous oval atrophic areas (necrobiosis lipoidica diabeticorum) on the anterior surfaces of the lower extremities frequently occur in children with diabetes. These areas are painless, but may persist and eventually ulcerate or become fibrotic. Injection of hydrocortisone into the lesion or the use of cortisone tape may be beneficial. This condition does not appear to be related to the degree of control and may precede glucose intolerance (as may granuloma annulare).[97] Xanthoma diabeticorum may be observed in patients with hyperlipemia, but is rare in children.

The presence of multiple joint contractures or limited joint mobility, primarily of the fingers, is relatively common.[98] Usually these findings are not functionally significant. There seems to be a relationship between the severity of limited joint mobility and the microvascular complications of diabetes. Documentation of joint abnormalities is important, and other complications need to be periodically carefully assessed.[99, 100]

Neuropathies

Abnormalities of the nervous system are common and may occur early in the course of diabetes mellitus.[101–103] Chemical changes such as altered myelin metabolism and a high accumulation of sorbitol and fructose have been documented.[39] Structural changes including segmental demyelinization of the peripheral nerve fiber occur. Interruption of the blood supply may be an important etiologic factor. How these features relate to the clinical signs and symptoms is not clear, but there is good evidence that significant nerve damage is more likely to occur in patients whose disease is inadequately controlled.[103, 104]

Clinical manifestations of neuropathy are variable. Symmetric sensory neuropathy is the most prevalent type in children. Neurologic changes may be subtle, with mild sensory loss (which can be measured with a tuning fork) and absent ankle jerks recognized during a routine examination,[103] or they may cause numbness, tingling, and burning pain. Symptoms generally are most severe distally in the lower extremities, although upper extremities can be involved.

Asymmetric motor neuropathies (diabetic amyotrophy) and isolated lesions of peripheral and cranial mononeuropathies also occur. Autonomic disorders such as bladder dysfunction predispose the patient to urinary tract infections because of urine retention. Gastrointestinal disturbances include intermittent diarrhea and delayed gastric emptying, but these are unusual problems in children. Impaired sweating, decreased beat-to-beat variation in heart rate, and postural hypotension are clinical findings of autonomic nervous system abnormalities.[103]

Motor conduction velocities, which are easily measured, may be impaired even in asymptomatic patients. In our clinic, 5% of randomly selected children with diabetes had delayed motor conduction velocities. This abnormality was found more frequently in patients with poorly controlled diabetes. Elevated cerebrospinal fluid protein has been reported in diabetics with or without peripheral neuropathies.[105]

The course of neuropathy is varied, but progression often can be halted and improvement may occur with better blood glucose control.[103, 104, 106]

Visual Abnormalities

Transient refractive changes in children with diabetes are common, particularly when there are periods of marked changes in blood glucose. The lens is like an osmometer, increasing and decreasing its refractive power level with changes of tonicity of the aqueous humor. Testing visual acuity at these times may lead to the erroneous conclusion that corrective lenses are indicated. Cataracts may occur early in the course of diabetes and are related to the accumulation of sorbitol in the lens and its consequent osmotic effect.[107] The incidence of diabetic retinopathy, as diagnosed by funduscopy, increases with duration of diabetes and the degree of hyperglycemia.[108] However, studies by Barta et al.[108] and Waltman et al.[110] demonstrated evidence of retinopathy by fluorescein angiography in children of all ages and in the earliest stages of diabetes.

Early retinopathy is characterized by punctate hemorrhages or microaneurysms. Sharply defined exudates (hard exudates) and increased tortuosity of the retinal veins indicate further progression. In this phase of diabetic retinopathy, all the changes are intraretinal and the main pathogenic mechanisms are vascular leakage and occlusion.[111] Macular edema may cause visual loss, but affects central vision only.

At some point, capillary endothelium may begin to proliferate at the periphery of areas of ischemia. The optic disk is the major site for new vessel formation, and disease in this location affords the worst prognosis (30% of patients are blind in 3 years with no treatment).[112] Hemorrhage, preretinal and intravitrial, which causes traction detachment of the retina, may occur. Spontaneous regression is infrequent. The most serious complication is neovascular glaucoma (rubeosis iridis).

The status of the retinal vasculature can be evaluated with the aid of fluorescein injected into an antecubital vein. Even in the earliest stages of retinopathy, fluorescein leakage may occur. This may be quantitated with the use of vitreous fluorophotometry.[110] Once vascular abnormalities are seen, the location and degree of leakage can be assessed by fluorescein angiography.[113]

A controlled clinical trial, the Diabetic Retinopathy Study, confirmed the benefits of "panretinal" photocoagulation in the treatment of proliferative diabetic retinopathy.[112] Positive effects of focal photocoagulation for background retinopathy with macular edema were reported in the Early Treatment in Diabetic Retinopathy Study (ETDRS).[114] The indications and benefits of vitrectomy to remove vitreous hemorrhages associated with severe retinopathy was evaluated in a randomized controlled clinical trial, the Diabetic Retinopathy Vitrectomy Study.[115] Aspirin (650 mg/day) is being tested in the ETDRS because it inhibits platelet aggregation.[114]

To ensure prompt recognition and treatment, all children should have periodic eye examinations by an ophthalmologist. These should begin 5 years after diagnosis or at puberty. It is important to maintain normal blood pressure levels. Evidence points to more rapid progression of retinopathy in persons with uncontrolled hypertension.

Strict metabolic control may reduce the frequency and delay the progression of retinopathy. However, caution must be taken in treating patients who have had prolonged poor control of diabetes. Rapid progression of vascular disease may occur, particularly retinopathy. A slow progressive return to euglycemia over 4 to 6 months is suggested.

Diabetic Nephropathy

Diabetic nephropathy (nephrosclerosis) is the major cause of mortality in adults with IDDM. Clinically, glomerulosclerosis usually occurs in about 30% to 40% of patients after IDDM has been present 10 to 15 years, but occasionally sooner.[108, 116, 117] The first clinical evidence of nephropathy is increased urinary albumin excretion (microalbuminuria). This test measures albumin excretion in the range of 25 to 250 mg/day. Dipstick-positive results indicate albumin excretion of more than 250 mg/day. Patients with diabetes and microalbuminuria are at a higher risk for renal insufficiency. Poor diabetes control, infection, stress, exercise, and hypertension may induce microalbuminuria; these factors must be excluded before interpreting the test results.

Clinically detectable proteinuria (250 mg/day) signals declining kidney function. Hypertension, edema, and renal insufficiency soon follow.[118, 119] There may be a decrease in insulin requirement, presumably because the kidney no longer degrades insulin efficiently.[120] If these signs occur in the younger child with diabetes, the diagnosis should be confirmed by renal biopsy. Renal transplantation is now considered feasible in children with diabetic nephropathy. Otherwise, therapy is essentially limited to vigorous treatment of hypertension and blood glucose control.

Patients with diabetes are at increased risk for acute renal failure after any procedure in which radiocontrast material is used. With judicious use of echography, radionuclide studies, and noncontrast computed tomographic scanning, radiocontrast studies are rarely necessary. If necessary, a minimum amount of contrast material should be injected, and there should be adequate hydration before and after the study. Mannitol can be used to maintain adequate excretion.

Large Vessel Disease

Accelerated atherosclerosis as manifested by coronary heart disease and peripheral vascular disease becomes an important cause of morbidity and mortality in adults who have had IDDM for more than 20 years or who have NIDDM. Lipid abnormalities, particularly decreased high-density lipoprotein (HDL) cholesterol concentrations, are thought to be significant risk factors for the development of macrovascular disease.[121] However, there is no characteristic lipoprotein or lipid abnormality specific for diabetes. Elevated levels of triglycerides and cholesterol are common during uncontrolled hyperglycemia and may be recognized by a lactescent serum. These abnormalities are corrected as normoglycemia is approached.[122] If hyperlipemia persists, familial hyperlipoproteinemia should be suspected. HDL cholesterol concentrations are abnormally low in adults with NIDDM, but are normal in those with IDDM. All children should have a lipid profile 6 months after the diagnosis of diabetes is made, and then every 2 years.

In addition to blood glucose control, a significant reduction in serum lipids is attained using diets restricted in cholesterol and saturated fats. However, multiple factors including genetic predisposition, stress, smoking, hormonal interactions, and physical fitness are associated with the process of atherogenesis. All must be considered in the assessment of results of treatment studies.[121]

Arterial calcifications (medial arteriosclerosis) may be an early complication in children with diabetes and are first visible by x-ray examination in the foot and leg. Large vessel changes and complications superimposed on microvascular disease accelerate the degenerative process of all organs.

SUMMARY OF CURRENT RESEARCH

Evidence that is being accumulated associates the development of microvascular complications with the degree and duration of hyperglycemia in persons with IDDM.[99, 104, 108, 122] The reversibility of many of the microvascular changes with intensive insulin therapy has not occurred, and in some studies there was a temporary worsening of retinopathy in the first 6 to 12 months[123, 124]; however, early changes may be reversed. The Diabetes Control and Complications Trial (DCCT), sponsored by the National Institutes of Health, was designed to determine whether intensive glycemic control can curtail microvascular complications already present. Completion of this study in the early 1990s should provide data for treatment decisions.

Recent research has centered on the development of alternative methods of delivering insulin, such as the closed-loop insulin pump (artificial pancreas with a glucose sensor), intranasal insulin,[125] and pancreas and islet cell transplants.[126]

Other areas of research pertinent to patient care include identification of persons at risk for diabetes and development of methods to prevent or delay its onset[6, 127, 128]; nutritional research, particularly on the use of high-fiber diets[129]; and a long-neglected area related to improving methods of health care delivery, including assessment and modification of factors affecting adherence.[130, 131]

APPENDIX I–A

Goals of Health Care Plan for Children With Insulin-Dependent Diabetes, and Criteria for Attainment

I. To achieve a metabolic state as normal as possible:
   A. Blood glucose goals:

      1. Premeal, 70–120 mg/dL.
      2. Postmeal, <180 mg/dL (<200 mg/dL in children younger than 5 years).
      3. 2:00–3:00 AM, 70–120 mg/dL.
  B. Absence of ketonuria.
  C. Hemoglobin A_1 or A_{1c} within 1% of normal.
  D. Normal growth rate and onset of puberty.
  E. Appropriate body weight.
  F. Normal lipid studies.
  G. Absence of severe hypoglycemic symptoms as defined by:
      1. Interference with normal activities.
      2. Loss of consciousness.
  H. Absence of hyperglycemic symptoms.
  I. Minimal neurologic and vascular complications.

II. To encourage a realistic attitude toward diabetes, recognizing that diabetes is a permanent condition, but one that can be controlled:
  A. Child resumes school or work schedule.
  B. Child resumes recreational activities.
  C. Child complies with the Health Care Plan.
  D. Child assumes self-care at the appropriate age.
  E. Child wears diabetes identification.
  F. Child is aware of potential complications at appropriate age.

III. To promote emotional well-being of the child and family:
  A. Child interacts appropriately with peers.
  B. Child interacts appropriately with family.
  C. Child matures psychologically at the normal rate.

IV. To provide the child and family with knowledge of diabetes to enable them to assume a primary role in daily diabetes management. The child and family should be able to:
  A. Define diabetes, possible causes, treatment, genetic implications, and long-term prognosis.
  B. Administer insulin correctly.
  C. Recognize the different kinds of insulin; know duration and peak of action, and proper storage.
  D. Test blood correctly with appropriate test materials; record and interpret results.
  E. Select meal patterns and adjust for changes in activity.
  F. Relate causes, symptoms, and treatment of hyperglycemia.
  G. Relate effect stress has on blood glucose.
  H. Relate causes, symptoms, and treatment of hypoglycemia.
  I. Engage in exercise regularly and make appropriate adjustments in health care plan.

V. To share responsibility for management of the diabetes appropriately
with health care providers:
A. Relate when and whom to ask for help.
B. Keep appointments.
C. Provide pertinent information bearing on diabetes control.

APPENDIX I–B

Insulin Preparations and Injection Technique

The insulins primarily used are short-acting (regular insulin), intermediate-acting (NPH or lente insulin), and long-acting (protamine zinc insulin or ultralente). These insulins are derived from bovine or porcine pancreas or are human insulin of semisynthetic or recombinant DNA origin. In most children therapy is begun with human insulin.

Regular insulin given subcutaneously begins to have some effect on blood glucose levels 15 to 30 minutes after injection; the effect peaks within 2 to 3 hours, and lasts 4 to 6 hours. This insulin is best used as a bolus to prevent the blood glucose level from rising too high with meals and to reduce it to the normal range within 3 to 4 hours. It should be given 15 to 30 minutes before meals.

NPH and lente insulin begin to be effective 1 to 2 hours after injection. The activity peaks within 8 to 12 hours, and lasts 18 to 24 hours. Because the effect is not immediate, these insulins can be given before or after a meal; however, they should be given at the same time each day. When NPH and regular insulin are administered together, the injection should be given before meals and at the same time each day.

NPH and lente insulin given before supper sometimes have a peak effect at 2:00 or 3:00 AM, causing hypoglycemia followed by rebound hyperglycemia.[53-58] Giving the intermediate insulin between 9:00 and 11:00 PM may alleviate this problem, yet provide more flexibility. Regular insulin is still given before supper and may be adjusted for activity level.

Ultralente insulin, derived from bovine or porcine pancreas, is given subcutaneously as basal insulin once or twice a day. It is active for 30 to 36 hours without a peak effect. Adjustments of ultralente insulin are based on fasting blood glucose levels and occasional tests at 2:00 to 3:00 AM.

Other preparations available are premixed and human ultralente insulins. Premixed insulins are not effective in managing labile type I diabetes because the amount of regular insulin cannot be adjusted. Human ultralente insulin has a definite peak and shorter duration of action than ultralente derived from beef or pork.

Insulin regimens include a single dose of intermediate or ultralente to provide basal insulin. Endogenous insulin must provide the mealtime boluses with this regimen. Occasionally children who are active and who eat small, frequent meals can maintain good control with a single dose of intermediate insulin.

Various intermediate or regular doses are shown in Table 1–3. In most instances children are started on a mixed insulin dose in the morning and before supper. After their response to this program is observed, another regimen that better fits their lifestyle may evolve.

When ultralente insulin is used, regular insulin is administered as a bolus before each meal. Up to 50% to 60% of the total daily amount is ultralente, given as a basal dose. Continuous subcutaneous insulin infusion (insulin pump) is similar to the ultralente and regular regimens. Between 40% and 60% is given as a basal infusion, and boluses are provided before meals and sometimes before snacks. The boluses are adjusted to eliminate excessive postprandial hyperglycemia and to attain the targeted blood glucose level before the next meal. The basal rate may need to be adjusted overnight, and most infusion devices can be preprogrammed at different infusion rates for specific time intervals.

In choosing an insulin regimen, use the simplest insulin program required at the time to attain the blood glucose level desired. Initially most children are given two injections of human mixed insulin a day. Many need only a single injection during the "honeymoon" period. As the pancreas secretes less insulin, exogenous insulin requirements will increase. What is the person with diabetes willing to do? Children who have been receiving only a single dose of insulin must be convinced that they need a second injection before starting them on three or four injections. It is also necessary to choose an insulin regimen that fits the person's daily schedule. Multiple insulin doses do allow for increased flexibility. Options for multiple insulin dose regimens include continuous subcutaneous insulin infusion (CSII). This regimen is particularly helpful when meals may be delayed, for example, in older adolescents and young adults.

Note that CSII does require close blood glucose monitoring. There is no long-acting insulin present, so any interruption in the system can lead to ketoacidosis in 4 to 6 hours. Use of this system is risky in young children because of their usual erratic and vigorous activity.

Insulin that is being used daily may be stored at room temperature in a kitchen cupboard or medicine cabinet. Extra bottles should be kept on a lower shelf in the refrigerator. On trips, care must be taken not to allow the insulin to become too warm.

Children older than 7 or 8 years, as well as both parents or significant others, are taught to give an insulin injection. The skin and subcutaneous tissue is pinched with one hand. The insulin syringe is held like a pencil so that the needle enters perpendicular to the skin. Appropriate injection sites are depicted in Figure 1–3.

The rate of insulin absorption is affected by the size of the dose, injection site, temperature changes, exercise, premixing of the insulin, and massage of the injection site.

APPENDIX I–C

Insulin Adjustment[132]

Changes in the basic, day-to-day insulin dose should be based on consistent

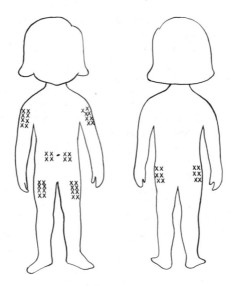

FIG 1–3.
Injection sites. Injections are given in the anterior thigh, abdomen, lateral aspect of the arm, and the buttock. Daily rotation of injection sites is encouraged.

blood glucose patterns. If a child's food intake and physical activity are relatively consistent and there are no major stresses, the following guidelines apply: First, establish premeal and postmeal blood glucose goals. Then look for a blood glucose pattern that is consistent for at least 3 days. If a clear pattern is present, determine which type of insulin is primarily responsible and adjust the dose by either an increase or a decrease of 1 to 2 U. Make only one adjustment at a time by small increments. For children receiving less than 10 U of insulin daily, adjust the dose by only one half a unit. For very young children, dilute the regular insulin dose to U50 or U20. Always try to prevent hypoglycemia before reacting to hyperglycemic episodes. Often an elevation in blood glucose level is secondary to excessive treatment of a low blood glucose level or to metabolic compensation. Finally, wait 3 days after each dose adjustment and reevaluate.

An example of insulin adjustment based on blood glucose patterns is shown in Table 1–5.

Once the basic insulin dose has been established, insulin supplements may be used. Insulin supplementation is part of an intensified insulin regimen. It involves a great deal of supervision by the health-care team and a lot of effort on the part of the patient. A careful balance of food intake, physical activity, and insulin use is essential. Self-monitoring of blood glucose four to seven times per day is required, as is self-adjustment of the insulin dose. It is especially important to test blood glucose after a supplement is given to assess whether it provided the desired effect. Monthly hemoglobin A_1 or A_{1c} testing helps in objectively evaluating the regimen.

TABLE 1-5.
Insulin Adjustment Based on Blood Glucose Patterns*

Breakfast		Lunch		Supper		Bedtime	
Insulin dose (U)	Blood glucose (mg/dL)	Insulin dose (U)	Blood glucose (mg/dL)	Insulin dose (U)	Blood glucose (mg/dL)	Insulin dose (U)	Blood glucose (mg/dL)
20 N/15 R	120	4 R	66†	18N/10 R	186†	...	104
20 N/15 R	96	4 R	54†	18N/10 R	112	...	86
20 N/15 R	85	4 R	69†	18N/10 R	153†	...	214†
20 N/14 R	117	4 R	83	18N/10 R	118	...	93

* N = NPH insulin, R = regular insulin. Maintaining fasting and preprandial blood glucose levels between 70 and 120 mg/dL is the goal.
† Level outside goal range.

Supplemental insulin doses must be recorded separately to ensure that the amount of the basic insulin dose is not forgotten. Supplementation should be individualized for the time of day and degree of activity. Supplements may be used when an extra large meal is anticipated or to compensate when the blood glucose level is high. Negative supplements are used when extra activity is anticipated.

The key to successful blood glucose control using supplementation is as follows: When supplements are needed for 3 consecutive days at a particular time of day, the basic insulin dose should be adjusted accordingly. In other words, use of a supplement can ensure that the blood glucose level does not remain elevated for a significant length of time, but the primary goal is to prevent elevations before they occur.

An example of insulin supplementation is shown in Table 1–6.

Changes in insulin should be made gradually. Initial blood glucose goals may need to be higher because of previous persistent hyperglycemia. A person who is used to having blood glucose values in the 200 to 300 mg/dL range will not feel well when their blood glucose levels are lowered into the normal range. They may have numbness, pain, and tingling, and symptoms of hypoglycemia when their blood glucose level is still elevated. Therefore blood glucose goals of 100 to 200 mg/dL may be chosen for the first 4 or 5 months, then gradually decreased.

APPENDIX I–D

Oral Glucose Tolerance Test

Procedure

A 5-hour oral glucose tolerance test (OGTT) usually is performed, particularly if reactive hypoglycemia is suspected. Glucose (1.75 g/kg up to a maximum of 75 g) is administered orally following an overnight fast of 8 to 9 hours. Blood samples for glucose and insulin are obtained at 0, 30, 60, 90, 120, 180, 240, and 300 minutes. (However, note that the most commonly used criteria for diabetes rely only on the first 2 to 3 hours for interpretation.) Urine is tested for glucose at 0, 1, and 2 hours.

Factors that influence test results include dietary preparation, physical activity, illness, and certain drugs (salicylates, diuretics, oral contraceptives, diphenylhydantoin). Differences in blood sampling techniques (venous vs. capillary, serum or plasma vs. whole blood) and methods of preservation and analysis of the blood sample must also be considered.

Current recommendations for standardization include:

1. Preparatory diet: 50% of calories as carbohydrate, or at least 150 g for 3 days preceding the test.
2. Delay of at least 2 weeks after a period of acute illness and discontinuance of hyperglycemic drugs prior to testing.

TABLE 1–6.
Insulin Supplementation Based on Blood Glucose Patterns*

Breakfast		Lunch		Supper		Bedtime	
Insulin dose (U)	Blood glucose (mg/dL)	Insulin dose (U)	Blood glucose (mg/dL)	Insulin dose (U)	Blood glucose (mg/dL)	Insulin dose (U)	Blood glucose (mg/dL)
22 N/10 R (1 R)	133†	⋯	96	8 R (2 R)	156†	8 N	83
22 N/10 R	79	⋯	110	8 R (1 R)	146†	8 N	95
22 N/10 R	103	⋯	93	8 R (2 R)	173†	8 N	117
24 N/10 R (1 R)	129†	⋯	72	8 R	115	8 N (3 R)	197†

* N = NPH insulin, R = regular insulin, ( ) = supplemental insulin. Maintaining fasting and preprandial blood glucose levels between 70 and 120 mg/dL is the goal.
† Level outside goal range.

3. *Quiet* activity permitted during the test. Insertion of indwelling scalp vein needle minimizes trauma.
4. Proper preservation of blood specimens and knowledge of the method for analysis (glucose oxidase, Nelson-Somogyi, or Autoanalyzer). Multiplying whole blood values by 1.15 and adding a constant of 6 mg/dL converts whole blood to plasma or serum glucose.[86]

Glucose Intolerance: Diagnostic Criteria for Children*

Diabetes Mellitus

I. Presence of classic symptoms plus a random plasma glucose greater than 200 mg/dL.

II. Asymptomatic with an elevated fasting glucose concentration on more than one occasion, an elevated 2-hour sample and one other elevated value between fasting and the 2-hour value during OGTT.
 A. Fasting:
  1. Venous plasma ≥140 mg/dL.
  2. Venous whole blood ≥120 mg/dL.
  3. Capillary whole blood ≥120 mg/dL.
 B. Two-hour OGTT and intervening value:
  1. Venous plasma ≥200 mg/dL.
  2. Venous whole blood ≥180 mg/dL.
  3. Capillary whole blood ≥200 mg/dL.

Impaired Glucose Tolerance†

I. Fasting:
 A. Venous plasma <140 mg/dL.
 B. Venous whole blood <120mg/dL.
 C. Capillary whole blood <120 mg/dL.

* Adapted from the National Diabetes Data Group. *Diabetes* 1979; 28:1039.
† Emphasis is on the fasting value.

APPENDIX I–E

Diabetes Diet Plan

It is the philosophy of our clinic that children with diabetes should be encouraged to adhere to a prescribed meal plan. Such a program will eliminate one variable in diabetes management, help to prevent wide fluctuations of blood glucose, and reduce the frequency of hypoglycemic episodes. Reduction of saturated fats, cholesterol, and simple sugars should have a favorable effect on serum lipids and ultimately upon large vessel disease. Few children with diabetes are obese; therefore, the diet is not designed for weight reduction, but must be adequate for normal growth.

A basic plan consists of 1,000 calories plus 100 calories/year of age up to 12 years. During adolescence girls generally need fewer calories than are provided by this formula, and boys more. Snacks are encouraged at midmorning, mid-afternoon, and bedtime. Calories are distributed as 50% carbohydrate, 20% protein, and 30% fat (at least one half polyunsaturated and low in cholesterol). Meals should be offered at approximately the same time each day, with the exception of the late evening snack, which can vary with the bedtime. Food is not weighed, but it is necessary for the family to have an accurate perception of a "normal" portion.

It is important to recognize that these general guidelines must often be modified to accommodate individual needs. Obviously, not all 10-year-old patients require exactly 2,000 calories. A dietary history provides insight into a child's eating habits prior to the onset of diabetes and allows a more rational basis for deviations from the basic program. When feasible, a patient's specific dietary habits and desires are accommodated as long as this does not interfere significantly with good diabetes management. In addition, an attempt is made to adjust the diet of the child to conform with the eating habits of the family, rather than to impose unpopular schedules on other family members. This approach helps in the family's adjustment to the treatment plan.

It may be necessary to modify the time of meals to allow for specific school or work schedules and extracurricular activities such as sports.

Parents usually ask about "dietetic" or "diabetic" foods that contain artificial sweeteners. As a general rule, carbonated beverages that have been made with these products may be used without restriction. However, most other "diabetic" foods, such as candy and cookies, may in fact contain some sugar in addition to an artificial sweetener and, in any case, they often contain a significant number of calories. Patients are discouraged from using these substitutes, as they tend to be considered "free" foods. If these products have been sanctioned for use, children become indiscriminate in their selection, with the ultimate result that a good dietary program is no longer followed. However, certain of these foods occasionally are allowed if the patient consults the physician or dietitian about a specific product, and the exact contents and equivalent substitution are clearly understood.

Presentation of the diet should be positive, with emphasis on the rationale for such a program. Poor understanding may be one reason for lack of adherence. It is stressed that the restrictions are not severe and that the diet actually differs little from that which would be considered desirable for any child. The younger the child, the easier it is for parents to encourage good nutritional habits. The whole family should participate. Nonetheless, it is this aspect of diabetic management that seems to be the most difficult for the child or adolescent to accept.

REFERENCES

1. Gorwitz K, Howen GG, Thompson T: Prevalence of diabetes in Michigan school-age children. *Diabetes* 1976; 25:122.
2. Kyllo DF, Nuttal FQ: Prevalence of diabetes mellitus in school-age children in Minnesota. *Diabetes* 1978; 27:57.
3. National Diabetes Data Group: Classifications and diagnosis of diabetes mellitus and other categories of glucose intolerance. *Diabetes* 1979; 28:1039.
4. Nerup J, Mandrup-Poulsen T, Molvig J: The HLA-IDDM Association: Implications for etiology and pathogenesis of IDDM. *Diabetes Metab Rev* 1987; 3:799–802.
5. Eisenbarth GS: Type I diabetes mellitus: A chronic autoimmune disorder. *N Engl J Med* 1986; 314:1360–1368.
6. Eisenbarth GS, Connelly J, Soeldner JS: The natural history of type I diabetes. *Diabetes Metab Rev* 1987; 3:873–892.
7. Fajans SS, Cloutier MC, Crowther RL: Clinical and etiologic heterogeneity of idiopathic diabetes mellitus. *Diabetes* 1978; 27:1112.
8. Winter WE, et al: Maturity-onset diabetes of youth in black Americans. *N Engl J Med* 1987; 285–291.
9. Finkelstein SM, Wielinski CL, Elliott GR: Diabetes mellitus associated with cystic fibrosis. *J Pediatr* 1988; 112:273–277.
10. Strock ES, Sandell JL: The ambulatory insulin program: Initiating insulin therapy in an outpatient setting. *Diabetes Educ* 1987; 14:338–345.
11. Nathan DM, et al: The clinical information value of the glycosylated hemoglobin assay. *N Engl J Med* 1984; 310:341–346.
12. Mogensen CE, Christiansen CK: Predicting diabetic nephropathy in insulin-dependent patients. *N Engl J Med* 1984; 311:89–93.
13. Krumlik JJ, Ehrlich RM: Insulin and sodium bicarbonate treatment of diabetic acidosis: A retrospective review. *J Pediatr* 1973; 83:268.
14. Lightner ES, Kappy MS, Reusin B: Low-dose intravenous insulin infusion in patients with diabetic ketoacidosis: Biochemical effect in children. *Pediatrics* 1977; 60:681.
15. Drop SLS, et al: Low-dose intravenous insulin injection: A controlled comparative study of diabetic ketoacidosis. *Pediatrics* 1978; 59:733.
16. Mosely J: Diabetic crises in children treated with small doses of intramuscular insulin. *Br Med J* 1975; 1:59.
17. Fort P, Waters SM, Lifshitz F: Low-dose insulin infusion in the treatment of diabetic ketoacidosis: Bolus versus no bolus. *J Pediatr* 1980; 96:36.
18. Finberg L: Management of the critically ill child with dehydration secondary to diarrhea. *Pediatrics* 1970; 45:1029.
19. Danowski TS: *Diabetes Mellitus: With Emphasis On Adults and Young Children.* Baltimore, Williams & Wilkins, 1957.
20. Podolsky S, Emerson K: Potassium depletion in diabetic keto acidosis (KA) and in hyperosmolar nonketotic coma (HNC). *Diabetes* 1973; 22 (suppl. 1):299.
21. Hockaday TO, Alberte KCMM: Diabetic coma. *Clin Endocrinol Metab* 1972; 1:751.
22. Zipf WB, et al: Hypocalcemia, hypomagnesemia, and transient hypoparathyroidism during therapy with potassium phosphate in diabetic ketoacidosis. *Diabetes Care* 1979; 2:265.
23. Keller V, Berger W: Prevention of hypophosphatemia by phosphate infusion during treatment of diabetic ketoacidosis and hyperosmolar coma. *Diabetes* 1980; 29:87.
24. Katz MA: Hyperglycemia-induced hyponatremia. Calculation of expected serum sodium depression. *N Engl J Med* 1973; 289:344.

25. Opie LH: Cardiac metabolism: The effect of some physiologic, pharmacologic, and pathologic influences. *Am Heart J* 1965; 69:401.
26. Assal J, et al: Metabolic effects of sodium bicarbonate in management of diabetic ketoacidosis. *Diabetes* 1974; 23:405.
27. Alberti KGMM, et al: 2,3-Diphosphoglycerate and tissue oxygenation in uncontrolled diabetes mellitus. *Lancet* 1972; 2:391.
28. Kanter Y, Gerson JR, Bessman AN: 2,3-Diphosphoglycerate, nucleotide phosphate, and organic and inorganic phosphate levels during the early phases of diabetic ketoacidosis. *Diabetes* 1977; 26:429.
29. Munk P, et al: Effect of bicarbonate on oxygen transport in juvenile diabetic ketoacidosis. *J Pediatr* 1974; 84:510.
30. Belmonte MM, et al: Nonketotic hyperosmolar diabetic coma in Down's syndrome. *J Pediatr* 1970; 77:879.
31. Rubin HM, Kramer R, Drash A: Hyperosmolality complicating diabetes mellitus in childhood. *J Pediatr* 1969; 74:177.
32. Duck SD, Wyatt DT: Factors associated with brain herniation in the treatment of ketoacidosis. *J Pediatr* 1988; 113:10.
33. Krane EJ, et al: Subclinical brain swelling in children during treatment of diabetic ketoacidosis. *N Engl J Med* 1985; 313:1147.
34. Arieff AI, Kleeman CR: Cerebral edema in diabetic comas. II: Effect of hyperosmolality, hyperglycemia and insulin in diabetic rabbits. *J Clin Invest* 1973; 52:571.
35. Cahill GF Jr, Etzwiler DD, Freinkel N: Blood glucose control in diabetes. *Diabetes* 1976; 25:237.
36. Camerini-Davalos RA, et al: Muscle capillary basement membrane width in genetic prediabetes. *J Clin Endocrinol Metab* 1979; 48:251.
37. Fajans SS, et al: Basement membrane thickening in latent diabetes, in Camerini-Davalos RA, Cole HS (eds): *Advances in Metabolic Disorders, Suppl. 2, Vascular and Neurological Changes in Early Diabetes*, Proc. 2d International Symposium on Early Diabetes, Curacao W.I., 1971. New York, Academic Press, 1973, pp 393–399.
38. Kilo C, Vogler N, Williamson JR: Muscle capillary basement membrane changes related to aging and diabetes mellitus. *Diabetes* 1972; 21:881.
39. Gabbay KH: The sorbital pathway and the complications of diabetes. *N Engl J Med* 1973; 288:831.
40. The DCCT Research Group: Are continuing studies of metabolic control and microvascular complications in insulin-dependent diabetes mellitus justified? *N Engl J Med* 1988; 318:246.
41. Traisman HS: Mauriac's syndrome. *Clin Pediatr* 1964; 3:520.
42. Tattersall RB, Pyke DA: Growth in diabetic children. *Lancet* 1973; 2:1105.
43. Evans N, Robinson VP, Lister J: Growth and bone age of juvenile diabetics. *Arch Dis Child* 1972; 47:589.
44. Jackson RL, et al: Growth and maturation of children with insulin-dependent diabetes mellitus. *Diabetes Care* 1978; 1:96.
45. Winter RJ, et al: Somatomedin activity and diabetic control in children with insulin-dependent diabetes. *Diabetes* 1979; 28:952.
46. Sussman RE: *Juvenile-Type Diabetes and Its Complications*. Springfield, Ill, Charles C Thomas, 1971, pp 388–389.
47. Speert DP, Silva J: Abnormalities of in vitro lymphocyte response to mitogens in diabetic children during acute ketoacidosis. *Am J Dis Child* 1978; 132:1014.
48. Berken A, Sherman AA: Reticuloendothelial system phagocytosis in diabetes mellitus. *Diabetes* 1974; 23:218.
49. Gardner LI, Reijersback GC: Brain damage in a juvenile diabetic patient associated with insulin hypoglycemia. *Pediatrics* 1951; 7:210.

50. Golden MP, et al: Longitudinal relationship of asymptomatic hypoglycemia to cognitive function in IDDM. *Diabetes Care* 1989; 12:89.
51. Bergada I: Severe hypoglycemia in IDDM children. *Diabetes Care* 1989; 12:239.
52. Amiel SA, et al: Effect of intensive insulin therapy on gylcemic thresholds for counterregularity hormone release. *Diabetes* 1988; 37:901.
54. Rosenbloom AL, Giordano B: Chronic overtreatment with insulin in children and adolescents. *Am J Dis Child* 1977; 131:881.
55. Bruck E, MacGillivray MH: Posthypoglycemic hyperglycemia in diabetic children. *J Pediatr* 1974; 84:672.
56. Clarke WL, Haymond MW, Santiago JV: Overnight basal insulin requirements in fasting insulin-dependent diabetics. *Diabetes* 1980; 29:78.
57. Schmidt MI, et al: Fasting hyperglycemia and associated free insulin and cortisol changes in "Somogyi-like" patients. *Diabetes Care* 1979; 2:457.
58. Stephenson JM, Schentheaner G: Dawn phenomenon and Somogyi effect in IDDM. *Diabetes Care* 1989; 12:245–251.
59. Guthrie RA, Murphy DYN, Womach W: Insulin resistance in diabetes in juveniles. *Pediatrics* 1967; 40:642.
60. Paulsen EP, Courtney JW, Duckworth WC: Insulin resistance caused by massive degradation of subcutaneous insulin. *Diabetes* 1979; 28:640.
61. Stern SP, Charles ES: Emotional factors in juvenile diabetes mellitus: A study of early life experience of eight diabetic children. *Psychosom Med* 1975; 37:237.
62. Koski ML: The coping processes in childhood diabetes. *Acta Pediatr Scand* 1969; 19 (suppl.):1.
63. Segal J:*Psychosomatic Diabetic Children and Their Families.* Mental Health Studies and Reports Branch, NIMH, 1977.
64. Hauser ST, et al: Ego development and self-esteem in diabetic adolescents. *Diabetes Care* 1979; 2:465.
65. Simonds JF: Psychiatric status of diabetic youth matched with a control group. *Diabetes* 1977; 26:921.
66. Baker L, et al: Beta adrenergic blockade and juvenile diabetes: Acute studies and longterm therapeutic trial. *J Pediatr* 1969; 75:19.
67. Parker L, Hunt GG, Spencer ML: Reducing diabetic ketoacidosis hospitalizations. *Diabetes* 1980; 29 (suppl. 2):106.
68. Sullivan B: Self-esteem and depression in adolescent diabetic girls. *Diabetes Care* 1978; 1:18.
69. Kaufman RV, Hersher B: Body images in teenage diabetics. *Pediatrics* 1971; 48:123.
70. Walsh CH, O'Sullivan DJ: Effect of moderate alcohol intake on control of diabetes. *Diabetes* 1974; 23:440.
71. McDonald J: Alcohol and diabetes. *Diabetes Care* 1980; 3:629.
72. Jovanovic L, Fuhrmann K, Peterson CM (eds): *Diabetes in Pregnancy: Teratology, Toxicology, and Treatment.* New York: Praeger, 1986.
73. Karlsson K, Kjellmer I: The outcome of diabetic pregnancies in relation to the mother's blood sugar level. *Am J Obstet Gynecol* 1972; 112:213.
74. Churchill JA, Berendes HW, Nemore J: Neuropsychological deficits in children of diabetic mothers. A report from the collaborative study for cerebral palsy. *Am J Obstet Gynecol* 1969; 105:257.
75. Jovanovic LB, et al: Feasibility of maintaining euglycemia in insulin dependent pregnant diabetic women. *Am J Med* 1980; 68:105.
76. Gillmer MDG, et al: Carbohydrate metabolism in pregnancy: I. Diurnal plasma glucose profile in normal and diabetic women. *Br Med J* 1975; 3:399.

77. Gabbe G: Management of diabetes mellitus in pregnancy. *Am J Obstet Gynecol* 1985; 153:824–828.
78. Pildes KS: Infants of diabetic mothers. *N Engl J Med* 1973; 289:902.
79. Sundell H, et al: Studies on infants with type II respiratory distress syndrome. *J Pediatr* 1971; 78:754.
80. Light IJ, et al: Impaired epinephrine release in hypoglycemic infants of diabetic mothers. *N Engl J Med* 1967; 277:394.
81. Martin FI, et al: Neonatal hypoglycemia in infants of insulin-dependent diabetic mothers. *Arch Dis Child* 1975; 50:472.
82. Tsang RC, et al: Hypocalcemia in infants of diabetic mothers. *J Pediatr* 1972; 80:384.
83. Brudenell M, Beard R: Diabetes in pregnancy. *J Clin Endocrinol Metab* 1972; 1:673.
84. Stebbens JA, Baker GL, Kitchell M: Outcome at age 1, 3, and 5 years of children born to diabetic women. *Am J Obstet Gynecol* 1977; 127:408.
85. Haworth JC, McRae KN, Dilling LA: Prognosis of infants of diabetic mothers in relation to neonatal hypoglycemia. *Dev Med Child Neurol* 1976; 18:471.
86. Klimt CC, et al: Standardization of the oral glucose tolerance. Report of the Committee on Statistics of the American Diabetes Association. June 14, 1968, *Diabetes* 1969; 18:299.
87. Martin MM, Martin ALA: Obesity, hyperinsulinism, and diabetes mellitus in childhood. *J Pediatr* 1973; 82:192.
88. Rosenbloom AL, et al: Age-adjusted analysis of insulin responses during normal and abnormal glucose tolerance tests in children and adolescents. *Diabetes* 1975; 24:820.
89. Paulsen EP: Experiences in sulfonylurea therapy. *Metabolism* 1973; 22:381.
90. Drash A: Treatment of the child with chemical diabetes mellitus. *Metabolsim* 1973; 22:377.
91. Rosenbloom A: Tolbutamide in chemical diabetes mellitus in children. *Metabolism* 1973; 22:399.
92. Pagliara AS, Karl IE, Kipnis DB: Transient neonatal diabetes: Delayed maturation of the pancreatic beta cell. *J Pediatr* 1973; 82:97.
93. Zarif M, Predes RS, Vidyasagar D: Insulin and growth hormone responses in neonatal hyperglycemia. *Diabetes* 1976; 25:428.
94. Schiff D, Colle E, Stern L: Metabolic and growth patterns in transient neonatal diabetes. *N Engl J Med* 1972; 287:119.
95. Gentz JCH, Cornblath M: Transient diabetes of the newborn. *Adv Pediatr* 1969; 16:345.
96. Greenwood RD, Traisman HS: Permanent diabetes mellitus in a neonate. *J Pediatr* 1971; 79:296.
97. Gouterman IH, Sibrack LA: Cutaneous manifestations of diabetes. *Cutis* 1980; 25:45.
98. Grgic A, et al: Joint contracture—common manifestations of childhood diabetes mellitus. *J Pediatr* 1976; 88:584.
99. Monnier VM, et al: Relation between complications of type I diabetes mellitus and collagen-linked fluorescence. *N Engl J Med* 1986; 314:403.
100. Rosenbloom AL: Skeletal and joint manifestations of childhood diabetes. *Pediatr Clin North Am* 1984; 31:569–589.
101. Chochinov RH, Ullyot GLE, Moorhouse JA: Sensory perception thresholds in patients with diabetes and their relatives. *N Engl J Med* 1972; 286:1233.
102. Fraser DM, et al: Peripheral and autonomic nerve function in newly diagnosed diabetes mellitus. *Diabetes* 1977; 26:546.

103. Clements RS: Diabetic neuropathy: Diagnosis and treatment. *Clin Diabetes* 1984; 2:73.
104. Greene DS, et al: Glucose-induced alterations in nerve metabolism: Current perspectives on the pathogenesis of diabetic neuropathy and future directions for research and therapy. *Diabetes Care* 1985; 8:290.
105. Kutt H, et al: Cerebrospinal fluid protein in diabetes mellitus. *Arch Neurol* 1961; 4:31.
106. Pietri A, Ehle AL, Raskin P: Changes in nerve conduction velocity after six weeks of glucoregulation with portable insulin infusion pumps. *Diabetes* 1980; 29:668.
107. Chylack LT Jr, Kinoshita JH: A biochemical evaluation of a cataract induced in a high-glucose medium. *Invest Ophthalmol* 1969; 8:401.
108. Pirart J: Diabetes mellitus and its degenerative complications: A prospective study of 4400 patients observed between 1947 and 1973. *Diabetes Care* 1978; 1:168, 252.
109. Barta L, Brooser G, Molnar M: Diagnostic importance of fluorescein angiography in infantile diabetes. *Acta Diabetol Lat* 1972; 9:290.
110. Waltman SR, et al: Quantitative vitreous fluorophotometry: A sensitive technique for measuring early breakdown of the blood-retinal barrier in young diabetic patients. *Diabetes* 1978; 27:85.
111. Burditt A, Caird F, Draper G: The natural history of diabetic retinopathy. *Q J Med* 1968; 37:303.
112. The Diabetic Retinopathy Study Research Group: Photocoagulation treatment of proliferative diabetic retinopathy. *Ophthalmology* 1978; 85:82.
113. Kohner EM, Dollery CT: Fluorescein angiography of the fundus in diabetic retinopathy. *Br Med Bull* 1970; 26:166.
114. Early Treatment Diabetic Retinopathy Study Research Group: Treatment techniques and clinical guidelines for photocoagulation of diabetic macular edema. *Ophthalmology* 1987; 94:761.
115. Diabetic Retinopathy Vitrectomy Study Research Group: Early vitrectomy for severe vitreous hemorrhage in diabetic retinopathy. *Arch Ophthalmol* 1985; 103:1644.
116. Balodimos MC, Legg MA, Bradley RF: Diabetic glomeruloscleroses in children. *Diabetes* 1971; 20:622.
117. Kussman MJ, Goldstein HH, Gleason RE: The clinical course of diabetic nephropathy. *JAMA* 1976; 236:1861.
118. Christiansen JS, et al: The natural history of diabetic nephropathy. *Diabetic Neuropathy* 1985; 4:104–106.
119. Viberti GC, Wiseman M, Redmond S: Microalbuminuria: Its history and potential for prevention of clinic nephropathy in diabetes mellitus. *Diabetic Nephropathy* 1984; 3:79–82.
120. Rubenstein AH, Spitz I: Role of the kidney in insulin metabolism and excretion. *Diabetes* 1968; 17:161.
121. Gotto A: Interactions with the major risk factors for coronary heart disease. *Am J Med* 1986; 80:48.
122. Lopes-Virella MF, et al: Effect of metabolic control on lipid, lipoprotein, and a polylipoprotein levels in 55 insulin dependent diabetic patients: A longitudinal study. *Diabetes* 1983; 32:20.
123. Ramsay RC, et al: Progression of diabetic retinopathy after pancreas transplantation for insulin-dependent diabetes mellitus. *N Engl J Med* 1988; 318:208.
124. Beck-Nielsen H, et al: Effect of insulin pump treatment for 1 year on renal function and retinal morphology in patients with IDDM. *Diabetes Care* 1985; 8:585.
125. Frauman AG, et al: Long-term use of intranasal insulin in insulin-dependent diabetic patients. *Diabetes Care* 1987; 10:573.

126. Hellerstrom C, et al: Experimental pancreatic transplantation in diabetes. *Diabetes Care* 1988; 11 (suppl 1):45.
127. Dupre J, et al: Clinical trials of cyclosporin in IDDM. *Diabetes Care* 1988; 11 (suppl 1):37.
128. Silverstein J, et al: Immunosuppression with azathioprine and prednisone in recent-onset insulin dependent diabetes mellitus. *N Engl J Med* 1988; 319:593.
129. Vinik AI, Jenkins DJA: Dietary fiber in management of diabetes. *Diabetes Care* 1988; 11:160.
130. Rodbard D: Potential role of computers in clinical investigation and management of diabetes mellitus. *Diabetes Care* 1988; 11(suppl 1):54.
131. Glasgow RE, McCaul KD, Schafer LC: Self-care behaviors and glycemic control in type I diabetes. *J Chronic Dis* 1987; 40:399.
132. Spencer ML: Type I diabetes: Control with individualized insulin regimens. *Postgrad Med* 1989; 85:201.

2

Hypoglycemia

Early diagnosis and treatment of hypoglycemia in children of any age is important. Brain damage occurs[1] and is apt to be more severe following hypoglycemia in the young infant. An appreciation of the many factors involved in maintaining normal blood glucose levels will allow a more logical approach to the complex problem of hypoglycemia.

CARBOHYDRATE HOMEOSTASIS

The major sources of blood glucose are the intestines (carbohydrate digestion and absorption) and the liver (glycogenolysis and gluconeogenesis). Adequate gluconeogenic substrates, primarily lactate, pyruvate, glycerol, and amino acids, are necessary to maintain normal blood glucose during fasting.[2] Functional hepatic enzymes for glycogenolysis and gluconeogenesis, and normal hormone action, are also critical. The endogenous control of glucose homeostasis has been summarized in an excellent review by Pagliara et al.[3] The reader is referred to this article for more detail. Glycogenolysis and gluconeogenesis are diagrammed in Figure 2–1.

Healthy children, in contrast to adults, become hypoglycemic when fasted for 24 to 48 hours.[4] Glycogen stores are sufficient to meet obligatory glucose requirements for 8 to 12 hours, but by 24 hours glucose is derived primarily by gluconeogenesis. Lipolysis provides free fatty acids that are oxidized to ketones which the brain can utilize.[5]

Insulin is the primary hormone regulating blood glucose levels. It promotes the storage of carbohydrates, fat, and protein. Just a minimal excess of insulin can suppress lipolysis and inhibit glucose release from the liver, whereas a greater concentration of insulin increases disposal of glucose into muscle and

40

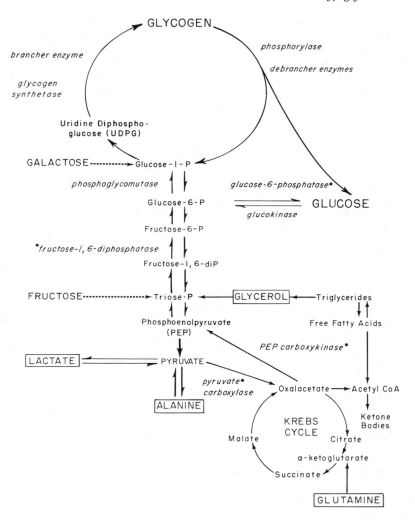

FIG 2–1.
Metabolic pathways for glycogen synthesis, glycogenolysis, and gluconeogenesis. Insulin stimulates glycogen synthetase and inhibits phosphorylase. Glucagon and epinephrine have the opposite effect. * = rate-limiting enzyme of gluconeogenesis. □ = principal gluconeogenic substrates.

adipose tissue cells.[6] This differential effect becomes important in the diagnosis of hyperinsulinism.[7]

Glucagon is the major hormone of fasting, while *growth hormone, glucocorticoids,* and *catecholamines* all tend to counteract the hypoglycemic effects of insulin and supply glucose and ketones to the brain and other tissues.[8] This is accomplished by inhibition of glucose uptake by muscle, mobilization of gluconeogenic amino acids (primarily alanine and glutamine), lipolysis, inhibition of insulin secretion, stimulation of glycogenolytic enzymes, and induction and activation of gluconeogenic enzymes. The hormonal effect on hepatic enzymes is mediated by cyclic adenosine 3',5' monophosphate.[9] Somatostatin and thyroid hormones do not seem to have a major effect on glucose homeostasis.

DEFINITION OF HYPOGLYCEMIA

A normal blood glucose level at birth is about 80% of the mother's blood glucose concentration, but falls rapidly during the first few hours of life. The normal range in a full-term infant is 30 to 120 mg/dL (mean, 50 to 60 mg/dL) for the first few days.

In a low birth weight infant the blood glucose may fall significantly lower (20 to 100 mg/dL) and remain low for 1 to 2 months.[10] More recently it is believed that these levels are too low and that any infant with blood glucose less than 40 mg/dL is at risk.[11]

Therefore, hypoglycemia can be defined as two or more sequential blood glucose values under 40 mg/dL. If clinical manifestations are present, but disappear after normalization of blood glucose, it can be assumed that symptomatic hypoglycemia exists.

Hypoglycemia is not a specific disease entity, but refers to an abnormal laboratory finding. Once hypoglycemia has been established on the basis of reliable blood glucose determinations, the cause must be determined. A classification of disorders associated with hypoglycemia is presented in Table 2–1.

TRANSIENT NEONATAL HYPOGLYCEMIA

Symptoms of hypoglycemia in the neonatal period include tremors, cyanosis, convulsions, apnea, limpness, unresponsiveness, and tachypnea. Unfortunately, these symptoms also are seen with central nervous system (CNS) disease, congenital heart disease, hypocalcemia, and other metabolic diseases. To add to the confusion, about 12% to 15% of infants with hypoglycemia also have hypocalcemia.[12] Only by noting the effects of treating each problem separately can we determine which factor is responsible for the symptoms.

Certain groups of newborn infants have been delineated as at risk for hypoglycemia. The incidence of hypoglycemia in *low birth weight infants* varies (5.7%[12] to 67%[13]) according to the criteria used for diagnosis, but most physicians agree that there is a direct relationship between blood glucose and body weight. The incidence of hypoglycemia increases as intrauterine growth retardation becomes more marked.[13, 14]

Hypoglycemia in the low birth weight infant usually occurs after the first

TABLE 2–1.
Classification of Disorders Associated With Hypoglycemia

I. Transient neonatal hypoglycemia
   A. Low birth weight infant
   B. "Hyperinsulinism"
      1. Infant of diabetic or gestational diabetic mother
      2. Infant with erythroblastosis
   C. Stresses in infant that may be associated with hypoglycemia
      1. Sepsis
      2. Cold injury
      3. Surgery
      4. Hyperalimentation
      5. Respiratory distress
II. Persistent hypoglycemia of infancy and childhood
   A. Inability to release adequate endogeneous glucose
      1. Hereditary enzyme deficiencies
         a. Glycogen storage diseases
            (1) Glucose-6-phosphatase (type I)
            (2) Debrancher enzyme complex (type III)
            (3) Phosphorylase abnormalities (type VI)
         b. Glycogen synthetase deficiency
         c. Fructose intolerance (decreased fructose-1-phosphate aldolase)
         d. Fructose-1,6-diphosphatase deficiency
         e. Galactose intolerance (galactose-1-phosphate uridyl transferase deficiency)
         f. Pyruvate carboxylase deficiency
         g. Phosphoenol pyruvate carboxykinase deficiency
         h. Amino acid disorders (cystinosis, maple syrup urine disease, tyrosinemia, arginosuccinic aciduria)
         i. Defects in fatty acid oxidation and ketogenesis (carnitine deficiency)
      2. Ketotic hypoglycemia
      3. Hormone abnormalities
         a. Panhypopituitarism
         b. Isolated growth hormone deficiency
         c. Glucocorticoid deficiency
             (1) Congenital adrenal hyperplasia
            (2) Addison's disease; ACTH unresponsiveness
            (3) Isolated adrenocorticotrophin deficiency
         d. Catecholamine abnormalities
         e. Thyroid hormone deficiency
      4. Liver disease
         a. Reye's syndrome
         b. Hepatitis, cirrhosis
      5. Malnutrition
   B. Increased or inappropriate insulin release
      1. Beta cell hyperplasia
      2. Nesidioblastosis
      3. Islet cell adenoma
      4. ? Functional hyperinsulinism
      5. Reactive hypoglycemia
      6. Beckwith-Wiedemann syndrome

continued.

TABLE 2–1 *(cont.)*

III. Miscellaneous disorders associated with hypoglycemia
    A. Extrapancreatic tumors
        1. Fibrosarcoma
        2. Wilms' tumor
        3. Hepatoma
        4. Neuroblastoma
    B. Malabsorption
    C. Poisons or toxins
        1. Salicylates
        2. Oral hypoglycemics
        3. Insulin
        4. Jamaican vomiting sickness
        5. TRIS buffer
        6. Propranolol
        7. Alcohol

24 hours. It is probably the result of decreased glycogen stores and increased utilization of carbohydrate because of the higher brain/liver ratio. Birth hypoxia, sepsis, and other stresses contribute to increased carbohydrate use. High levels of alanine and other substrates have been found in these infants, which suggests immaturity of the hepatic gluconeogenic enzyme system as a possible cause of hypoglycemia.[15] Decreased corticosteroid production[16] and inability to increase epinephrine secretion[17] also have been implicated in the pathogenesis of hypoglycemia in low birth weight infants. Free fatty acid levels and ketone bodies in the blood of those infants who become hypoglycemic are lower than in normoglycemic low birth weight infants.[18] However, it is likely that there is no single cause and that multiple factors interplay to cause hypoglycemia in an already vulnerable infant.

Immature infants who have appropriate weight for gestational age usually are not hypoglycemic unless additional stresses, such as *respiratory distress syndrome* or sepsis, are present.[19]

Excessive birth weight for gestational age also carries a greater risk of hypoglycemia. This category includes the *infant of a diabetic mother* (IDM) and the *infant of a gestational diabetic mother* (IGDM). The incidence of hypoglycemia in the IDM varies with the criteria used, reported as 16% (blood glucose <20 mg/dL) and 44% (blood glucose <30 mg/dL).[20] The frequency of hypoglycemia in the IGDM is about 20% (blood glucose <30 mg/dL).[20] Only 10% to 20% of the infants in both groups who have a blood glucose in the hypoglycemic range are symptomatic.[13]

The IDM and IGDM are clinically similar. Both have increased body fat and glycogen secondary to *hyperinsulinism*. Islet cell hyperplasia is present at autopsy.[10] In addition, decreased catecholamine response to hypoglycemia has been reported.[21]

Hypoglycemia tends to occur within the first few hours of life. Recurrent hypoglycemia is a hazard if glucose infusion is abruptly stopped. Normal development usually occurs if no other congenital anomalies are present.[22, 23] This syndrome can be prevented by meticulous blood glucose control during the last trimester of pregnancy.

Infants with *erythroblastosis fetalis* develop hypoglycemia. The incidence is related to the severity of the primary disease, for example, an incidence of 17.8% with the cord hemoglobin less than 10 gm/dL, and only 1.9% with the cord hemoglobin greater than 10 gm/dL.[24] Autopsy and serum insulin measurements confirm hyperinsulinism as the cause of hypoglycemia.[24, 25] Reactive hypoglycemia is also a problem, particularly if ACD blood is used for the exchange transfusion.[26]

Infants with *sepsis, CNS hemorrhage*, or *anomalies*, or those exposed to *cold injury*,[27] are prone to hypoglycemia, as are infants subjected to *hyperalimentation* or *surgery*.[28] A positive relationship between *gram-negative sepsis* and hypoglycemia has been noted,[29] as well as increased peripheral utilization of glucose in neonatal sepsis.[30]

The effect of hypoglycemia on the future development of infants is not well documented. It is not always clear whether neurologic damage is the result of the low blood glucose level, or of a primary neurologic disorder that might be responsible for the hypoglycemia.[22] A study by Griffiths and Bryant[31] compares the neurologic status of a group of children who were hypoglycemic during the neonatal period with that of matched controls. Evidence of cerebral damage at the mean age of 51 months occurred in 14.6% of those who had been hypoglycemic and in 2.2% of controls. The difference was not statistically significant. In addition, infants with asymptomatic hypoglycemia had no evidence of brain damage. Prognosis is reported to be worse if the infant was symptomatic with convulsions.[32]

PERSISTENT HYPOGLYCEMIA OF INFANCY AND CHILDHOOD

In 1954 McQuarrie described a group of infants with fasting hypoglycemia of unknown cause.[33] There was a high incidence of neurologic sequelae, and treatment with diet alone frequently was unsuccessful. Subsequently, the term idiopathic hypoglycemia was used to classify any patient with low blood glucose of undetermined cause, regardless of severity. With improved laboratory techniques, it is now possible to identify a specific abnormality of carbohydrate homeostasis in most cases.

Hereditary Enzyme Deficiencies

Hypoglycemia due to hereditary enzyme deficiencies sometimes is apparent in the newborn period, depending upon the severity of the defect. The *glycogen storage diseases* associated with low blood glucose—types I, III, and VI—are caused by abnormalities of glucose-6-phosphatase, debrancher enzymes, and phosphorylase, respectively. They share the features of growth retardation, hepatomegaly, cushingoid appearance, and significant hypoglycemia that may be asymptomatic. Type I usually is the most severe and is characterized by hyperlipidemia, hyperuricemia, and lactic acidosis. In all types, hypoglycemia is a result of inability to release glucose from the liver.[34]

Glycogen synthetase deficiency is a rare cause of hypoglycemia in which hepatomegaly is not a prominent feature. Absent or decreased glycogen is demonstrated by liver biopsy in addition to an abnormal glucagon test in a fasted state.[35]

The presenting symptom in *galactosemia* usually is not hypoglycemia. Patients have jaundice, cataracts, vomiting, hepatosplenomegaly with cirrhosis, failure to thrive, and mental retardation, as well as mellituria and aminoaciduria. Hypoglycemia, when present, is thought to be secondary to the accumulation of galactose-1-phosphate, which may inhibit phosphoglucomutase, resulting in acute inhibition of glycogenolysis.[36] The defect is a deficiency of galactose-1-phosphate uridyl transferase. Avoidance of galactose prevents progression of symptoms and permits normal growth and development.[37]

Fructose intolerance (decreased fructose-1-phosphate aldolase) is manifested by symptoms of hypoglycemia and vomiting following feedings containing fructose. Hepatomegaly, failure to thrive, and renal tubular acidosis also may be present. Hypoglycemia is secondary to the accumulation of fructose-1-phosphate.[38] *Fructose-1,6-diphosphatase deficiency* has been described in patients with hepatomegaly, fasting hypoglycemia, lactic acidosis, and increased pyruvate levels in the blood. These children are unable to convert alanine, fructose, or glycerol to glucose.[39]

Hyperlactemia, hyperpyruvemia, and hypoglycemia have also been observed with inactivity of pyruvate carboxylase, which converts pyruvate to oxaloacetate.[40]

Deficiency of phosphoenol pyruvate carboxykinase has also been reported.[41] Inactivity of this enzyme blocks the Cori cycle and causes hypoglycemia associated with elevated levels of lactate and pyruvate.

The presence of hypoglycemia in *maple syrup urine disease* (abnormal excretion of the amino acids valine, leucine, and isoleucine) was reported in 1961. The cause of hypoglycemia is thought to be defective gluconeogenesis.[42] Hypoglycemia may occur in other amino acid disorders such as tyrosinemia, cystinosis, and argininosuccinicaciduria.

Carnitine is a vitamin and cofactor important in the oxidation of long-chain fatty acids. Hereditary carnitine deficiency may present in infancy or early childhood with hypoglycemia, vomiting, coma, seizures, and no urine ketones.[43]

Ketotic Hypoglycemia

The most frequent type of symptomatic hypoglycemia occurring in childhood probably is ketotic hypoglycemia.[44] It is characterized by early morning ketosis, vomiting, and hypoglycemic seizures. Frequently, these episodes follow brief periods of food deprivation or infection.

In 1964 Colle and Ulstrom[45] demonstrated that a low calorie, high fat diet provoked ketosis and hypoglycemia in some children with "idiopathic hypoglycemia." However, since that time it has been established that all children on a ketogenic diet, followed by a prolonged fast, become equally ketotic and hypoglycemic.[46] In fact, Chaussain[4] found a large overlap in mean blood sugar levels and degree of ketosis after a 24-hour fast both in children with ketotic hypoglycemia and in healthy children. Glucagon unresponsiveness during hypoglycemia is the common finding.[45]

Hypofunction of the adrenal medulla has been implicated in ketotic hypoglycemia,[47, 48] but has not been confirmed by all investigators.[49] Growth hormone, cortisol, and insulin responses are appropriate during hypoglycemia.[4, 46] The coincidence of ketosis and hypoglycemia may occur in a number of disorders as a result of specific enzyme or hormone deficiencies. However, in a majority of children, it probably represents an exaggeration of the normal tendency to respond to starvation with ketonuria and a fall in blood glucose. Alanine has been reported to be low in these children.[47, 50] This may reflect either a decrease in glucose-derived pyruvate[51] or a true deficiency.[50] Ketotic hypoglycemia is typically seen in small, thin children who presumably would have limited glycogen stores and gluconeogenic precursors. There could be an association between catecholamine insufficiency and low gluconeogenic amino acids as the cause of hypoglycemia in these children.

Hormone Deficiencies

Growth hormone, cortisol, catecholamines, and to a lesser extent *thyroxine* normally act as insulin antagonists with respect to carbohydrate homeostasis. Children with congenital adrenal hyperplasia, Addison's disease, or growth hormone deficiency are particularly prone to hypoglycemia when there is a decrease of carbohydrate intake.[52-54] The presence of microphallus and hypoglycemia at birth should alert one to the possibility of hypothalamic-pituitary insufficiency.[55] These endocrine deficiency states are dangerous in patients with diabetes mellitus because of the increased risk of severe hypoglycemia following insulin administration.[56] A few cases of glucagon deficiency have been reported to be associated with hypoglycemia in children, but these are not well documented.[57]

Liver Disease

In view of the central role of the liver in blood glucose regulation, it is readily understood that *acute* and *chronic liver disease* may interfere with carbohydrate metabolism. Hepatic glycogen synthesis and gluconeogenesis may be impaired in *acute viral hepatitis*, causing fasting hypoglycemia.[58] *Cirrhosis, biliary disease,* and *hepatotoxins* may also be responsible for hypoglycemia. *Reye's syndrome* (encephalopathy with fatty degeneration of the liver) is associated with hypoglycemia, particularly in the younger child.[59, 60]

Malnutrition

Severely malnourished children exhibit an accelerated decline in blood glucose concentrations on fasting. Insulin levels are appropriate.[61] Decreased liver glycogen and gluconeogenic substrates are the most likely explanations for this finding.

Hyperinsulinism

Hyperinsulinism, or inappropriate insulin secretion, is observed in some children with hypoglycemia. *Leucine sensitivity* was first described by Cochrane et al. in 1956.[62] They noted an increased number of seizures when some children with idiopathic hypoglycemia were placed on a high protein, low carbohydrate diet. The onset of symptoms usually was early in the 1st year of life when milk is the primary food.

Leucine stimulates insulin secretion in all people[63]; however, certain children show an exaggerated release of insulin with an associated fall of blood glucose. A high correlation between leucine sensitivity and insulinomas has been noted both in children[64] and in adults.[65] It now appears that leucine sensitivity should not be considered a diagnosis per se, but rather an indication of hyperinsulinism, which in turn may be caused by an islet cell tumor, beta cell hyperplasia, nesidioblastosis, or abnormal secretion of insulin without histologic abnormality.

Beta cell adenomas (insulinomas) are uncommon in children and even less frequent among those under 1 year of age.[66] Although rare, an insulinoma is a potentially curable cause of hypoglycemia. Unfortunately, brain damage frequently occurs before the tumor is removed, emphasizing the need for early diagnosis. Most children are first seen with persistent severe hypoglycemia unresponsive to medical therapy. Insulin levels alone have not been diagnostic, but the glucose-insulin ratio may be of some value.[67] (See the section Diagnosis of Hypoglycemia.) Elevated plasma proinsulin has been noted in adults with insulinomas.[68]

Inappropriately low concentrations of β-hydroxybutyrate and free fatty acids in the presence of hypoglycemia are evidence of hyperinsulinism in infants and young children.[69] Chaussain et al.[70] reported the association of low blood glucose and low concentrations of branched-chain amino acids (valine, leucine, isoleucine) with hyperinsulinism in infancy. In children, the tolbutamide tolerance test has not been useful because both false positive and false negative responses occur.[71] The leucine tolerance test, when performed, has been positive in most patients.[65, 72, 73] However, it is not possible to differentiate insulinomas from other causes of hyperinsulinism on the basis of the glucose:insulin ratio or the response to leucine administration.

Nesidioblastosis[74, 75] refers to a proliferation of beta cells along the pancreatic ducts and can therefore be considered an extension of an embryologic process. Unlike classic beta cell hyperplasia, histologic demonstration of nesidioblastosis may require the use of special histochemical staining techniques.

Although hyperinsulinism resulting from beta cell adenoma would not be expected to resolve spontaneously, neither the natural history nor the frequency of beta cell hyperplasia or nesidioblastosis in children is known.

Reactive hypoglycemia associated with mild carbohydrate intolerance sometimes is seen in children. Attacks of hypoglycemia occur approximately 3 to 5 hours after meals. During a glucose tolerance test, such individuals often have normal or slightly elevated fasting blood glucose levels, an elevated 1-hour blood glucose, a delay in the return of blood glucose to normal, and then a sudden fall to hypoglycemic levels. A delayed but exaggerated insulin response has been found.[76] Patients commonly complain of headaches, fainting spells, or lethargy in the late morning or late afternoon.

Infant giants (Beckwith-Wiedemann syndrome) are children with increased birth weight, excessive growth, omphalocele or umbilical hernia, macroglossia, hepatomegaly, and renal enlargement. Neonatal hypoglycemia occurs and persists in a variable number of these infants (20% to 50%).[77] Hyperinsulinism and pancreatic islet cell hyperplasia have been documented.[78]

MISCELLANEOUS DISORDERS ASSOCIATED WITH HYPOGLYCEMIA

In addition to tumors of the beta cells of the pancreas, a variety of *extrapancreatic neoplasms* have been associated with hypoglycemic symptoms.[79] There are reports of recurrent hypoglycemia in patients with *fibrosarcomas, Wilms' tumor, hepatomas,* and *neuroblastomas,* although these are rare in children.[80] The cause for the hypoglycemia may be the production of an insulin-like substance, decreased insulin degradation, increased glucose use, or the presence of an insulin-stimulating substance.

Malabsorption syndromes, whether caused by congenital enzyme deficiencies or secondary to infection or allergy, may have associated hypoglycemia due to starvation or to excess stimulation of insulin.[81]

A drug history should be obtained in all patients with hypoglycemia. *Salicylate intoxication* more commonly causes hyperglycemia and glycosuria, though hypoglycemia has been reported, especially in the younger child.[82] The effect of salicylates on carbohydrate metabolism is not well understood. *Oral hypoglycemic agents* are responsible for severe, protracted hypoglycemia. Maternal ingestion of these agents may result in hypoglycemia in the newborn infant,[83] and severe hypoglycemia also may follow the use of chlorpropamide in the treatment of diabetes insipidus.[84] Other toxic or drug-associated episodes of hypoglycemia include ingestion of unripe akee fruit *(Jamaican vomiting sickness),* *TRIS buffer* (tromethamine), or *propranolol.*[85]

Acute alcohol ingestion has been reported with increased frequency in children. Hypoglycemia is a frequent complication and is due to decreased hepatic gluconeogenesis.[86]

Factitious hypoglycemia may occur in older children. Insulin being used in the household should alert one to the possibility.

DIAGNOSIS OF HYPOGLYCEMIA

Investigation of hypoglycemia in children requires an individualized approach. Not all metabolic studies need to be done on all children. This is particularly true in the infant less than 6 months of age. An infant's small blood volume limits the number of tests. Furthermore, in patients with severe hypoglycemia, the blood glucose may be so difficult to control that studies of carbohydrate metabolism are impossible to perform or interpret, and the high risk of permanent brain damage necessitates prompt and continuous treatment.

Figure 2–2 is an outline of a diagnostic/management approach in an infant with symptoms of hypoglycemia; Figure 2–3 depicts evaluation of hypoglycemia in a child. The history and physical examination are most important in defining which aspect of carbohydrate homeostasis needs investigation. Details such as age at onset, frequency, and temporal relationship of symptoms to meals are significant in addition to any family history of carbohydrate abnormalities. All medications received by a child (or in the case of a newborn, the mother) should be noted. Each child's height and weight should be carefully plotted on growth curves and the size of the liver recorded. Hepatomegaly suggests that liver function should be the first area thoroughly studied.

Studies of Carbohydrate Metabolism

Proper preparation of the patient is important for metabolic studies. Although not always feasible, optimum results are obtained when the child is quiet, adequately nourished, and free of emotional stress. Drugs known to affect carbohydrate tolerance, such as salicylates, diuretics, and diphenylhydantoin,[87, 88] should be avoided if possible. In all studies, serum insulin determinations, as well as blood glucose measurements should be obtained.

Serial blood glucose determinations with simultaneous insulin levels in the fasting state are helpful in determining the pattern and severity of the hypoglycemia. These measurements may have to be continued over 18 to 24 hours. The fast is terminated if significant hypoglycemia occurs. During this time, urine is tested for ketones. The glucose-insulin ratio may establish the presence of relative hyperinsulinism even when insulin values appear low. This ratio in the normal fasting subject is roughly 5:1 or 10:1; absolute insulin values usually range from about 5 to 15 μU/ml.[89, 67] Concentrations of β-hydroxybutyrate and free fatty acids seem to be sensitive indicators of the suppressive effect of insulin on lipolysis even in the presence of normal insulin levels in the peripheral blood.[7] Branched-chain amino acid levels also parallel β-hydroxybutyrate concentrations.[70] Growth hormone and cortisol levels should also be obtained during fasting and may help to eliminate the possibility of hypopituitarism as a cause of hypoglycemia. However, if pituitary deficiency is strongly considered on clinical grounds, a more extensive evaluation should be conducted (see Chapter 3). Elevated lactate and other gluconeogenic substrates point to a defect in hepatic

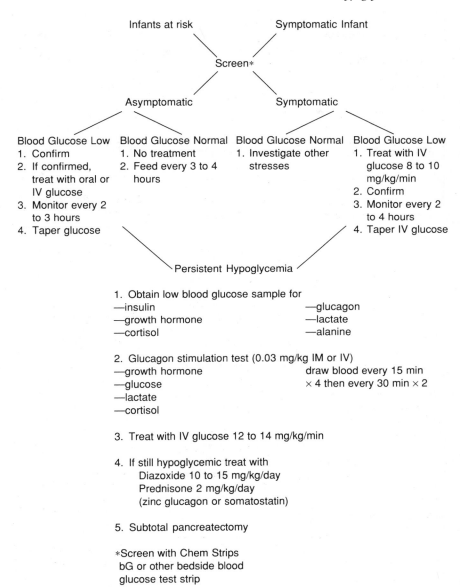

Infants at risk   Symptomatic Infant

Screen*

Asymptomatic   Symptomatic

Blood Glucose Low
1. Confirm
2. If confirmed,
   treat with oral or
   IV glucose
3. Monitor every 2
   to 3 hours
4. Taper glucose

Blood Glucose Normal
1. No treatment
2. Feed every 3 to 4
   hours

Blood Glucose Normal
1. Investigate other
   stresses

Blood Glucose Low
1. Treat with IV
   glucose 8 to 10
   mg/kg/min
2. Confirm
3. Monitor every 2
   to 4 hours
4. Taper IV glucose

Persistent Hypoglycemia

1. Obtain low blood glucose sample for
   —insulin   —glucagon
   —growth hormone   —lactate
   —cortisol   —alanine

2. Glucagon stimulation test (0.03 mg/kg IM or IV)
   —growth hormone   draw blood every 15 min
   —glucose   × 4 then every 30 min × 2
   —lactate
   —cortisol

3. Treat with IV glucose 12 to 14 mg/kg/min

4. If still hypoglycemic treat with
   Diazoxide 10 to 15 mg/kg/day
   Prednisone 2 mg/kg/day
   (zinc glucagon or somatostatin)

5. Subtotal pancreatectomy

*Screen with Chem Strips
bG or other bedside blood
glucose test strip

FIG 2–2.
Diagnostic/management approach to neonatal hypoglycemia.

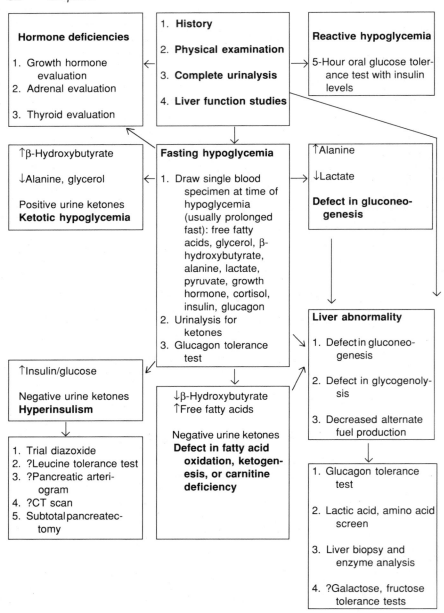

FIG 2–3.
Diagnostic approach to childhood hypoglycemia. Information gained from the initial history, physical examination, and laboratory studies define specific areas of carbohydrate metabolism that require further investigation.

gluconeogenesis. Low β-hydroxybutyrate with elevated free fatty acids may indicate a defect in fatty acid oxidation, ketogenesis, or carnitine deficiency.

An *oral glucose tolerance test* (see Appendix 1–D) is frequently performed, but responses are variable and sometimes of little diagnostic value. Patients with hyperinsulinism have been reported to have a diabetic curve as a result of the Somogyi phenomenon[90] (see Chapter 1). Malabsorption may cause a flat or diabetic curve depending on the defect and transit time. A glucose concentration of 40 mg/dL or less at 3 to 5 hours suggests reactive hypoglycemia; levels of 40 to 50 mg/dL are suspicious, particularly if associated with symptoms. Delayed and excessive insulin secretion also is common in reactive hypoglycemia.[76]

An *intravenous glucose tolerance test* has been used primarily in infants to determine the rate of glucose disappearance (K_1). An elevated K_1 value (over 2) has been reported in infants with low birth weight,[91] infants with neonatal infection,[30] and a miscellaneous group of infants[92] with symptomatic hypoglycemia. Hyperinsulinism and increased peripheral utilization for various reasons could increase the K_1 rate. Beard et al.[93] suggested using the intravenous glucose tolerance test therapeutically; for example, a K_1 value of over 3 in an infant with symptomatic hypoglycemia is an indication that hydrocortisone, in addition to intravenous glucose, should be given.

Leucine stimulates the release of insulin from the beta cells of the pancreas. A positive *leucine tolerance test* in a child less than 1 year of age indicates hyperinsulinism resulting from either a functional sensitivity to leucine, nesidioblastosis, beta cell hyperplasia, or an adenoma. In the older child with recent onset of symptoms, a positive test is particularly suggestive of an adenoma. (Suggested procedure for the leucine test and other tolerance tests is outlined in Appendix 2.)

Glucagon stimulates glucose release from the liver by activating the phosphorylase system and glycogenolysis. A normal response to the *glucagon tolerance test* indicates both adequate stores and normal enzyme activity. Excessive hyperglycemia can be seen in patients with hyperinsulinism as well as a reactive hypoglycemia.[94] This test may also be used as a stimulus to the release of both growth hormone and glucocorticoids if prolonged to 3 hours.[95]

Tolbutamide causes insulin release in healthy subjects. In adults, an exaggerated response to the *tolbutamide tolerance test* occurs in the presence of an insulinoma.[96] However, in children, tolbutamide causes significant hypoglycemia in any entity with hyperinsulinism and is not a specific diagnostic test for insulinoma.[71] Therefore, because of the severe clinical hypoglycemic response seen with tolbutamide, leucine probably is a safer stimulus to assess hyperinsulinism.

Specific tests for *thyroid, growth hormone,* and *adrenal function* (see Chapters 3, 6, and 7) should be performed if there is clinical evidence of deficiency.

Pancreatic arteriograms have been suggested for localization of insulinomas. Accurate detection appears possible in about 50% of patients, but experience in younger children is limited.[88, 97]

Percutaneous transhepatic selective pancreatic venous catheterization for venous sampling for insulin assay may facilitate localization of occult insulinomas at surgery.[98]

TREATMENT

Immediate

An acute hypoglycemic episode must be treated initially with *intravenous* (IV) *glucose*, even if the exact cause is not known. A 50% glucose solution (1 to 2 mL/kg), diluted with an equal volume of sterile water, is administered by rapid infusion, followed by a 10% to 15% glucose solution. The rate of infusion and the concentration of glucose may gradually be reduced over the next few days.

If intravenous treatment is not possible, aqueous *glucagon* (0.03 mg/kg, up to a maximum dose of 1 mg) or *epinephrine* 1:1,000 (0.01 mL/kg) could be used intramuscularly or subcutaneously. Because of the short action of these drugs, oral feedings must follow once the patient is alert. Many children vomit, either secondary to hypoglycemia or to the glucagon, but this alone may help to raise blood glucose. Glucagon probably will be of little value in patients with decreased glycogen stores, defective liver glycogenolysis, or gluconeogenesis (e.g., glycogen storage disease or low birth weight).

If the symptoms of hypoglycemia persist, *hydrocortisone* (5 mg/kg/day) or *prednisone* (2 mg/kg/day) may be added. However, *diazoxide* (5 to 15 mg/kg/day), a benzothiadiazine that suppresses insulin secretion and also increases blood glucose by stimulating glucose release from the liver,[99] is more specific if hyperinsulinism is suspected.

Contrary to the experience in adults, there has been only one reported case of beta cell adenoma in a child that responded to diazoxide.[100] Therefore, therapeutic failure increases the likelihood that an insulinoma is present. The predominant side effects are hypertrichosis and hyperglycemia, which are dose related. Other problems reported in children are anorexia; hyperuricemia; sodium retention; and, rarely, hematologic abnormalities and skin rash.

Our experience with diazoxide showed that 13 of 17 children with persistent hypoglycemia responded to diazoxide (5 to 10 mg/kg) within 48 hours. The pathologic diagnoses in the four infants who failed to respond were islet cell adenoma (two children) and nesidioblastoma (two).[101] Maximum duration of treatment was 11 years. Treatment was discontinued in three children, all of whom remained asymptomatic in spite of continued laboratory evidence of hyperinsulinism. Addition of a thiazide diuretic may potentiate the hyperglycemic effect of diazoxide and prevent fluid retention.

Phenytoin, which inhibits insulin release,[87] has been reported effective in some cases of hypoglycemia and may be considered an alternative to diazoxide. A long-acting somatostatin analog has been used to control hypoglycemia in refractory cases.[102] Surgical exploration and *subtotal pancreatectomy* are necessary if medical treatment continues to be unsuccessful.[103] This should not be delayed unnecessarily.

Maintenance

Adequate substitution therapy with *glucocorticoids, growth hormone,* or *thyroid* should be provided for patients with these deficiencies. Routine use of thyroid or growth hormone is not indicated for other causes of hypoglycemia. Long-term therapy with steroids may cause growth arrest and other expected undesirable side effects.

Infants at special risk for hypoglycemia should be fed initially at 4 to 6 hours of age and every 2 to 3 hours thereafter. *Frequent high-carbohydrate feedings* with additional sugar when a child becomes ketotic prevents most episodes of hypoglycemia in children with ketotic hypoglycemia. In addition, parents can be taught to monitor their child's blood glucose level. A *diabetic diet* consisting of 20% protein and 50% carbohydrate, (primarily complex) divided into six feedings is beneficial in reactive hypoglycemia. Most children with congenital metabolic disorders also respond to dietary measures. Avoidance of galactose in galactosemia and fructose in fructose intolerance improves the prognosis and symptoms.

Frequent feedings of glucose and avoidance of fructose, sucrose, and lactose improves the growth of children with type I glycogen storage disease and decreases the number of episodes of lactic acidosis. Creation of a *portacaval shunt* reduces hyperlipidemia and improves the growth rate in these patients.[104] Significant benefit has also been noted in patients treated with continuous nocturnal intragastric feeding[105, 106]; in fact, this regimen is probably as effective, and certainly less traumatic, than the portacaval shunt.

Low protein, low leucine diets have been used for infants displaying leucine sensitivity (hyperinsulinism). However, these generally are of little value, and lack of this essential amino acid causes poor growth. Long-acting preparations such as *zinc glucagon* and *epinephrine* in suspension have largely been replaced by *diazoxide* in the treatment of children with severe hypoglycemia. *Ephedrine* has been used in some children with ketotic hypoglycemia when dietary therapy failed.[48, 49]

Abdominal exploration and *subtotal pancreatectomy* have been advocated for the treatment of intractable hypoglycemia. This operation is curative in patients with beta cell adenoma, but about 25% of children with hyperinsulinism for other reasons require supplemental drug therapy following surgery.[100, 101]

In summary, hypoglycemia is a relatively frequent finding in infants and children. It is usually associated with a transient imbalance of glucose production and utilization. With a thorough history and careful laboratory evaluation, persistent hypoglycemia may be classified as due to increased insulin production, decreased substrate availability, or inability to produce or release endogenous glucose. This approach will facilitate treatment and may prevent neurologic sequelae.

APPENDIX 2

Leucine Tolerance Test

Procedure

After the patient has fasted 4 to 8 hours, 150 mg/kg of L- leucine is dissolved in a dilute alkaline solution, flavored and sweetened with saccharine, and administered orally. A nasogastric tube may have to be used. Blood for glucose and insulin is obtained at 0, 15, 30, 45, 60, and 90 minutes. If possible, blood for assessing growth hormone, glucagon, and corticoid levels should also be obtained.

Response

A positive test shows a decrease in blood glucose to 50% of the fasting value.[63] This usually occurs between 20 and 45 minutes, often precipitating symptoms. The results cannot be interpreted unless the fasting blood glucose level is more than 40 mg/dL and the glucose pattern of the patient while fasting is known (sham leucine test).

Glucagon Tolerance Test

Procedure

Following a fast of 6 to 8 hours, blood is obtained for glucose. Glucagon, 0.03 mg/kg (not more than 1 mg), is given intramuscularly. Specimens are collected at 0, 2, 5, 10, 20, 30, 60, 90, and 120 minutes. If glycogen storage disease is suspected, blood lactic acid should be determined. For evaluation of growth hormone and cortisol response, the test should be extended to 180 minutes, with blood samples obtained at 120 and 180 minutes for these hormones.[95]

Response

A rise in blood glucose of 25 to 50 mg/dL normally is found within 15 to 45 minutes. If hyperglycemia does not occur, the test should be repeated 3 hours after a meal. Under these conditions patients with type III glycogen storage disease usually respond positively, but those with type I do not. A rise in lactic acid during the test also is more frequently seen in type I glycogen storage disease.[34]

Intravenous Glucose Tolerance Test

Procedure

After the patient has fasted 3 to 4 hours without glucose infusion for at least 30 minutes, 50% glucose, 1 g/kg,[92] is injected rapidly. Blood for glucose and insulin is obtained at 0, 2, 5, and 10 minutes and every 10 minutes thereafter for 1 hour. (A dose of 0.5 g/kg of glucose also has been used.)

Glucose Disappearance Rate (K₁)

Blood glucose values are plotted against time on semilogarithmic paper, and the percentage disappearance rate/minute is calculated as a constant, K_1. A K_1 value greater than 2 is indicative of abnormality.[92] ($K_1 = \dfrac{0.693}{t^{1/2} \text{ (min)}} \times 100$.)

Prolonged Fast

Procedure

After the patient has fasted 4 to 8 hours, monitor blood glucose and urine ketones every 2 hours. At 18 to 24 hours, or when the blood glucose drops below 40 mg/dL, collect blood to test for glucose, lactate, pyruvate, glycerol, alanine, β-hydroxybutyrate, free fatty acids, insulin, cortisol, and growth hormone. Glucagon may be given at the end of this test (see Glucagon Tolerance Test earlier in this appendix).

Response

Results should be interpreted as illustrated in Figure 2–3. Increased β-hydroxybutyrate and decreased alanine and glycerol are consistent with ketotic hypoglycemia. Increased lactate and alanine indicates a defect in hepatic gluconeogenesis. Decreased β-hydroxybutyrate with increased free fatty acids and negative urine ketones indicates a defect in fatty acid oxidation, ketogenesis, or carnitine deficiency. Low cortisol or growth hormone response with hypoglycemia points to primary adrenal insufficiency or hypopituitarism. A decreased glucose-insulin ratio of less than 5:1 or an absolute fasting insulin level of greater than 15 μU/mL leads one to suspect hyperinsulinism. C peptide and proinsulin levels may also be helpful in this instance.

REFERENCES

1. Ingram TTS, Stark GD, Blackhorn K: Ataxia and other neurological disorders as sequels of severe hypoglycemia in childhood. *Brain* 1967; 90:851.
2. Felix P: The glucose-alanine cycle. *Metabolism* 1973; 22:179.
3. Pagliara AS, et al: Hypoglycemia in infancy and childhood. *J Pediatr* Part I, 1973; 82:365; Part II, 1973; 82:588.
4. Chaussain JL: Glycemic response to 24 hour fast in normal children and children with ketotic hypoglycemia. *J Pediatr* 1973; 82:438.
5. Owen OE, et al: Brain metabolism during fasting. *J Clin Invest* 1967; 46:1589.
6. Zierler KL, Rabinowitz D: Effect of small concentrations of insulin on forearm metabolism. Persistence of its action on potassium and free fatty acids without its effect on glucose. *J Clin Invest* 1964; 43:950.
7. Wolfsdorf JI, Senior B: The diagnosis of insulinoma in a child in the absence of fasting hyperinsulinemia. *Pediatrics* 1979; 64:496.
8. Liljenquist J, et al: Evidence for an important role of glucagon in the regulation of hepatic glucose production in normal man. *J Clin Invest* 1977; 59:369.
9. Exton JH: Gluconeogenesis. *Metabolism* 1972; 21:945.

10. Cornblath M, Schwartz R: *Disorders of Carbohydrate Metabolism in Infancy*. Philadelphia, WB Saunders Co, 1966.
11. Sexson WR: Incidence of neonatal hypoglycemia: A matter of definition. *J Pediatr* 1984; 105:149.
12. Pildes R, et al: Incidence of neonatal hypoglycemia. A completed survey. *J Pediatr* 1967; 70:76.
13. Lubchenco LQ, Bard H: Incidence of hypoglycemia in newborn infants classified by birth weight and gestational age. *Pediatrics* 1971; 47:831.
14. Haworth JC, Duling L, Younoszai MK: Relation of blood glucose to haematocrit, birth weight, and other body measurements in normal and growth-retarded newborn infants. *Lancet* 1967; 2:901.
15. Haymond MW, Karl IE, Pagliara AS: Increased gluconeogenic substrates in the small-for-gestational-age infant. *N Engl J Med* 1974; 291:322.
16. Cathro DM, Forsyth CG, Cameron J: Adrenocortical response to stress in newborn infants. *Arch Dis Child* 1969; 44:88.
17. Stern L, Sourkes TL, Raiha N: The role of the adrenal medulla in the hypoglycemia of foetal malnutrition. *Biol Neonate* 1967; 11:129.
18. deLeeuw R, deVries IJ: Hypoglycemia in small-for-dates newborn infants. *Pediatrics* 1976; 58:18.
19. Beard AG, et al: Perinatal stress and the premature neonate. Effect of fluid and caloric deprivation on blood glucose. *J Pediatr* 1966; 68:329.
20. Raivio KO, Hallman N: Neonatal hypoglycemia: I. Occurrence of hypoglycemia in patients with various neonatal disorders. *Acta Paediatr Scand* 1968; 57:517.
21. Stern L, Ramos A, Leduc J: Urinary catecholamine excretion in infants of diabetic mothers. *Pediatrics* 1968; 42:598.
22. Knobloch H, et al: Prognostic and etiologic factors in hypoglycemia. *J Pediatr* 1967; 70:876.
23. Farquhar JW: Prognosis for babies born to diabetic mothers in Edinburgh. *Arch Dis Child* 1969; 44:36.
24. Raivio KO, Osterlund K: Hypoglycemia and hyperinsulinemia associated with erythroblastosis fetalis. *Pediatrics* 1969; 43:217.
25. Falurni A, et al: Glucose metabolism, plasma I, and GH secretion in newborn infants with erythroblastosis fetalis compared with normal newborns and those born to diabetic mothers. *Pediatrics* 1972; 49:682.
26. Schiff D, et al: Metabolic effects of exchange transfusions. I: Effect of citrated and of heparinized blood on glucose, nonesterified fatty acids, 2-(4 hydroxybenzeneazo) benzoic acid binding, and insulin. *J Pediatr* 1971; 78:603.
27. Mann TP, Elliot RIK: Neonatal cold injury due to accidental exposure to cold. *Lancet* 1957; 1:229.
28. Henderson BM, et al: Hypoglycemia with hepatic glycogen depletion: A post operative complication of pyloric stenosis. *J Pediatr Surg* 1968; 3:309.
29. Yeung CY: Hypoglycemia in neonatal sepsis. *J Pediatr* 1970; 77:812.
30. Yeung CY, Lee VWY, Yeung CM: Glucose disappearance rate in neonatal infection. *J Pediatr* 1973; 82:486.
31. Griffiths AD, Bryant GM: Assessment of effects of neonatal hypoglycemia: A study of 41 cases with matched controls. *Arch Dis Child* 1971; 46:819.
32. Koivisto M, Blanco-Sequeiros M, Krause V: Neonatal symptomatic and a symptomatic hypoglycaemia: A followup study of 151 children. *Dev Med Child Neurol* 1972; 14:603.
33. McQuarrie I: Idiopathic spontaneously occurring hypoglycemia in infants. *Am J Dis Child* 1954; 87:399.

34. Spencer-Peet J, et al: Hepatic glycogen storage disease. Clinical and laboratory findings in 23 cases. *Q J Med* 1971; 40:95.
35. Dykes IRW, Spencer-Peet J: Hepatic glycogen synthetase deficiency. *Arch Dis Child* 1972; 47:558.
36. Segal S: Disorders of galactose metabolism, in Stanbury JB, Wyngaarden JB, Frederickson DS (eds): *The Metabolic Basis of Inherited Disease*. New York, McGraw-Hill, 1972, p 174.
37. Hsia DYY, Walker FA: Variability in the clinical manifestations of galactosemia. *J Pediatr* 1961; 59:872.
38. Cornblath M, et al: Hereditary fructose intolerance. *N Engl J Med* 1963; 269:1271.
39. Baker L, Winegrad AI: Fasting hypoglycaemia and metabolic acidosis associated with deficiency of hepatic fructose-1,6-diphosphatase activity. *Lancet* 1970; 2:13.
40. Ter heggen HG, Lowenthal A, Walker P: Lactic acidosis due to pyruvate carboxylase deficiency (abstract). *Pediatr Res* 1977; 11:1016.
41. Hommes FA, et al: Two cases of phosphoenol pyruvate carboxykinase deficiency. *Acta Paediatr Scand* 1976; 65:233.
42. Haymond MW, Ben-Galim E, Strobel KE: Glucose and alanine metabolism in children with maple syrup urine disease. *J Clin Invest* 1978; 62:398.
43. Slonim AE, et al: Nonketotic hypoglycemia: An early indicator of systemic carnitine deficiency. *Neurology* 1985; 33:29.
44. Kogut MO, Blaskovics M, Donnell GN: Idiopathic hypoglycemia: A study of 26 children. *J Pediatr* 1969; 74:853.
45. Colle F, Ulstrom RA: Ketotic hypoglycemia. *J Pediatr* 1964; 64:632.
46. Senior B, Loriden L: Gluconeogenesis and insulin in the ketotic variety of childhood hypoglycemia and in control children. *J Pediatr* 1969; 74:529.
47. Sizonenko PC, et al: Response to 2-deoxy-d-glucose and to glucagon in "ketotic hypoglycemia" of childhood: Evidence for epinephrine deficiency and altered alanine availability. *Pediatr Res* 1973; 7:983.
48. Court JM, Dunlap ME, Boulton TJC: Effect of ephedrine in ketotic hypoglycemia. *Arch Dis Child* 1974; 49:63.
49. Rosenbloom AL, Tiwary CM: Ketotic (idiopathic glucagon unresponsive) hypoglycaemia, catecholamine excretion and effects of ephedrine therapy. *Arch Dis Child* 1972; 47:924.
50. Haymond MW, Pagliara AS: Ketotic hypoglycemia. *Clinical Endocrinol Metab* 1983; 12:447.
51. Chang TW, Goldberg AL: The origin of alanine produced in skeletal muscle. *J Biol Chem* 1978; 253:367.
52. Hanna CE, et al: Detection of congenital hypopituitary hypothyroidism: Ten years' experience in the Northwest regional screening program. *J Pediatr* 1986; 109:959.
53. Underwood LE, et al: Islet cell function and glucose homeostasis in hypopituitary dwarfism: Synergism between growth hormone and cortisone. *J Pediatr* 1973; 82:28.
54. Hopwood NJ, et al: Hypoglycemia in hypopituitary children. *Am J Dis Child* 1975; 129:918.
55. Cacciara E, et al: Congenital hypopituitarism associated with neonatal hypoglycemia and microphallus: Effect of GH therapy. *Helv Paediatr Acta* 1976; 31:481.
56. DiRaimondo VC, Earll JM: Remarkable sensitivity to insulin in a patient with hypopituitarism and diabetic acidosis. *Diabetes* 1968; 17:147.
57. Vidnes J, Oyasaeter S: Glucagon deficiency causing severe neonatal hypoglycemia in a patient with normal insulin secretion. *Pediatr Res* 1977; 11:943.
58. Felig P, et al: Glucose homeostasis in viral hepatitis. *N Engl J Med* 1970; 283:1436.

59. Huttenlocher PR: Reye's syndrome: Relation of outcome to therapy. *J Pediatr* 1972; 80:850.
60. Glasgow AM, Cotton RB, Dhienshiri K: Reye's syndrome. III: The hypoglycemia. *Am J Dis Child* 1973; 125:809.
61. Kerr DS, et al: Hypoglycemia and the regulation of fasting glucose metabolism in malnutrition, in Gardner LI, Amacher P (eds): *Endocrine Aspects of Malnutrition.* Santa Ynez Calif, Kroc Foundation, 1973.
62. Cochrane WA, et al: Familial hypoglycemia precipitated by amino acids. *J Clin Invest* 1956; 35:411.
63. Fajans SS: Leucine-induced hypoglycemia. *N Engl J Med* 1965; 23:1224.
64. Mann JR, Rayner PHH, Gourevitch A: Insulinoma in childhood. *Arch Dis Child* 1969; 44:435.
65. Floyd JC, Jr, et al: Plasma insulin in organic hyperinsulinism. Comparative effects of tolbutamide, leucine, and glucose. *J Clin Endocrinol Metab* 1964; 24:747.
66. Fischer GW, et al: Neonatal islet cell adenoma: Case report and literature review. *Pediatrics* 1974; 53:753.
67. Fajans SS, Floyd JC, Fij SK: Differential diagnosis of spontaneous hypoglycemia, in Krysten LJ, Shaw RA (eds): *Endocrinology and Diabetes: The Thirtieth Hahnemann Symposium.* New York, Grune & Stratton, 1975.
68. Gutman RA, et al: Circulating proinsulin-like material in patients with functioning insulinomas. *N Engl J Med* 1971; 284:1003.
69. Stanley CA, Baker L: Hyperinsulinism in infancy: Diagnosis by demonstration of abnormal response to fasting hypoglycemia. *Pediatrics* 1976; 57:702.
70. Chaussain JL, et al: Serum branched-chain amino acids in the diagnosis of hyperinsulinism in infancy. *J Pediatr* 1980; 96:923.
71. Schotland MG, Kaplan SL, Grumbach MM: The tolbutamide tolerance test in the evaluation of childhood hypoglycemia. *Pediatrics* 1967; 39:838.
72. Garces LY, Drash A, Kenny FM: Islet cell tumor in the neonate: Studies in carbohydrate metabolism and therapeutic response. *Pediatrics* 1968; 41:789.
73. Grant DB, Barbor PRH: Islet-cell tumour causing hypoglycaemia in a newborn infant. *Arch Dis Child* 1970; 45:434.
74. Yakovac WC, Baker L, Hummeler K: Beta cell nesidioblastosis in idiopathic hypoglycemia of infancy. *J Pediatr* 1971; 79:226.
75. Heitz PV, et al: Nesidioblastosis: The pathologic basis of persistent hyperinsulinemic hypoglycemia in infants. Morphologic and quantitative analysis of seven cases based on specific immunostaining and electron microscopy. *Diabetes* 1977; 26:632.
76. Hofeldt FD, et al: Are abnormalities in insulin secretion responsible for reactive hypoglycemia? *Diabetes* 1974; 23:589.
77. Sotelo-Avila C, Singer DB: Syndrome of hyperplastic fetal visceromegaly and neonatal hypoglycemia (Beckwith's syndrome). A report of seven cases. *Pediatrics* 1970; 46:240.
78. Schiff D, et al: Metabolic aspects of the Beckwith-Wiedemann syndrome. *J Pediatr* 1973; 82:258.
79. Nissan S, Bar-Maor A, Shafrir E: Hypoglycemia associated with extrapancreatic tumors. *N Engl J Med* 1968; 278:177.
80. Loutfi AH, et al: Hypoglycemia with Wilms' tumor. *Arch Dis Child* 1964; 39:197.
81. Lifshitz F, Coello-Ramirez P, Gutierrez-Topete G: Monosaccharide intolerance and hypoglycemia in infants with diarrhea. II: Metabolic studies in 23 infants. *J Pediatr* 1970; 77:604.

82. Barrett HL, et al: Salicylate intoxication in infants and children. *J Pediatr* 1942; 21:214.
83. Zucher P, Simon G: Prolonged symptomatic neonatal hypoglycemia associated with maternal chlorpropamide therapy. *Pediatrics* 1968; 42:824.
84. Kuhn LR, et al: Chlorpropamide-induced hypoglycemia in a child with diabetes insipidus (letter). *JAMA* 1969; 210:907.
85. Kallen RJ, Mohler JH, Lin HL: Hypoglycemia: A complication of treatment of hypertension with propranalol. *Clin Pediatr* 1980; 19:567.
86. Madison LL: Ethanol-induced hypoglycemia. *Adv Metab Disord* 1968; 3:85.
87. Malherbe C, et al: Effect of diphenylhydantoin on insulin secretion in man. *N Engl J Med* 1972; 286:339.
88. Ginsberg-Fellner F, Rayfield EJ: Metabolic studies in a child with a pancreatic insulinoma. *Am J Dis Child* 1980; 134:64.
89. Pagliara AS, et al: Hypoalaninemia: A concomitant of ketotic hypoglycemia. *J Clin Invest* 1972; 51:1440.
90. Somogyi M: Diabetogenic effect of hyperinsulinism. *Am J Med* 1959; 26:192.
91. Gentz J, Persson B, Zetterstrom R: On the diagnosis of symptomatic neonatal hypoglycemia. *Acta Paediatr Scand* 1969; 58:449.
92. Pildes RS, Patel DA, Nitzan M: Glucose disappearance rate in symptomatic neonatal hypoglycemia. *Pediatrics* 1973; 52:75.
93. Beard A, et al: Neonatal hypoglycemia: A discussion. *J Pediatr* 1971; 79:314.
94. Kumar D, Mehtalia SD, Miller LV: Diagnostic use of glucagon-induced insulin response: Studies in patients with insulinoma or other hypoglycemic conditions. *Ann Intern Med* 1974; 80:697.
95. Vanderschueren-Lodeweyckx M, et al: The glucagon stimulation test: Effect on plasma growth hormone and on immunoreactive insulin, cortisol and glucose in children. *J Pediatr* 1974; 85:182.
96. Fajans SS, et al: The diagnostic value of sodium tolbutamide in hypoglycemic states. *J Clin Endocrinol Metab* 1969; 21:371.
97. Epstein HY, et al: Angiographic localization of insulinomas: High reported success rate and two additional cases. *Ann Surg* 1969; 169:349.
98. Millan VG, et al: Localization of occult insulinoma by superselective pancreatic venous sampling for insulin assay through percutaneous transhepatic catheterization. *Diabetes* 1979; 28:249.
99. Smith HM (ed): Diazoxide and treatment of hypoglycemia. *Ann NY Acad Sci* 1968; 150:191.
100. Balsam MJ, et al: Beta cell adenoma in a child with hypoglycemia controlled with diazoxide. *J Pediatr* 1972; 80:788.
101. Spencer ML: Hyperinsulinism in infants and children. Response to diazoxide. *Pediatr Res* 1981; 15:1568.
102. Jackson JA, et al: Long-term treatment of refractory neonatal hypoglycemia with long-acting somatostatin analog. *J Pediatr* 1987; 111:548.
103. Fonkalsrud EW, et al: Idiopathic hypoglycemia in infancy. *Arch Surg* 1974; 108:801.
104. Starzl TE, et al: Portal diversion for the treatment of glycogen storage disease in humans. *Ann Surg* 1973; 178:525.
105. Greene HL, et al: Nocturnal intragastric feeding for type I glycogen storage disease. *N Engl J Med* 1976; 294:423.
106. Burr IM, et al: Comparison of the effects of total parenteral nutrition, continuous intragastric feeding, and portacaval shunt on a patient with type I glycogen storage disease. *J Pediatr* 1974; 85:792.

3

Abnormal Growth

REGULATION OF GROWTH

Regulation of growth is a complex process involving the interaction among a number of genetic, hormonal, and environmental factors.[1-8]

Fetal growth appears to be influenced significantly by the physical size of the mother, but also by other maternal factors such as nutrition, illness, and exposure to toxic agents (e.g., alcohol, hydantoins). Insulin may be an important hormonal regulator of intrauterine growth. Infants with congenital hypothyroidism or growth hormone (GH) deficiency are typically of normal size at birth, although thyroid hormone is necessary for normal skeletal maturation in utero.

During the first several years of life, it is not unusual for a child's height to cross percentile lines on the growth chart as genetic makeup, based largely on the combined size of the parents (i.e., mid-parental height), assumes greater importance. Thyroxine, GH, insulin, and adequate nutrition contribute to normal growth during childhood, and it is now well known that psychosocial factors also exert an influence (see Chapter 4). The gonadal sex hormones (which, like thyroxine and GH, are under hypothalamic-pituitary control) contribute to the pubertal growth spurt, although synergism with GH appears to be important. Adrenal androgens may also have a relatively modest role. Normal growth may be inhibited at any time by intercurrent illness, but adequate compensatory growth is usually observed unless the severity or chronicity of the condition is marked.

Somatomedin-C (Sm-C), probably identical to insulin-like growth factor (IGF-I), is a small polypeptide secreted by the liver and apparently has a direct stimulatory effect on skeletal growth, both prenatally and postnatally. There is considerable evidence that Sm-C in turn is the common denominator by which the effects of many other growth determinants are mediated; for example, its production appears to be enhanced by GH, insulin, and the sex steroids and diminished by malnutrition and estrogen treatment (dose dependent?), and possibly by corticosteroids. The relationship between linear growth and serum concentration of Sm-C is not always consistent, however. The rapid growth rate during infancy is associated with increased production of GH but low serum levels of Sm-C, suggesting a negative feedback system; likewise, relatively high Sm-C concentrations persist into late adolescence, when growth rate is decelerating.

DWARFISM

Because there are so many causes of dwarfism (Table 3–1), the choice of appropriate diagnostic studies may be difficult. In an attempt to facilitate the evaluation and management of the short child, this section will include (1) a description of the more common varieties of dwarfism, (2) a suggested scheme of evaluation, and (3) a discussion of the currently available forms of treatment. A review of diagnostic procedures is presented in the appendix.

Systemic Diseases (Other Than Skeletal and Endocrine)

Mental retardation and other types of cerebral dysfunction frequently are associated with short stature. The cause of dwarfism in these patients is not clear, although injury to the hypothalamus in experimental animals does lead to growth failure.[9] It could be speculated that a central nervous system disorder might affect hypothalamic-pituitary regulation in human beings. In one report[10] serum GH response to stimuli was reported to be blunted in some patients with "cerebral dwarfism." However, other studies indicate that GH concentrations are normal in both the fasting state[11] and following insulin-induced hypoglycemia.[12]

Children with *congenital heart disease* (CHD) as a group are shorter than their healthy peers.[13] In one study, 69% of 107 patients with CHD were below the 10th percentile.[14] Growth tends to be poorest in children with cyanotic CHD,[14, 15] but the degree of cyanosis does not appear to be a factor.[15] An increased growth rate often follows surgical correction of the defect.[13]

The small size of these patients does not appear to be directly related to tissue anoxia, infection, pulmonary hypertension, or poor nutrition.[15] Concentrations of GH in fasting children with CHD do not differ from those in healthy subjects.[14]

Relative malnutrition may be largely responsible for the short stature of some patients with *chronic pulmonary disease*. Treatment with steroids further retards growth in children with severe asthma. In *cystic fibrosis*, growth is compromised by malabsorption, but primarily by lung disease. Fasting GH levels

TABLE 3–1.

Causes of Dwarfism in Children

Systemic disease (other than skeletal and endocrine)
  Central nervous system
    Mental retardation
    Neurofibromatosis
  Cardiovascular
    Congenital heart disease
    Acquired (rheumatic) heart disease
  Pulmonary
    Cystic fibrosis
    Asthma
    Tuberculosis
  Gastrointestinal
    Malabsorption
    Deprivation syndromes
  Renal
    Chronic insufficiency
    Tubular acidosis
  Hematologic
    Chronic anemias
Skeletal
  Osteochondrodysplasia
  Rickets
  Pseudohypoparathyroidism and pseudo-
    pseudohypoparathyroidism
Genetic
  Familial
  Chromosomal
    Monogolism
    Trisomies
    Turner's syndrome
Primordial
  Without associated anomalies
  With associated anomalies
Constitutional delayed growth
Endocrine disorders
  Hypothyroidism
  Panhypopituitarism
  Isolated growth hormone deficiency and variants
    (e.g.; Laron)
  Adrenal disorders
    Congenital adrenal hyperplasia
    Cushing's syndrome, including iatrogenic type
Psychosocial (deprivation) dwarfism

tend to be high, but further increases following artificial stimulation are minimal,[16] suggesting that the pituitary is responding maximally under basal conditions. Nutritional deficiencies are responsible for the short stature of patients with the various *malabsorption syndromes*, such as giardiasis, gluten sensitivity, and deficiency of disaccharidases. Growth failure attributable to celiac disease, even when the condition is asymptomatic, has been reported.[17]

McCaffrey et al.[18] reported severe growth retardation (< 3rd percentile) in 22 of 130 children with *inflammatory bowel disease*. Short stature was attributed to secondary hypopituitarism in many cases. Conversely, Tenore et al. reported excessive rather than impaired GH responses in their patients.[19] However, it is most likely that nutritional insufficiency is primarily responsible for the stunted growth, at least in patients with Crohn's disease.[20, 21]

The point is made that growth may be impaired prior to the onset of obvious bowel symptoms.[22] Growth is enhanced by successful steroid therapy[19] in some patients, even when high doses are required,[22] or following surgical intervention[22, 23] if performed prior to puberty.[23]

Whereas many systemic illnesses responsible for small size may be readily recognized by the classic physical features of the primary disorder, this may not be the case in *renal disease*. An exception is the association of congenital urinary tract defects with malformation of the external ear. In one series, 23 of 27 children with abnormal external ears were found to have urinary tract anomalies.[24] The cause of growth failure in uremic renal disease is probably related to several factors: acidosis; chronic malnutrition; and renal rickets.[25-27] Renal tubular acidosis (RTA) is also associated with short stature in addition to increased thirst, frequent urination, and nephrolithiasis.

Chronic anemias such as Cooley's anemia[28] have been associated with small size, although the degree of retardation may be more closely related to anatomic anomalies than to reduced hemoglobin. Impaired growth hormone response to GH-releasing hormone has been reported in thalassemia major.[29]

Severe *zinc deficiency* is more common in countries where inadequate nutrition is prevalent. However, a mild form, manifested by anorexia and poor growth, has been reported in infants and children in the United States.[30] Likewise, while overt *lead poisoning* is seen less frequently than in the past, Schwartz et al.[31] have found a positive correlation between decreased stature and higher blood levels of lead, even levels within the accepted normal range.

Skeletal Abnormalities

The term osteochondrodysplasia denotes an abnormality of cartilage and/ or bone growth and development. These types of short stature usually can be characterized by the disproportionate nature of the dwarfism, the extremities being noticeably affected, and the remainder of the skeleton being involved to a lesser extent, if at all. The correct diagnosis in these patients usually will be suggested by the physical appearance and confirmed by radiographic skeletal survey. Some representative disorders are described here and reviewed in detail elsewhere.[32]

Achondroplasia

Patients with achondroplasia are dwarfed because of insufficient growth of epiphyseal cartilage. Extremities are short, frequently with bowing of the legs and incomplete extension at the elbows. Megalocephaly (relative or absolute) is present with frontal bossing. Final height is invariably less than 5 ft, and usually nearer 4 ft. Typical radiographic features consist of short, broad tubular bones, with irregularities at the epiphyseal ends of the shafts. The base of the skull is short, and the pelvis is characterized by a small sciatic notch and flat acetabular roof.

Achondroplasia is inherited as a dominant trait. Matings between achondroplastic individuals and those not carrying the trait should result in about 50% affected offspring. However, approximately 90% of cases represent fresh mutations, both parents being genetically normal.[33] There is evidence that children of two achondroplastic parents tend to have multiple malformations in addition to dwarfism, possibly a result of a double dose of achondroplastic genes.[34]

Metaphyseal Dysostosis

This abnormality[35, 36] is characterized by dominant inheritance and inadequate mineralization of the primary zones of calcification in the metaphyses. Radiographically, the metaphyseal irregularities are similar to rickets, but the shafts of the bones are spared. This condition is further differentiated from achondroplasia by the normal size and appearance of the head and by the lack of typical radiographic changes in the skull, spine, and pelvis. Metaphyseal dysostosis may be classified as the Jansen or Schmid type, the former being more severe.

Hypochondroplasia

Another dominantly transmitted type of short-limbed dwarfism, hypochondroplasia,[37] like metaphyseal dysostosis, can be distinguished from achondroplasia by the relatively normal appearance of the patient's skull. Roentgenograms of the long bones reveal marked shortening, but the typical metaphyseal irregularities of metaphyseal dysostosis are not present.

Cartilage-Hair Hypoplasia

Cartilage-hair hypoplasia (CHH)[38] (Fig 3–1) is usually considered a variant (McKusick type) of metaphyseal dysostosis, because the radiographic appearance is similar. This condition is characterized by fine or sparse hair in addition to short extremities. These children tend to have abnormal susceptibility to varicella infection, apparently as a result of a cellular immune defect. Lux et al.[39] reported two children whose immunoglobulin levels were normal or elevated, but who demonstrated lymphopenia, reduced lymphocyte response to phytohemagglutinin, and diminished delayed skin hypersensitivity. Subsequently, an infant with CHH and severe combined immunodeficiency has been described.[40] It is important to differentiate CHH from achondroplasia and from the other types

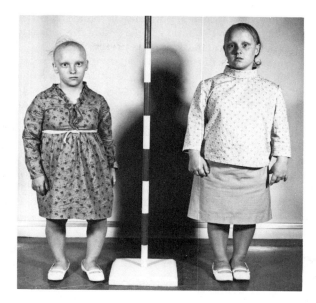

FIG 3–1.
Two sisters, aged 15 and 17 years, with cartilage-hair hypoplasia, a form of osteochon-drodysplasia. Note sparse scalp hair and disproportionate shortening of extremities relative to trunk.

of metaphyseal dysostosis, as the mode of inheritance is autosomal recessive rather than dominant.

Rickets, Pseudohypoparathyroidism, and Pseudo-Pseudohypoparathyroidism

Rickets of any type may cause short stature. These conditions are discussed in Chapter 11.

The chemical abnormalities in *pseudohypoparathyroidism* (PHP)[41] are the same as those found in hypoparathyroidism (i.e., low calcium and high phosphorus), although alkaline phosphatase levels also are occasionally elevated. The metabolic defect is not a result of primary hypofunction of the parathyroid gland, but rather an inability of the renal tubule to respond to parathormone. Parathormone levels tend to be high.

The characteristic physical features of PHP are a round face and short extremities, the hands and feet being particularly affected. The shortened fourth and fifth metacarpals result in decreased prominence of the corresponding knuckles when the hand is made into a fist. Some degree of mental retardation may be present. None of these associated clinical features appears to be related to the chemical defect.

The attenuated fourth and fifth metacarpals are a prominent radiographic feature of PHP, although a similar abnormality is found in Turner's syndrome. Calcification may be found in the basal ganglia and in the subcutaneous tissues. Osteoporosis and lenticular cataracts may be present.

PHP, also referred to as Albright's hereditary osteodystrophy (AHO), has now been further classified as PHP type Ia.[42] Additional forms of PHP currently recognized are type Ib and type II, which typically are not associated with short stature and the other physical features of AHO. All three types have in common the lack of end-organ response to PTH, resulting in low levels of serum calcium and high levels of phosphorus, but are apparently caused by different biochemical defects (see Chapter 11).

The physical features of *pseudo-PHP*[41] are the same as those found in PHP type Ia, but there are no chemical abnormalities. In some patients serum calcium and phosphorus concentrations vary intermittently from normal to abnormal levels. Thus, it is probable that the presumed differences between these two conditions are more apparent than real.

Genetic Dwarfism

It is well known that the stature of children tends to be related to parental height. Thus, it should not be too surprising for two parents whose height falls within the low normal range to produce a child whose stature is sufficiently affected to place him or her below the arbitrary limits of normal. The small size in such a case is probably *familial*, but this diagnosis must be made with caution, particularly if the patient has several siblings of normal size. When the discrepancy is great, it is prudent to consider other causes of short stature, even though it is possible that none will be found.

Turner's syndrome (Fig 3–2) may be associated with a 45,XO chromosome complement or with one of a number of mosaic patterns such as XX/XO. The frequency of the anomalies associated with these two karyotypes is listed in Table 3–2.[43]

Other abnormalities sometimes seen include a narrow palate; small mandible; anomalous auricles; ocular anomalies such as strabismus and inner canthal folds; increased carrying angle of the arms; cardiovascular defects,[44] particularly bicuspid aortic valve and coarctation of the aorta; renal anomalies such as horseshoe or multicystic kidney[45]; and perceptive hearing impairment. It has been reported that the observation of wide-spaced nipples in Turner's syndrome cannot be confirmed by actual measurements.[46]

The incidence of thyroid abnormalities such as thyroiditis is higher in these girls than in the general population,[47] as is the frequency of diabetes mellitus and Addison's disease. Some degree of osteoporosis is commonly present, presumably related to estrogen deficiency.[48] There is evidence that some of these girls may have a relative deficiency of GH.[49]

The diagnosis may be suggested in the newborn period in an infant with edematous hands or feet (Bonnevie-Ullrich syndrome); this problem resolves during infancy. Birth weight tends to be lower than average.[50] In children with

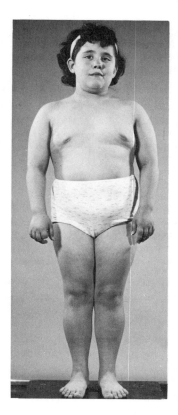

FIG 3–2.
Thirteen-year-old girl with Turner's syndrome, with short stature, wide neck, broad chest, and lack of breast development. The anomalies in this girl are less severe than in some patients. Chromosome count revealed an unusual mosaic pattern, XX/X-iso-X (long arm on one X chromosome).

relatively few anomalies Turner's syndrome sometimes is not diagnosed until puberty, when they seek attention because of short stature and lack of secondary sexual characteristics.

Patients with Turner's syndrome have dysplastic ovaries, usually represented by fibrous "streaks." Vagina and uterus are present, but infantile. Some patients develop varying amounts of pubic hair, but axillary hair is minimal. Absence of breasts is also the rule, but moderate pretreatment development (5.4% in one large series[50]) and menarche occasionally occur, particularly in mosaics or in patients with partial short arm deletions of the X chromosome.[51] There has even been one report of precocious puberty in a child with an XO/XX karyotype.[52]

The generalization that girls with Turner's syndrome have mental retardation is no longer tenable, although a higher incidence of specific deficits in spatial

TABLE 3–2.
Relative Frequency (%) of Abnormalities
Associated With XO and XO/XX Turner's
Syndrome*

Abnormality	XO	XO/XX
Short stature	100	80
Streak gonads	92	90
Shield chest	80	75
Hypoplastic nails	77	55
Short fourth metacarpal	58	44
Webbed neck	54	16
Pigmented nevi	52	37
Lymphedema	39	12
Congenital heart disease	21	7
Menstruation	8	21
Severe mental defect	8	6
Phallic hypertrophy	3	5

* Modified from Ferguson-Smith.[43] MA: Karyotype = genetic
correlations in gonadal dysgenesis and their bearing on
the pathogenesis of malformations. *J Med Genet* 1965;
2:142.

ability, particularly in nonmosaics, has been reported.[53] A recent study confirms normal or above normal verbal IQs; however, although an impairment in visual memory was demonstrated, spatial deficits were not present if the patient's intelligence was normal.[54]

Ultimate height in patients with Turner's syndrome usually is between 54 and 58 inches. Adequate secondary sexual characteristics and menses can be achieved with estrogen replacement therapy, but with rare exceptions,[55] these patients are sterile.

There are several interesting variants of Turner's syndrome. One group ("pure" gonadal dysgenesis) consists of patients with ovarian agenesis but normal height and none of the usual stigmata other than sexual immaturity.[56] The chromosome pattern is frequently XY. This condition resembles the testicular feminization syndrome, in which the chromosomes also are XY. However, the latter is characterized by an absent uterus with vagina ending in a blind pouch, histologically normal intra-abdominal testes with no ovarian component, and adequate breast development (see Chapter 8). Both conditions can be familial.

Another variant in girls consists of streak gonads and other typical features of Turner's syndrome, but with a normal 46,XX chromosome pattern (sometimes identified as XX Turner phenotype).[57] Finally, some patients with the stigmata of Turner's syndrome are phenotypic males, usually with a normal XY karyotype (XY Turner phenotype). The genitalia of these patients may be normal or may demonstrate various abnormalities such as infantilism, hypospadias, and cryptorchism. The term Noonan's syndrome has been applied to both the XX and XY Turner's phenotype.[58] Brosnan et al. have described two girls with 46,XY phenotype with anomalies of ectodermal and mesodermal structures.[59]

Primordial Dwarfism

Children with primordial dwarfism do not reach normal height as adults, but have normal endocrine function. They differ from the group with primary skeletal abnormalities in that growth retardation affects the entire body. As a result, the small size is relatively proportional. The exception may be head circumference, which tends to correspond more closely with chronologic age (CA) unless mental retardation is present.[60] However, this does not appear to be true in children with the rubella syndrome, whose head circumference correlates better with stature than with intellect.[61]

Usually, patients with primordial short stature are small for gestational age (SGA) at birth. Conversely, many SGA infants remain small, although catch-up growth is possible.[62-65] The cause of intrauterine growth retardation is not always apparent, but maternal ingestion of cytotoxic agents (e.g., medications, alcohol) or congenital viral infections (e.g., rubella) can sometimes be implicated.

Patients with primordial dwarfism (and also those with familial short stature), in contrast to those with constitutional delayed growth, typically have a bone age (BA) consistent with CA rather than height age (HA). However, BA may be more similar to HA (and therefore misleading) in early childhood.

Some patients with primordial dwarfism appear essentially normal except for their small size. They have normal intelligence and sexual maturation and are miniatures of unaffected children their own age. Ultimate height varies considerably, but may not exceed 4 ft in extreme cases. (It is possible that some of these otherwise unclassified patients actually have very mild forms of Silver-Russell syndrome.)

Other patients have obvious physical anomalies in addition to their small size; their conditions often bear the name of the investigator(s) who first described it (e.g., Seckel's syndrome, Fig 3–3; Silver-Russell syndrome, Fig 3–4). Some have mental retardation as well. Descriptions of most of the recognizable primordial forms of short stature may be found elsewhere.[66]

Among the most frequently encountered forms of primordial short stature is the *Silver-Russell syndrome* (Fig 3–4), which has been reviewed in depth by Tanner et al.[67] In addition to SGA, these patients have small, triangular facies, small mandibles, and short, incurved fifth fingers. Significant asymmetry of the extremities (Silver syndrome) was present in one third of Tanner's patients. In the remainder, the limbs were essentially of equal length, consistent with the condition originally described by Russell. However, there appears to be no bimodality, but rather a spectrum of limb length differences from none to marked. Therefore, it is suggested that the term Silver-Russell syndrome be applied to all patients who have the typical features, with or without asymmetry.

As with some other types of primordial short stature, BA tends to be delayed in early childhood, but approaches the CA as the patients get older. Puberty occurs at the usual time, and ultimate height is usually about 3 SD below the mean. Intelligence is usually normal. The condition typically occurs sporadically.

In a more recent study, some exceptions to the typical features were reported: 3 of 15 patients with the classic features of Silver-Russell syndrome had

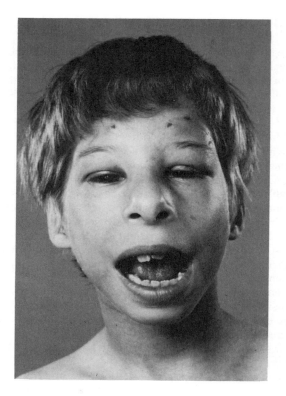

FIG 3–3.
Boy with Seckel's syndrome, a form of primordial short stature with associated anomalies (sometimes referred to as "bird-headed" dwarfism). Note microcephaly with hypoplastic facies and prominent nose.

normal birth weight, and 5 of 15 exhibited late catch-up growth and reached a final height between the 10th and 40th percentile.[68]

There is no satisfactory treatment for Silver-Russell syndrome. However, it is of interest that an associated GH deficiency has been reported in at least five patients with Silver-Russell syndrome.[69]

Another condition being recognized with increasing frequency is *fetal alcohol syndrome*,[70] a form of prenatal and postnatal growth deficiency secondary to maternal alcoholism. Facial characteristics and abnormalities include short palpebral fissure, short upturned nose, hypoplastic philtrum, thinned upper vermilion border, ptosis, strabismus, epicanthal folds, microphthalmia, posteriorly rotated ears, cleft lip or palate, and small teeth. Other relatively common features are microcephaly, mental retardation, developmental delay, hyperactivity, and speech problems. There is an increased incidence of cardiac, urogenital, and skeletal malformations. Impaired ability to acidify the urine has also been observed,[71] as well as low levels of plasma zinc.[72]

Constitutional Delayed Growth

Constitutional delayed growth is particularly common in boys and is the most prevalent type of short stature among children. These patients do not have true endocrine deficiencies, but are slow in attaining their ultimate height, which usually is within the normal range. These children are of normal size at birth, but typically begin to experience deceleration of growth rate at the age of 3 to 6 months.[73] This process may continue for several years, at which time the growth rate frequently becomes normal again. Ultimate height is not compromised, but its attainment is delayed beyond the usual time.

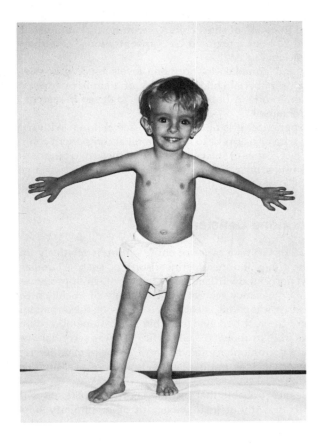

FIG 3–4.
Boy with Silver-Russell syndrome, characterized by intrauterine growth retardation, triangular facies, relatively small mandible, and in this patient significant asymmetry of the extremities.

The BA of children with constitutional delayed growth is retarded and characteristically consistent with HA. Sexual maturation likewise is delayed. (The term delayed maturation syndrome sometimes is used interchangeably with constitutional delayed growth.)

Studies of thyroid function and of the hypothalamic-pituitary-adrenal axis are normal, and in general, serum GH levels rise normally after stimulation.[74] However, some prepubertal children with delayed growth and maturation appear to have transient partial deficiency of GH.[75] Response to testing becomes normal following estrogen or androgen priming, or after the onset of puberty, suggesting a physiologic role of sex hormones on GH secretion during the prepubertal years. Therefore, a blunted GH response to appropriate stimuli in this age group would not be diagnostic of permanent deficiency in an unprimed patient. Likewise, a neuroregulatory defect may be present in some cases; Zadik et al. reported that 45% of short children with normal stimulated GH responses had decreased 24-hour integrated GH concentrations[76] (see the section Growth Hormone Deficiency).

Pituitary and gonadal sex hormone levels tend to be low, as would be expected in a prepubertal child. A history of a similar pattern of slow growth and maturation in one or both parents (e.g., delayed menarche in the mother) frequently is obtained.

In our experience, it is not unusual to see children with constitutional delayed growth who also appear to have a familial component contributing to their small size. In fact, Lanes et al.[77] concluded that these two groups do not distribute into distinct entities, but rather represent a continuum or two largely overlapping populations.

Growth Hormone Deficiency

Deficiency of GH as a cause of short stature is relatively uncommon compared with the group of nonendocrine disorders, such as familial, constitutional delay, or psychosocial dwarfism (see Chapter 4). In approximately 80% of patients with GH deficiency seen at the University of Michigan the disorder has been classified as idiopathic; nearly two thirds of these patients had isolated deficiency, and the rest had evidence that at least one other pituitary hormone was lacking as well. In about 10% GH deficiency was secondary to an intracranial tumor, usually a craniopharyngioma, and in the remainder represented miscellanous causes, such as trauma, septo-optic dysplasia, and irradiation of the head and neck.

It now seems probable that in the majority of patients with *idiopathic GH deficiency*, with or without insufficiency of other pituitary hormones, lack of hypothalamic GH-releasing hormone is the primary problem.[78] Although "idiopathic" implies unknown cause, a high incidence of perinatal problems has been documented in these patients.[79] These include excessive vaginal bleeding during gestation, prolonged or unusually short labor, intrapartum distress and asphyxia, and breech delivery.

Hypoglycemia is not unusual in infants with isolated GH deficiency; babies with multiple pituitary hormone deficiencies may also have micropenis. Either of these conditions should alert the physician to the possibility of hypothalamic-pituitary dysfunction.[80–82] A neonatal hepatitis syndrome has also been reported in these infants, although the reason for this association is not clear.[83]

Patients with isolated GH deficiency tend to have high-pitched voices, immature facies, and relative adiposity of the breast and abdominal areas particularly (Fig 3–5). Skeletal maturation usually is delayed, with an average BA/CA ratio of about 0.75,[84] although we have observed great variability among our patients.

If there is associated deficiency of gonadotrophins, normal puberty will not occur spontaneously. Even when GH deficiency occurs alone, puberty is usually delayed and genitalia appear small relative to CA; however, sexual maturation progresses consistent with BA.

Isolated GH deficiency may be present in more than one family member. Inheritance may be autosomal recessive,[85, 86] autosomal dominant, or X-linked recessive[87]; these familial cases are now referred to as types I, II, and III, respectively. A subgroup, type I-A, has also been described, characterized by diminished length at birth, early appearing clinical features, and GH antibodies.[88, 89]

Craniopharyngioma[90] is the most common space-occupying central nervous system lesion causing short stature; multiple pituitary deficiencies are often present, including vasopressin. Patients frequently give a history of headache, vomiting, or visual disturbance. Examination may reveal papilledema, visual field defects, or neurologic signs. Either weight loss or excessive gain may occur. Lateral skull roentgenograms show intracranial calcification or abnormalities of the sella turcica (enlargement, distortion) in the majority of patients.

As expected, patients with craniopharyngioma continue to manifest evidence of hypopituitarism following surgery and radiation therapy. Jenkins et al. reported deficiencies of GH and gonadotrophin in essentially all patients, and pituitary-adrenal dysfunction in half.[91] In addition, most had evidence of hypothyroidism. Prolactin was sometimes increased.

Richards et al. described four children with space-occupying lesions of the head who had clinical and laboratory evidence of hypothalamic-pituitary deficiencies which did not become apparent until several years after therapeutic irradiation.[92] However, an immediate suppressive effect of radiation therapy on GH secretion is also possible. The endocrine sequelae of chemotherapy or irradiation for head and neck malignancies have been studied by several investigators.[93–96]

Other demonstrable abnormalities of the central nervous system associated with GH deficiency and short stature include *septo-optic dysplasia*,[97] *vascular malformation* of the hypothalamus,[98] *empty-sella syndrome*,[99, 100] and *histocytosis X*.

In some patients, short stature appears to result from inability to generate somatomedin(s) (see the section Regulation of Growth). *Laron dwarfs*[101–103] are similar in appearance to GH-deficient children, but serum GH levels are elevated. Somatomedin-C is low and does not respond to exogenous GH, suggesting a

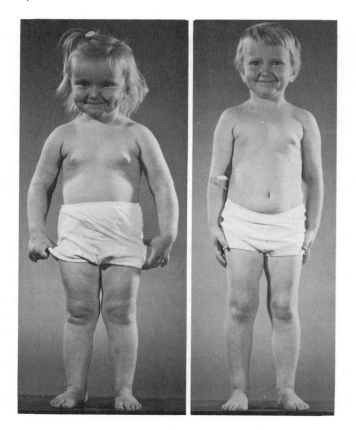

FIG 3–5.
Two sisters, aged 6 and 10 years, with isolated growth hormone deficiency. Note immature facies and tendency to adiposity.

defect in GH receptors. The condition is probably autosomal recessive.

More recently there has been considerable interest in a group of normal appearing short children who have adequate GH levels and low Sm-C; however, unlike Laron dwarfs, they respond to administered GH with a rise in Sm-C and an increase in growth rate, suggesting that the endogenous GH is immunoassayable but biologically inactive.[104] This condition has been called *"growth hormone–dependent growth failure,"*[105] or *"normal variant short stature."*[106, 107] Rudman et al.[108] reported that about half of a group of hyposomatomedic short children had normal GH responses to sleep and provocative testing. It is not clear how many of these patients actually have inactive GH, because Sm-C levels can be influenced by factors other than GH, such as nutrition.

There has also been a report of a short adolescent who has normal levels of GH and elevated Sm-C, suggesting a possible defect in Sm-C responsiveness.[109] Huseman et al.[110] described an interesting group of short patients whose apparent GH deficiency may be a result of impaired GH release secondary to an endogenous dopaminergic disorder.

Likewise, more patients are being recognized such as those described by Zadik et al.[76] (see the section Constitutional Delayed Growth earlier in this chapter), who respond to provocative testing but not to physiologic stimuli and therefore have low 12- or 24-hour integrated GH concentrations. These subjects are functionally GH deficient, and can be referred to as having *neurosecretory dysfunction* (see the section Scheme of Evaluation later in this chapter).

Short Stature as a Result of Other Endocrinopathies

Primary *hypothyroidism* is discussed in Chapter 6. Secondary (thyroid-stimulating hormone–deficient) hypothyroidism is less common, and generally occurs in association with other hypothalamic-pituitary deficiencies. Patients with *congenital adrenal hyperplasia* (see Chapter 7), if untreated, are large as children, but become short adults as a result of early fusion of the epiphyses secondary to increased androgen production. Growth is delayed in *Cushing's syndrome* as a result of antagonism of growth hormone action by cortisol at the growth centers of the long bones. Skeletal maturation also is retarded; therefore, catch-up growth is possible following treatment. Note that in some cases short stature may be the only obvious clinical sign of Cushing's syndrome.[111] Children with *Addison's disease* may have mildly delayed growth due to lack of adrenal androgens. Children with *diabetes insipidus* may grow poorly if excessive water drinking compromises adequate caloric intake.

Scheme of Evaluation

The decision as to which short children require evaluation, and to what extent, often is difficult. Arbitrarily, the 5th (or 3rd) percentile for height (approximately 2 SD below the mean) is considered the dividing line between normal and abnormal. However, several other factors help to determine the need for diagnostic evaluation. These include the degree of shortness, recent growth rate, and stature of family members. For example, intensive evaluation may be justifiably delayed in some patients in whom (1) height is minimally below the 5th percentile, (2) recent growth *rate* is normal, and (3) parents are relatively short (methods are available for determining normal heights based on the stature of the parents).[112] Procrastination sometimes is rewarded because the most common cause of proportional short stature, constitutional delayed growth, carries a good prognosis without treatment. However, in general, the following minimum investigation should be carried out in any child with a chief complaint of short stature whose height is below the 5th percentile:

1. History, particularly birth length and weight; growth rate from past mea-

surements; chronic illnesses; drugs (e.g., steroids); family heights; psychosocial environment.

2. Physical examination.
3. Bone age roentgenogram.
4. Roentgenogram of lateral skull.
5. Serum thyroxine or other thyroid function studies.
6. Screening test for growth hormone, and Sm-C.
7. Evaluation of renal function by blood urea nitrogen, creatinine, and/or urinalysis testing with specific gravity. Renal disease is an unlikely cause of dwarfism if the specific gravity is 1.015 or greater.[113] Electrolytes may also be helpful, particularly if urine is alkaline; hyperchloremia and hypokalemia are consistent with RTA.

Considerable information may be gained from these few procedures. A severely retarded BA (BA less than HA) suggests hypothyroidism. BA in patients with panhypopituitarism or isolated GH deficiency varies, but usually is less retarded than in primary hypothyroidism. Children with constitutional delayed growth typically have a BA consistent with HA. A BA equal to CA suggests primordial short stature, but BA in these patients may be retarded early in life. Features suggestive of Turner's syndrome or PHP may also be evident on roentgenograms of the hand.[114]

The skull roentgenogram usually is abnormal in children with craniopharyngioma,[90, 115] and sella turcica volume may be diminished in patients with growth hormone deficiency,[116] or increased in those with primary hypothyroidism.[117]

Chest roentgenogram, complete blood count, and serum calcium and phosphorus may be obtained, but are not likely to reveal the cause of short stature if physical examination is normal. Likewise, a sedimentation rate might identify children with inflammatory bowel disease before the clinical manifestations become obvious, but the yield will be very low.

Short girls who fail to mature at the expected time can be screened for possible gonadal dysgenesis by measuring serum gonadotrophins [follicle stimulating hormone (FSH) and luteinizing hormone (LH)], which should be abnormally high by about the age of 12 years.[118] A buccal smear is less reliable, as it may be normal in mosaicism such as XX/XO. In any case, confirmation of diagnosis is by chromosome count.

As the mechanisms controlling growth and the secretory dynamics of GH and Sm-C have become better understood, the precise diagnosis of GH deficiency has become more complex. It has long been known that a single fasting growth hormone determination is of limited value, since low levels frequently are found in normal children. A fasting growth hormone concentration of 7 (or even 5) ng/mL is highly suggestive of normal GH reserve without further study,[119] but the chance of obtaining such a level in an isolated sample is probably not more than 25%. Growth hormone–deficient patients tend to have fasting concentrations less than 1 ng/mL,[119] but this generalization cannot be relied on for definitive diagnosis.

A number of screening tests for GH deficiency have been devised in an effort to avoid the more definitive but also more cumbersome tests. A method sometimes used in children with suspected GH deficiency is the exercise test.[120–123] Following 20 minutes of vigorous activity (e.g., running, exercise bike), a single serum sample for GH is obtained. A level of 5 to 7 ng/mL or more is usually considered a normal response. This test enables detection of the great majority (up to 98% in one series!)[122] of children with normal GH reserve. It is beneficial if the patient is fasting, but this is not critical.

However, some short children who respond to a provocative GH stimulus (e.g., exercise, arginine,[124] insulin[125]) may not have a normal *integrated concentration of GH* (IC-GH). These children, in whom standard tests would be non-diagnostic, probably have functional GH deficiency secondary to *neurosecretory dysfunction*.[126, 127] Likewise, the fallibility of the provocative tests is emphasized by the reverse situation, in which nonresponders have normal IC-GH.[127] The IC-GH, which would include a stage III/IV sleep segment (physiologic stimulus for GH release), is probably the most reliable of all procedures.

These diagnostic dilemmas have not been entirely solved by determination of Sm-C, as had once been hoped. Significant discordance has been found between Sm-C and GH concentrations following provocative testing, making interpretation uncertain.[128] If on outpatient screening both the Sm-C and exercise GH are normal, or even if only the Sm-C is *clearly* within the normal range, it is probable that the patient does not have GH deficiency. However, continued deceleration of growth rate, or subnormal levels of both GH and Sm-C on initial testing, is an indication for further evaluation on an inpatient basis.

Note that in addition to the exercise test, several other provocative tests, for example, arginine, may be performed on an outpatient basis if appropriate facilities and personnel are available. However, the insulin test is not recommended for the ambulatory setting because of the potential for significant hypoglycemia.

Inpatient studies should include:

1. Complete blood count, urinalysis.
2. Serum electrolytes, BUN, creatinine, calcium, phosphorus, cholesterol, total protein, and sedimentation rate.
3. Serum thyroxine or other thyroid function studies.
4. Growth hormone studies, e.g., sequential arginine-insulin tolerance test (which will also evaluate the pituitary/adrenal axis); IC-GH (see Appendix 3); Sm-C.
5. X-ray examination of lateral skull, chest, and hands for BA.
6. In patients with delayed puberty, serum gonadotrophins, testosterone (in boys), estradiol, karyotype (in girls).

The combined arginine-insulin tolerance test reduces the failure rate to about 2% or 3%, even though roughly 15% of subjects fail to respond to either test alone. The oral L-dopa test appears to be an appropriate substitute,[129–132] in terms of GH, for either arginine or insulin, and will also stimulate a cortisol response. However, nausea is a prominent side effect. Other provocative tests, which are probably not quite so reliable, include the glucose tolerance test, during which GH often rises by 4 hours after ingestion,[133] and the glucagon tolerance test,[134, 135] which will stimulate the release of both GH and cortisol if carried out to 3 hours. Clonidine may also be a useful agent.[136] However, in view of the foregoing discussion regarding the reliability of Sm-C and provocative GH testing,[128, 137] it is probable that a 12- or 24-hour IC-GH is the procedure of choice if facilities and personnel are available.[138, 139] On the other hand, not even this study is infallible diagnostically.

Patients in whom an intracranial neoplasm is suspected on the basis of clinical or radiographic features can be further evaluated by computed tomography[140, 141] or magnetic resonance imaging.[142]

Treatment

For many years, *growth hormone deficiency* was treated with GH extracted from human pituitary glands. To ensure that the limited supply of GH was available to patients with a legitimate need, pituitary glands were collected by the National Hormone and Pituitary Program (NHPP), a federal agency, and the GH was distributed to endocrinologists, who administered the hormone according to research protocols. However, in 1985 it was learned that three men, all young adults who had previously received pituitary GH, had died of apparent Creutzfeldt-Jakob disease, a "slow-virus" affecting the nervous system. Since this condition in the general population is extremely rare, it was strongly suspected that the GH had been contaminated with the virus, and further distribution of the hormone was curtailed. Because of the nature of the infection, it may take years to determine with reasonable certainty if pituitary GH was in fact responsible for the deaths.[143]

Meanwhile, the GH that was being manufactured biosynthetically from *Escherichia coli* by recombinant DNA technology proved effective. It has subsequently been approved by the FDA—although only for use in children with documented GH deficiency—and thus can be obtained commercially by prescription; it is recommended, however, that treatment be under the direction of an endocrinologist. (The NHPP is not regulating the distribution of synthetic GH.)

A typical program consists of 0.06 to 0.1 mg/kg of body weight, administered intramuscularly or subcutaneously (by the patient or parents) three times a week until growth ceases or satisfactory height is achieved, or indefinitely if hypoglycemia is a problem. However, because the supply is no longer limited, it is probable that higher doses, with the likelihood of greater growth response, will be used in the future.

Treatment can be of some value up until the epiphyses fuse, but ideally should be instituted at the earliest possible time, when the remaining growth potential is greatest. However, note that the short-term Sm-C response to GH does not appear to predict clinical benefit with accuracy.[144]

The effect of GH can be enhanced when used in conjunction with androgen therapy.[145] However, it is possible that this combination might stimulate excessive skeletal maturation in some cases and therefore may not be indicated unless the patient is a boy with significant delay of maturation. Undue advance of BA is not a problem when GH is used alone.[146]

Even with treatment, the final height of patients with GH deficiency is often not optimal.[146] This may be related to delayed onset of therapy, noncompliance, excessive steroid replacement in a child with adrenocorticotrophic hormone (ACTH) deficiency, the undetected onset of hypothyroidism, or (rarely) the development of a significant titer of anti-GH antibodies. The use of Sm-C or GH-releasing hormone has been suggested as a possible alternative to GH in the future, but at present these modes of treatment are not practical.[147] It has also been reported that some GH-deficient children will respond to L-dopa or bromcriptine.[148]

Pituitary deficiencies in addition to GH deficiency (e.g., TSH, FSH/LH, ACTH) are treated with appropriate hormonal replacement, in conjunction with GH, as described in other chapters.

Other treatable causes of short stature include such entities as inflammatory bowel disease and congenital heart disease, in which growth rate usually improves if correction of the underlying defect is possible. Treatment of primary hypothyroidism is reviewed in Chapter 6; that of psychosocial dwarfism, in Chapter 4.

Other types of short stature (e.g., familial, primordial, "short-limbed") have generally been considered refractory to treatment, although in previous years limited trials of pituitary GH in patients with intrauterine growth retardation,[149] achondroplasia,[150] and gonadal dysgenesis have resulted in transient improvement of growth velocity in some cases. Now that the supply of synthetic GH is more plentiful, experimental protocols are being developed to treat some of these forms of dwarfism with this hormone. Early results in Turner's syndrome suggest possible benefit.[151-153]

The question has also arisen as to whether "short-normal" children would respond to GH with an increase in final height as well as growth rate.[154, 155] It can be argued that it is unlikely that an individual could exceed his or her "genetic potential"; on the other hand, this thesis is refuted by the examples of pituitary gigantism. As experimentation continues and more data are collected, it appears possible that physicians, and society in general, might be faced with the ethical issue of GH therapy in relatively short but otherwise healthy children who wish their stature augmented for athletic or social reasons. The risk-benefit ratio in such cases must also be considered: although treatment with physiologic doses of synthetic GH currently appears very safe, it has been speculated that its use in non-GH-deficient children (probably in pharmacologic amounts) could possibly result in diabetes mellitus, disproportionate growth, and even the formation of GH antibodies that might blunt the effect of the patient's own endogenous GH.

Surgery is the treatment of choice for craniopharyngioma,[90] but removal is not always possible, and long-term prognosis is guarded.[156] Postoperative irradiation is of questionable value. Replacement therapy with vasopressin, thyroid hormone, and glucocorticoids usually is necessary following operation. Following surgery some patients experience an accelerated growth rate without administration of GH. The cause of this "catch-up" growth is not clear, but it may be related to hyperinsulinism.[157, 158] If catch-up growth does not occur, treatment with growth hormone may be considered for patients who do not demonstrate evidence of further progression of the tumor.

Patients with *Turner's syndrome* usually are given estrogens at age 12 to 14 years. A typical program would consist of ethinyl estradiol (Estinyl), 10 to 20 μg/day. Medication is frequently given 3 weeks each month, or may be taken continuously until "breakthrough" bleeding occurs. Other suitable hormone preparations are conjugated estrogens (Premarin) or micronized estradiol (Estrace). Menses frequently begin during the first 6 months of treatment, and there is gradual development of secondary sexual characteristics during this time. A modest growth spurt may be expected,[159] but there is no evidence that ultimate height is improved. Since estrogens also stimulate skeletal maturation, it is prudent to obtain BA roentgenograms at yearly intervals. However, advance in BA in excess of the increment in height has not been a problem in our clinic.

Children whose menses are irregular or whose sexual development is not satisfactory may benefit from the addition of medroxyprogesterone (Provera), 2.5 to 10 mg daily, during week 3 of the cycle. Contraceptive agents would provide a similar combination. There is some evidence that progestins may decrease the possibility of estrogen-induced uterine malignancy.[160–162]

An alternative treatment program consists of the use of synthetic androgens, fluoxymesterone (Halotestin),[163] or preferably oxandrolone (Anavar) for 6 to 12 months, or until growth has stopped, at which time estrogen therapy is begun. Recommended dose is 2 to 5 mg daily of fluoxymesterone or 0.1 to 0.2 mg/kg/day of oxandrolone. Treatment in these amounts minimizes the androgenic side effects and probably does not cause excessive skeletal maturation. There is some evidence that this form of treatment may actually improve the ultimate height of patients with Turner's syndrome,[163, 164] although controversy exists.[165] There has also been recent interest in the use of low doses of estrogen at an early age in an attempt to promote growth,[166] and as noted earlier, GH has been tried experimentally with some success.[151–153]

The synthetic androgens also may be used in patients with *constitutional delayed growth*.[167–172] The dosage varies depending upon the desirability of stimulating sexual maturation as well, but the maximum usually is about 10 mg/day of fluoxymesterone or 0.2 mg/kg/day of oxandrolone. The goal of therapy is a growth spurt earlier than that which would occur naturally. In optimum doses it is not likely that ultimate height is significantly affected adversely or favorably,[173] nor does gonadotrophin suppression persist after withdrawal.[173] One report describes a disproportionate stimulation of skeletal maturation.[171] This generally has not been the experience of others, but an unfavorable result appears more likely when treatment is instituted in younger children.[171] Therefore, androgen therapy should be limited to children whose skeletal age is approximately 10 years or more. Conversely, the increase in growth velocity does not appear to be as great in patients treated after about 13 years.[170]

Treatment of this condition is justifiable if delayed growth is sufficiently severe to cause psychological problems,[174, 175] but BA must be monitored and hepatitis is a rare complication. Methyltestosterone has generally been avoided because of concern about its effect on skeletal maturation, but at least one report suggests that these fears may be exaggerated.[176]

EXCESSIVE HEIGHT

Children who are too tall for their age (above the 95th percentile) may fall into one of the following categories: (1) cerebral gigantism, (2) pituitary gigantism, or (3) a normal variant (familial).

Cerebral Gigantism

Patients with cerebral gigantism (Sotos' syndrome)[177–181] are large at birth and continue to grow rapidly during early childhood. Thereafter, the growth rate tends to decrease, and final height may not be above the normal range. Facies are characteristic, with large skull, prominent forehead, antimongoloid slant of the eyes, and large jaw. Hands and feet are large. Mental retardation usually is present.

Endocrine function studies, including growth hormone and somatomedin activity, are normal, although a paradoxic rise in growth hormone following glucose administration has been reported. Radiographically, the skull is large, with dilated ventricles. BA is advanced, consistent with HA.

The cause of cerebral gigantism is not known, but it is thought to represent a congenital abnormality of the hypothalamus. There is evidence for an autosomal dominant mode of inheritance. There is no treatment.

Pituitary Gigantism

Pituitary gigantism[182] usually is caused by an eosinophilic adenoma of the pituitary. The increase in growth rate is proportional, and typically there are no distinguishing facial features, as in cerebral gigantism. Fasting growth hormone levels are elevated and not suppressible by glucose, but response to stimuli is blunted. BA is normal or advanced. If the tumor becomes active after the epiphyses have fused, the clinical features of acromegaly will be present. Pituitary gigantism may be treated with various types of irradiation or by surgery, but no therapy is ideal. Results of external irradiation have been particularly disappointing. Fortunately, pituitary gigantism appears to be a rare condition.

Normal Variant (Familial or Constitutional)

Many children with height above the 95th percentile for their CA do not demonstrate any endocrine abnormality or other cause for their excessive growth. Usually these children have relatively tall parents, and the problem can be attributed to a genetic trait. In other patients, it may be more difficult to attribute the excessive height to a familial tendency, in which case the term "constitutional tall stature" can probably be applied. (If BA is advanced, the situation is essentially the converse of "constitutional delayed growth"). Increased levels of Sm-C/IGF-I have been found in these patients,[183] and paradoxical increases in GH following oral glucose loading.[184]

Suggested minimal diagnostic studies include fasting GH determination and x-ray examination of the skull and hands. If BA is advanced, growth potential is limited and ultimate height may be satisfactory. A final height prediction can be made from tables on the basis of current HA and BA.[185] If the height prediction in a girl indicates that final stature will be unacceptable (generally greater than 6 feet), therapy may be attempted. This consists of estrogen,[186–189] for example, conjugated estrogens, in gradually increasing amounts until a daily dose of 5 to 10 mg is reached, or ethinyl estradiol, 250 to 300 μg/day. The purpose is to stimulate skeletal maturation and cause early epiphyseal fusion, but an initial growth spurt frequently occurs. The patient should be prepared for the onset of menses and the development of secondary sex characteristics.

High doses of estrogen cause nausea in some patients. Another occasional complication is temporary amenorrhea following cessation of therapy, presumably a result of suppression of gonadotrophins. Although it is theoretically possible, we are not aware of permanent amenorrhea following this form of treatment. Finally, the risk of thrombosis and endometrial carcinoma is an important consideration.[162, 190]

There is general agreement that therapy should be initiated by the time BA is 12 years, but even then there is considerable controversy concerning its effectiveness. Because of the potential hazards and questionable benefit of therapy, it is justified only in patients whose height prediction is clearly unsatisfactory. However, it is true that the limit of acceptability depends to some extent on the attitude of the patient and her parents; they should be made fully aware of the limitations of therapy before a decision is made. Once begun, treatment ideally should be continued until the epiphyses have fused.

The use of bromcriptine, 2.5 mg twice daily, has also been suggested[191] as therapy for tall stature. The beneficial effect of this long-acting dopamine agonist is apparently mediated through inhibition of GH secretion.

Other Conditions Associated With Excessive Height

These include Marfan's syndrome, neurofibromatosis, and homocystinuria, descriptions of which may be found in standard pediatric texts. Patients with sexual precocity (see Chapter 9) and untreated congenital adrenal hyperplasia (see Chapter 7) are tall as children, but adult height is compromised because of early epiphyseal fusion. Patients with Beckwith-Wiedemann syndrome are large as infants.[192]

APPENDIX 3

Arginine Tolerance Test (ATT) for Growth Hormone (GH)[124]

Begin at 8 to 9 AM with the patient taking nothing by mouth after midnight. Arginine HCl, 0.5 g/kg not to exceed 20 g, is given intravenously over a period of 30 minutes. Samples for GH are obtained prior to infusion, and at 30, 60, and 90 minutes following the start of infusion.

A GH concentration of 7 to 10 ng/mL or higher at any time during the study generally is considered a normal response. Most patients with GH deficiency do not have levels over 2 ng/mL. Peak concentrations between 2 and 7 ng/mL may suggest partial GH deficiency.

Insulin Tolerance Test (ITT) for Growth Hormone[125]

Conditions, time of samples, and interpretation are the same as for the ATT. Dose of insulin is 0.1 U/kg, diluted to 1 U/mL by mixing 20 units of U100 regular insulin (0.2 mL) with 19.8 mL of sterile water just prior to injection. Insulin solution is given rapidly intravenously following the 0-minute blood sample.

Blood glucose determinations are obtained with each sample; a fall to 50% of the 0-minute level is considered adequate hypoglycemia. Otherwise, results of the test are of questionable validity if GH fails to rise. A level greater than 7 to 10 ng/mL is a normal response.

Note that this is a potentially dangerous test,[193] and should be terminated with 50% glucose intravenously (must be at bedside) if significant symptoms of hypoglycemia occur. A saline IV drip should be kept open during the test. A physician must be present.

In patients with known hypoglycemia, an L-dopa test or a glucagon tolerance test (see Chapter 2) with GH levels may be substituted for the ITT.

Combined Arginine-Insulin Tolerance Test for Growth Hormone[194]

Because of the possibility of false negative tests, an abnormal response to at least two provocative tests is necessary. This may be accomplished by combining the ATT and ITT as follows: a routine ATT is performed as described, and insulin is injected following the 90-minute sample. This sample serves as the 0-minute sample for the ITT, which is then performed in the usual manner. Time required for the combined test is 3 hours.

L-Dopa Tolerance Test for Growth Hormone[131, 132, 195]

This test stimulates the release of cortisol, prolactin, and glucagon, as well as GH. It is often used in combination with the ATT, substituting for the ITT. The patient is fasted, except for water, after midnight. L-Dopa is administered orally according to body weight: <15 kg–125 mg, 15 to 30 kg–250 mg, >30 kg–500 mg. Serum samples are obtained at 30, 45, 60, 90, and 120 minutes. A peak GH concentration of ≥7 ng/mL is a normal response.

Exercise Screening Test for Growth Hormone[120–123]

The patient is exercised on a stationary bicycle, by climbing stairs, or by brisk walking with intermittent jogging as tolerated, for 20 minutes. A single serum sample for GH is obtained after a 10-minute rest. A level of ≥5 to 7 ng/mL is indicative of normal pituitary reserve. Ideally, the patient should be fasting, but this is not critical.

Priming Prior to Provocative Testing

It appears that the GH response to stimuli may be increased by pretreatment with estrogens,[196, 197] and propranolol has been reported to augment the response to exercise[198, 199] or L-dopa.[200, 201] However, estrogen administration requires additional time (2 or 3 days) and may produce nausea, and use of propranolol has been associated with hypotension, bradycardia, and hypoglycemia.[202] Also, many are of the opinion that a primed provocative test requires a higher GH concentration for a normal response, thereby diluting the value of this procedure. For these reasons, pretreatment currently is not frequently used, although priming with androgens or estrogens may still be indicated in the prepubertal child with suspected constitutional delay who has a blunted response to routine provocative testing.[75]

Integrated Concentration of Growth Hormone (IC-GH)[76, 127, 139, 203]

Most reports have described serum sampling every 20 to 30 minutes, by means of a constant withdrawal pump or indwelling catheter, for a 24-hour period. It is difficult to provide absolute interpretive guidelines: reported results differ somewhat depending on the source; there is also age dependency (highest GH values between 15 and 20 years), and some overlap between presumed GH-deficient and non-GH-deficient children. However, an IC-GH of approximately

3 ng/mL appears to be the dividing line between GH-deficient patients, including those with neurosecretory dysfunction, and healthy subjects. Bercu et al.[127] reported the following IC-GH results: classic GH-deficient patients—mean GH 1.5 ng/mL (range, 0.5 to 3.3); NSD—2.0 (<1.0 to 3.0); controls—5.7 (3.0 to 12.2).

Twenty-four hour IC-GH results have also been compared with various day or night segments of shorter duration. Of these, a 12-hour nighttime (8 PM to 8 AM) IC-GH appears to be the most reliable and is probably a reasonable substitute for the 24-hour IC-GH. Because of the usual contribution of the stage III-IV sleep segment, mean concentrations are higher: Bercu et al.[127] reported 2.0 ng/mL (0.5 to 4.6) for GH deficiency, 2.8 (1.0 to 4.7) for neurosecretory dysfunction, and 8.0 (3.3 to 18.6) for controls. The reader is referred to the original reports for further details.

Tests of Other Pituitary-Target Organ Systems

Because a significant number of GH-deficient children also have deficiency of other trophic hormones, it is important to rule out these conditions as well. The rise in serum cortisol during the ITT (or L-dopa or glucagon) test may be used to assess pituitary-adrenal responsiveness. An increase of 10 μg/dL from the 0-minute sample, or a maximum concentration of over 20 μg/dL, can be considered indicative of normal function, but ideally interpretive guidelines should be established for each laboratory. A Metopirone (metyrapone) test can also be performed if desired (see Chapter 7). Gonadotrophin testing is described in Chapter 9; however, it may be justifiable to postpone this evaluation in order to determine if sexual development will occur spontaneously at the expected time of puberty.

Tests of thyroid function are discussed in Chapter 5. Minimal screening (e.g., $T_4 + T_3$ resin uptake, or free T_4) is usually adequate to rule out thyroid deficiency in a child with suspected GH deficiency unless laboratory results are not consistent with clinical evidence. Note also that GH responsiveness may be blunted in a hypothyroid child; therefore, thyroid replacement therapy in these patients must be initiated before GH results can be considered valid.

Additional Sources Not Cited In The Text

A comprehensive review by Frasier[204] was written relative to pituitary GH therapy but summarizes many studies that are also applicable to the use of synthetic GH, and is recommended for further reading. Older reviews that still contain much useful information include a summary of tests of GH reserve, also compiled by Frasier,[205] and Part II of an inclusive discussion of short stature (etiology and evaluation) by Rimoin and Horton.[206]

Informative articles appearing more recently include a narrative of the sequence of events leading to the suspicion that contaminated pituitary GH was responsible for the deaths from Creutzfeldt-Jakob disease,[207] and a review of the therapeutic and ethical questions raised by the current ready availability of human GH.[208]

REFERENCES

1. Rimoin DL, Horton WA: Short stature: Part I. *J Pediatr* 1978; 92:523.
2. Garn SM, Shaw HA, McCabe KD: Birth size and growth appraisal. *J Pediatr* 1977; 90:1049.
3. Dahlmann N, Petersen K: Influences of environmental conditions during infancy on final body stature. *Pediatr Res* 1977; 11:695.
4. Hill DJ, Milner RDG: Insulin as a growth factor. *Pediatr Res* 1985; 19:879.
5. Widdowson EM, McCance RA: A review: New thoughts on growth. *Pediatr Res* 1975; 9:154.
6. Johnson JD: Regulation of fetal growth. (Presidential address, Society for Pediatric Research, May 1984.) *Pediatr Res* 1985; 19:738.
7. D'ercole AJ, et al: Tissue and plasma somatomedin-C/insulin-like growth factor: I. concentrations in the human fetus during the first half of gestation. *Pediatr Res* 1986; 20:253.
8. Rosenfield RI, Furlanetto R, Bock D: Relationship of somatomedin-C concentrations to pubertal changes. *J Pediatr* 1983; 103:723.
9. Reichlin S: Growth and the hypothalamus. *Endocrinology,* 1960; 67:760.
10. Castells S, et al: Cerebral dwarfism: Association of brain dysfunction with growth retardation. *J Pediatr* 1974; 85:36.
11. Lowrey GH, et al: Fasting growth hormone levels in mentally retarded children of short stature. *Am J Ment Defic* 1968; 73:474.
12. Frasier SD, Hilburn JM, Smith FG, Jr: Dwarfism and mental retardation: The serum growth hormone response to hypoglycemia. *J Pediatr* 1970; 77:136.
13. Mehrizi A, Drash A: Growth disturbance in congenital heart disease. *J Pediatr* 1962; 61:418.
14. Bacon GE, et al: Growth hormone levels in children with congenital heart disease. *Am Heart J* 1969; 78:280.
15. Linde LM, et al: Growth in children with congenital heart disease. *J Pediatr* 1967; 70:413.
16. Green OC, Fefferman R, Nair S: Plasma growth hormone levels in children with cystic fibrosis and short stature. Unresponsiveness to hypoglycemia. *J Clin Endocrinol Metab* 1967; 27:1059.
17. Cacciari E, et al: Short stature and celiac disease: A relationship to consider even in patients with no gastrointestinal tract symptoms. *J Pediatr* 1983; 103:708.
18. McCaffrey TD, et al: Severe growth retardation in children with inflammatory bowel disease. *Pediatrics* 1970; 45:386.
19. Tenore A, et al: Basal and stimulated serum growth hormone concentrations in inflammatory bowel disease. *J Clin Endocrinol Metab* 1977; 44:622.
20. Motil KJ, et al: The effect of disease, drug, and diet on whole body protein metabolism in adolescents with Crohn disease and growth failure. *J Pediatr* 1982; 101:345.
21. Rosenthal SR, et al: Growth failure and inflammatory bowel disease: Approach to treatment of a complicated adolescent problem. *Pediatrics* 1983; 72:481.
22. Berger M, Gribetz D, Koreilitz BI: Growth retardation in children with ulcerative colitis: The effect of medical and surgical therapy. *Pediatrics* 1975; 55:459.
23. Homer DR, Grand RJ, Colodny AH: Growth, course, and prognosis after surgery for Crohn's disease in children and adolescents. *Pediatrics* 1977; 59:717.
24. Hilson D: Malformation of ears as sign of malformation of genitourinary tract. *Br Med J* 1957; 2:785.
25. Holliday MA: Calorie deficiency in children with uremia: Effect upon growth. *Pediatrics* 1972; 50:590.

26. Betts PR, Mann MD, Wolfsdorf J: Growth and nutrition of uremic piglets. *Pediatr Res* 1976; 10:937.
27. Stickler GB, Bergen BJ: A review: Short stature in renal disease. *Pediatr Res* 1973; 7:978.
28. Logothetis J, et al: Body growth in Cooley's anemia (homozygous betathalassemia) with a correlative study as to other aspects of the illness in 138 cases. *Pediatrics* 1972; 50:92.
29. Pintor C, et al: Impaired growth hormone (GH) response to GH-releasing hormone in thalassemia major. *J Clin Endocrinol Metab* 1986; 62:263.
30. Hambridge KM, et al: Low levels of zinc in hair, anorexia, poor growth, and hypogeusia in children. *Pediatr Res* 1971; 6:868.
31. Schwartz J, Angle C, Pitcher H: Relationship between childhood blood lead levels and stature. *Pediatrics* 1986; 77:281.
32. Bailey JA: *Disproportionate Short Stature—Diagnosis and Management.* Philadelphia, WB Saunders Co, 1973.
33. Zellweger H, Taylor B: Genetic aspects of achondroplasia. *Lancet* 1965; 85:8.
34. Morgan BC, Aase JM, Graham CB: Homozygosity for achondroplasia? Report of a possible case, with congenital heart disease and severe mental deficit. *Pediatrics* 1970; 45:112.
35. Gordon SL, et al: Jansen's metaphyseal dysostosis. *Pediatrics* 1976; 58:556.
36. Rosenbloom AL, Smith DW: The natural history of metaphyseal dysostosis. *J Pediatr* 1965; 66:857.
37. Walker BA, et al: Hypochondroplasia. *Am J Dis Child* 1971; 122:95.
38. McKusick VA, et al: Dwarfism in the Amish: II. Cartilage-hair hypoplasia. *Johns Hopkins Med J* 1965; 116:285.
39. Lux SE, et al: Chronic neutropenia and abnormal cellular immunity in cartilage-hair hypoplasia. *N Engl J Med* 1970; 282:231.
40. Steele RW, et al: Severe combined immunodeficiency with cartilage-hair hypoplasia: in vitro response to thymosin and attempted reconstitution. *Pediatr Res* 1976; 10:1003.
41. Mann JB, Alterman S, Hills AG: Albright's hereditary osteodystrophy comprising pseudohypoparathyroidism and pseudo-pseudohypoparathyroidism. With a report of two cases representing the complete syndrome occurring in successive generations. *Ann Intern Med* 1962; 56:315.
42. Levine MA, Jap T, Hung W: Infantile hypothyroidism in two sibs: An unusual presentation of pseudohypoparathyroidism type Ia. *J Pediatr* 1985; 107:919.
43. Ferguson-Smith MA: Karyotype-genetic correlations in gonadal dysgenesis and their bearing on the pathogenesis of malformations. *J Med Genet* 1965; 2:142.
44. Miller MJ, et al: Echocardiography reveals a high incidence of bicuspid aortic valve in Turner syndrome. *J Pediatr* 1983; 102:47.
45. Rahal F, Young RB, Mammunes P: Gonadal dysgenesis associated with a multicystic kidney. *Am J Dis Child* 1973; 126:505.
46. Collins E: The illusion of widely spaced nipples in the Noonan and the Turner syndromes. *J Pediatr* 1973; 83:557.
47. Pai GS, et al: Thyroid abnormalities in 20 children with Turner syndrome. *J Pediatr* 1977; 91:267.
48. Brown DM, et al: Osteoporosis in ovarian dysgenesis. *J Pediatr* 1974; 84:816.
49. Ross JL, et al: Growth hormone secretory dynamics in Turner syndrome. *J Pediatr* 1985; 106:202.
50. Park E, Bailey JD, Cowell CA: Growth and maturation of patients with Turner's syndrome. *Pediatr Res* 1983; 17:1.

51. Kalousek D, et al: Partial short arm deletions of the X chromosome and spontaneous pubertal development in girls with short stature. *J Pediatr* 1979; 94:891.
52. Huseman CA: Mosaic Turner syndrome with precocious puberty. *J Pediatr* 1983; 102:892.
53. Bender B, et al: Cognitive development of unselected girls with complete and partial X monosomy. *Pediatrics* 1984; 73:175.
54. Lahood BJ, Bacon GE: Cognitive abilities of adolescent Turner's syndrome patients. *J Adolesc Health Care* 1985; 6:358.
55. Lajborek-Czyz I: A 45,X woman with a 47,XY, G+ son. *Clin Genet* 1976; 9:113.
56. Shoval AR: The syndrome of pure gonadal dysgenesis. *Am J Med* 1965; 38:615.
57. Nora JJ, Sinha AK: Direct familial transmission of the Turner phenotype. *Am J Dis Child* 1968; 116:343.
58. Collins E, Turner G: The Noonan syndrome—A review of the clinical and genetic features of 27 cases. *J Pediatr* 1973; 83:941.
59. Brosnan PG, et al: A new familial syndrome of 46,XY gonadal dysgenesis with anomalies of ectodermal and mesodermal structures. *J Pediatr* 1980; 97:586.
60. O'Connell EJ, Feldt RH, Stickler BG: Head circumference, mental retardation and growth failure. *Pediatrics* 1965; 36:62.
61. Macfarlane DW, et al: Intrauterine rubella, head size, and intellect. *Pediatrics* 1975; 55:797.
62. Warkany J, Monroe BB, Sutherland BS: Intrauterine growth retardation. *Am J Dis Child* 1961; 102:249.
63. Beck GJ, van den Berg BJ: The relationship of the rate of intrauterine growth of low-birth-weight infants to later growth. *J Pediatr* 1975; 86:504.
64. Fitzhardinge PM, Steven EM: The small-for-date infant: I. Later growth patterns. *Pediatrics* 1972; 49:671.
65. Vohr BR, Oh W: Growth and development in preterm infants small for gestational age. *J Pediatr* 1983; 103:941.
66. Smith DW: *Recognizable Patterns of Human Malformation*, ed 3. Philadelphia, WB Saunders Co, 1982.
67. Tanner JM, Lejarraga H, Cameron N: The natural history of the Silver-Russell syndrome: A longitudinal study of thirty-nine cases. *Pediatr Res* 1975; 9:611.
68. Saal HM, Pagon RA, Pepin MG: Reevaluation of Russell-Silver syndrome. *J Pediatr* 1985; 107:733.
69. Draznin MB, Stelling MW, Johanson AJ: Silver-Russell syndrome and craniopharyngioma. *J Pediatr* 1980; 96:887.
70. Iosub S, et al: Fetal alcohol syndrome revisited. *Pediatrics* 1981; 68:475.
71. Assadi FK, Ziai M: Impaired renal acidification in infants with fetal alcohol syndrome. *Pediatr Res* 1985; 19:850.
72. Assadi FK, Ziai M: Zinc status of infants with fetal alcohol syndrome. *Pediatr Res* 1986; 20:551.
73. Horner JM, Thorsson AV, Hintz RL: Growth deceleration patterns in children with constitutional short stature: An aid to diagnosis. *Pediatrics* 1978; 62:529.
74. Frohman LA, Aceto T, Jr, MacGillvray MH: Studies of growth hormone secretion in children: Normal, hypopituitary and constitutional delayed. *J Clin Endocrinol Metab* 1967; 27:1409.
75. Gourmelen M, Pham-Huu-Trung MT, Girard F: Transient partial hGH deficiency in prepubertal children with delay of growth. *Pediatr Res* 1979; 13:221.
76. Zadik Z, et al: Do short children secrete insufficient growth hormone? *Pediatrics* 1985; 76:355.

77. Lanes R, et al: Are constitutional delay of growth and familial short stature different conditions? *Clin Pediatr* 1980; 19:31.
78. Schriock EA, et al: Effect of growth hormone (GH)-releasing hormone (GRH) on plasma GH in relation to magnitude and duration of GH deficiency in 26 children and adults with isolated GH deficiency or multiple pituitary hormone deficiencies: Evidence for hypothalamic GRH deficiency. *J Clin Endocrinol Metab* 1984; 58:1043.
79. Craft WH, Underwood LE, Van Wyk JJ: High incidence of perinatal insult in children with idiopathic hypopituitarism. *J Pediatr* 1980; 96:397.
80. Lovinger RD, Kaplan SL, Grumbach MM: Congenital hypopituitarism associated with neonatal hypoglycemia and microphallus: four cases secondary to hypothalamic hormone deficiencies. *J Pediatr* 1975; 87:1171.
81. Johnson JD, et al: Hypoplasia of the anterior pituitary and neonatal hypoglycemia. *J Pediatr* 1973; 82:634.
82. Hopwood NJ, et al: Hypoglycemia in hypopituitary children. *Am J Dis Child* 1975; 129:918.
83. Herman SP, Baggenstoss AH, Cloutier MD: Liver dysfunction and histologic abnormalities in neonatal hypopituitarism. *J Pediatr* 1975; 87:892.
84. Soyka LF, et al: Effectiveness of long-term human growth hormone therapy for short stature in children with growth hormone deficiency. *J Clin Endocrinol Metab* 1970; 30:1.
85. Rimoin DL, Merimee TJ, McKusick VA: Growth hormone deficiency in man: An isolated, recessively inherited defect. *Science* 1966; 152:1635.
86. Sheikholislam BM, Stempfel RS, Jr: Hereditary isolated somatotrophin deficiency: Effects of human growth hormone administration. *Pediatrics* 1972; 49:362.
87. Zipf WB, Kelch RP, Bacon GE: Variable X-linked recessive hypopituitarism with evidence of gonadotropin deficiency in two prepubertal males. *Clin Genetics* 1977; 11:249.
88. Rivarola MA, et al: Phenotypic heterogeneity in familial isolated growth hormone deficiency type I-A. *J Clin Endocrinol Metab* 1984; 59:34.
89. Illig R, et al: Hereditary prenatal growth hormone deficiency with increased tendency to growth hormone antibody formation (A type of isolated growth hormone deficiency). *Acta Pediatr Scand* 1970; 60:607.
90. Banna M, et al: Craniopharyngioma in children. *J Pediatr* 1973; 83:781.
91. Jenkins JS, Gilbert CJ, Ang V: Hypothalamic-pituitary function in patients with craniopharyngiomas. *J Clin Endocrinol Metab* 1976; 43:394.
92. Richards GE, et al: Delayed onset of hypopituitarism: Sequelae of therapeutic irradiation of central nervous system, eye, and middle ear tumors. *J Pediatr* 1976; 89:553.
93. Bajorunas DR, et al: Endocrine sequelae of antineoplastic therapy in childhood head and neck malignancies. *J Clin Endocrinol Metab* 1980; 50:329.
94. Romshe CA, et al: Evaluation of growth hormone release and human growth hormone treatment in children with cranial irradiation-associated short stature. *J Pediatr* 1984; 104:177.
95. Thomsett MJ, et al: Endocrine and neurologic outcome in childhood craniopharyngioma: Review of effect of treatment in 42 patients. *J Pediatr* 1980; 97:728.
96. Oberfield SE, et al: Long-term endocrine sequelae after treatment of medulloblastoma: Prospective study of growth and thyroid function. *J Pediatr* 1986; 108:219.
97. Huseman CA, et al: Sexual precocity in association with septo-optic dysplasia and hypothalamic hypopituitarism. *J Pediatr* 1978; 92:748.
98. Russell JD, Wise PH, Rischbieth HG: Vascular malformation of hypothalamus: A cause of isolated growth hormone deficiency. *Pediatrics* 1980; 66:306.

99. LaFranchi SH, Hanna CE, Krainz PL: Primary hypothyroidism, empty sella, and hypopituitarism. *J Pediatr* 1986; 108:571.
100. Shulman DI, et al: Hypothalamic-pituitary dysfunction in primary empty sella syndrome in childhood. *J Pediatr* 1986; 108:540.
101. Elders MJ, et al: Laron's dwarfism: Studies on the nature of the defect. *J Pediatr* 1973; 83:253.
102. Clemons RD, Costin G, Kogut MD: Laron dwarfism: Growth and immunoreactive insulin following treatment with human growth hormone. *J Pediatr* 1976; 88:427.
103. Jacobs LS, et al: Receptor-active growth hormone in Laron dwarfism. *J Clin Endocrinol Metab* 1976; 42:403.
104. Bright GM, et al: Short stature associated with normal growth hormone and decreased somatomedin-C concentrations: Response to exogenous growth hormone. *Pediatrics* 1983; 71:576.
105. Frazer T, et al: Growth hormone-dependent growth failure. *J Pediatr* 1982; 101:12.
106. Rudman D, et al: Normal variant short stature: Subclassification based on responses to exogenous human growth hormone. *J Clin Endocrinol Metab* 1979; 49:92.
107. Rudman D, et al: Further observations on four subgroups of normal variant short stature. *J Clin Endocrinol Metab* 1980; 51:1378.
108. Rudman D, Kutner MH, Chawla RK: The short child with subnormal plasma somatomedin-C[1]. *Pediatr Res* 1985; 19:975.
109. Lanes R, et al: Dwarfism associated with normal serum growth hormone and increased bioassayable, receptorassayable, and immunoassayable somatomedin. *J Clin Endocrinol Metab* 1980; 50:485.
110. Huseman CA, Hassing JM, Sibilia MG: Endogenous dopaminergic dysfunction: A novel form of human growth hormone deficiency and short stature. *J Clin Endocrinol Metab* 1986; 62:484.
111. Lee PA, Weldon VV, Migeon CJ: Short stature as the only clinical sign of Cushing's syndrome. *J Pediatr* 1975; 86:89.
112. Garn SM, Rhomann CG: Interaction of nutrition and genetics in the timing of growth and development. *Pediatr Clin North Am* 1966; 13:353.
113. West CD, Smith WC: An attempt to elucidate the cause of growth retardation in renal disease. *Am J Dis Child* 1956; 91:460.
114. Poznanski AK, et al: The pattern of shortening of the bones of the hand in PHP and PPHP—a comparison with brachydactyly E, Turner syndrome, and acrodysostosis. *Radiology* 1977; 123:707.
115. Kurnick JE, et al: Abnormal sella turcica: A tumor board review of the clinical significance. *Arch Intern Med* 1977; 137:111.
116. Underwood LE, et al: Assessment of the sella turcica volume in dwarfed children. *J Clin Endocrinol Metab* 1973; 36:734.
117. Yamada T, et al: Volume of sella turcica in normal subjects and in patients with primary hypothyroidism and hyperthyroidism. *J Clin Endocrinol Metab* 1976; 42:817.
118. Boyar RM, et al: Twenty-four-hour luteinizing and follicle-stimulating hormone secretory patterns in gonadal dysgenesis. *J Clin Endocrinol Metab* 1973; 37:521.
119. Kaplan SL, et al: Growth and growth hormone: I. Changes in serum level of growth hormone following hypoglycemia in 134 children with growth retardation. *Pediatr Res* 1968; 2:43.
120. Okaka Y, et al: Human growth hormone secretion after exercise and oral glucose administration in patients with short stature. *J Clin Endocrinol Metab* 1972; 34:1055.
121. Keenan BS, Killmer LB, Jr, Sode J: Growth hormone response to exercise: A test of pituitary function in children. *Pediatrics* 1972; 50:760.

122. Johanson AJ, Morris GL: A single growth hormone determination to rule out growth hormone deficiency. *Pediatrics* 1977; 59:467.

123. Eisenstein E, et al: Evaluation of the growth hormone exercise test in normal and growth hormone-deficient children. *Pediatrics* 1978; 62:526.

125. Frasier SD: The serum growth hormone response to hypoglycemia in dwarfism. *J Pediatr* 1967; 71:625.

126. Spiliotis BE, et al: Growth hormone neurosecretory dysfunction: A treatable cause of short stature. *JAMA* 1984; 251:2223.

127. Bercu BB, et al: Growth hormone (GH) provocative testing frequently does not reflect endogenous GH secretion. *J Clin Endocrinol Metab* 1986; 63:709.

128. Rosenfeld RG, et al: Insulin-like growth factors I and II in evaluation of growth retardation. *J Pediatr* 1986; 109:428.

129. Root AW, Russ RD: Effect of L-dihydroxyphenylalanine upon serum growth hormone concentrations in children and adolescents. *J Pediatr* 1972; 81:808.

130. Chakmakjian ZH, Marks JF, Fink CW: Effect of levodopa (L-dopa) on serum growth hormone in children with short stature. *Pediatr Res* 1973; 7:71.

131. Weldon VV, et al: Evaluation of growth hormone release in children using arginine and L-dopa in combination. *J Pediatr* 1975; 87:540.

132. Becker DJ, Villalpando S, Drash AL: L-dopa as a screening test of hypothalamo-pituitary adrenal and pancreatic function in children. *Pediatr Res* 1976; 10:336. (Abstract)

133. Streeto JM: Late post-glucose rise in plasma growth hormone as a test of pituitary function. *J Clin Endocrinol Metab* 1970; 31:85.

134. Vanderschueren-Lodeweyckx M, et al: The glucagon stimulation test: Effect on plasma growth hormone and on immunoreactive insulin, cortisol, and glucose in children. *J Pediatr* 1974; 85:182.

135. AvRuskin TW, et al: The glucagon infusion test and growth hormone secretion. *J Pediatr* 1975; 86:102.

136. Lanes R, Hurtado E: Oral clonidine—an effective growth hormone-releasing agent in prepubertal subjects. *J Pediatr* 1982; 100:710.

137. Reiter EO, Lovinger RD: The use of a commercially available somatomedin-C radioimmunoassay in patients with disorders of growth. *J Pediatr* 1981; 99:720.

138. Plotnick LP, et al: Comparison of physiological and pharmacological tests of growth hormone function in children with short stature. *J Clin Endocrinol Metab* 1979; 48:811.

139. Chalew SA, et al: Growth hormone (GH) response to GH-releasing hormone in children with subnormal integrated concentrations of GH. *J Clin Endocrinol Metab* 1986; 62:1110.

140. Ferry PC: Computed cranial tomography in children. *J Pediatr* 1980; 96:961.

141. Smith SP, et al: Value of computed tomographic scanning in patients with growth hormone deficiency. *Pediatrics* 1986; 78:601.

142. Leonard JC, et al: Nuclear magnetic resonance: An overview of its spectroscopic and imaging applications in pediatric patients. *J Pediatr* 1985; 106:756.

143. Underwood LE, et al: Degenerative neurologic disease in patients formerly treated with human growth hormone. (Report of the Committee on Growth Hormone Use of the Lawson Wilkins Pediatric Endocrine Society, May 1985.) *J Pediatr* 1985; 107:10.

144. Plotnick LP, Van Meter QL, Kowarski AA: Human growth hormone treatment of children with growth failure and normal growth hormone levels by immunoassay: Lack of correlation with somatomedin generation. *Pediatrics* 1983; 71:324.

145. Romshe CA, Sotos JF: The combined effect of growth hormone and oxandrolone in patients with growth hormone deficiency. *J Pediatr* 1980; 96:127.
146. Joss E, et al: Final height of patients with pituitary growth failure and changes in growth variables after long term hormonal therapy. *Pediatr Res* 1983; 17:676.
147. Borges JLC, et al: Stimulation of growth hormone (GH) and somatomedin C in idiopathic GH-deficient subjects by intermittent pulsatile administration of synthetic human pancreatic tumor GH-releasing factor. *J Clin Endocrinol Metab* 1984; 59:1.
148. Huseman CA, Hassing JM: Evidence for dopaminergic stimulation of growth velocity in some hypopituitary children. *J Clin Endocrinol Metab* 1984; 58:419.
149. Lanes R, Plotnick LP, Lee PA: Sustained effect of human growth hormone therapy on children with intrauterine growth retardation. *Pediatrics* 1979; 63:731.
150. Escamilla RF, et al: Achondroplastic dwarfism: Effects of treatment with human growth hormone. *Calif Med* 1966; 105:104.
151. Ross JL, et al: Growth response relationship between growth hormone dose and short term growth in patients with Turner's syndrome. *J Clin Endocrinol Metab* 1986; 63:1028.
152. Rosenfeld RG, et al: Methionyl human growth hormone and oxandrolone in Turner syndrome: Preliminary results of a prospective randomized trial. *J Pediatr* 1986; 109:936.
153. Raiti S, et al: Growth-stimulating effects of human growth hormone therapy in patients with Turner syndrome. *J Pediatr* 1986; 109:944.
154. Gertner JM, et al: Prospective clinical trial of human growth hormone in short children without growth hormone deficiency. *J Pediatr* 1984; 104:172.
155. Milner RDG: Which children should have growth hormone therapy. *Lancet* 1986; 1:483.
156. Lyen KR, Grant DB: Endocrine function, morbidity, and mortality after surgery for craniopharyngioma. *Arch Dis Child* 1982; 57:837.
157. Kenny FM, et al: Prolactin and somatomedin in hypopituitary patients with "catch-up" growth following operations for craniopharyngioma. *J Clin Endocrinol Metab* 1973; 36:378.
158. Costin G, et al: Craniopharyngioma: The role of insulin in promoting postoperative growth. *J Clin Endocrinol Metab* 1976; 42:370.
159. Rosenfield RL, Fang VS: The effects of prolonged physiologic estradiol therapy on the maturation of hypogonadal teen-agers. *J Pediatr* 1974; 85:830.
160. Smith DC, et al: Association of exogenous estrogen and endometrial carcinoma. *N Engl J Med* 1975; 293:1164.
161. Ziel HK, Finkle WC: Increased risk of endometrial carcinoma among users of conjugated estrogens. *N Engl J Med* 1975; 293:1167.
162. New MI, et al: Report on the Conference in Estrogen Treatment of The Young. *Pediatrics* 1978; 62(suppl 6).
163. Johanson AJ, Brasel JA, Blizzard RM: Growth in patients with gonadal dysgenesis receiving fluoxymesterone. *J Pediatr* 1969; 75:1015.
164. Moore DC, et al: Studies of anabolic steroids: VI. Effect of prolonged administration of oxandrolone on growth in children and adolescents with gonadal dysgenesis. *J Pediatr* 1977; 90:462.
165. Sybert VP: Adult height in Turner syndrome with and without androgen therapy. *J Pediatr* 1984; 104:365.
166. Ross JL, et al: Effect of low doses of estradiol on 6-month growth rates and predicted height in patients with Turner syndrome. *J Pediatr* 1986; 109:950.

167. Zangeneh F, Steiner MM: Oxandrolone therapy in growth retardation of children. *Am J Dis Child* 1967; 113:234.
168. Bettmann HK, et al: Oxandrolone treatment of short stature: Effect on predicted mature height. *J Pediatr* 1971; 79:1018.
169. Marti-Henneberg C, Niirianen AK, Rappaport R: Oxandrolone treatment of constitutional short stature in boys during adolescence: Effect on linear growth, bone age, pubic hair, and testicular development. *J Pediatr* 1975; 86:783.
170. Moore DC, et al: Studies of anabolic steroids: V. Effect of prolonged oxandrolone administration on growth in children and adolescents with uncomplicated short stature. *Pediatrics* 1976; 58:412.
171. Jackson ST, et al: Use of oxandrolone for growth stimulation in children. *Am J Dis Child* 1973; 126:481.
172. Blethen SL, Gaines S, Weldon V: Comparison of predicted and adult heights in short boys: Effect of androgen therapy. *Pediatr Res* 1984; 18:467.
173. Hopwood NJ, et al: The effect of synthetic androgens on the hypothalamic-pituitary-gonadal axis in boys with constitutional delayed growth. *J Pediatr* 1979; 94:657.
174. Gordon M, et al: Psychosocial aspects of constitutional short stature: Social competence, behavior problems, self-esteem, and family functioning. *J Pediatr* 1982; 101:477.
175. Richards GE, Marshall RN, Kreuser IL: Effect of stature on school performance. *J Pediatr* 1985; 106:841.
176. Kaplan JG, et al: Constitutional delay of growth and development. The effects of treatment with androgens. *J Pediatr* 1973; 82:38.
177. Sotos JF, et al: Cerebral gigantism in childhood. A syndrome of excessively rapid growth with acromegalic features and a non-progressive neurologic disorder. *N Engl J Med* 1964; 271:109.
178. Poznanski AK, Stephenson JM: Radiographic findings in hypothalamic acceleration of growth associated with cerebral atrophy and mental retardation (cerebral gigantism). *Radiology* 1967; 88:446.
179. Stephenson JM, Mellinger RD, Manson G: Cerebral gigantism. *Pediatrics* 1968; 41:130.
180. Saenger P, et al: Somatomedin in cerebral gigantism. *J Pediatr* 1976; 88:155.
181. Zonana J, et al: Dominant inheritance of cerebral gigantism. *J Pediatr* 1977; 91:251.
182. Lopis S, Rubenstein AH, Wright AD: Measurements of serum growth hormone and insulin in gigantism. *J Clin Endocrinol Metab* 1968; 28:393.
183. Gourmelen M, et al: Serum levels of insulin-like growth factor (IGF) and IGF binding protein in constitutionally tall children and adolescents. *J Clin Endocrinol Metab* 1984; 59:1197.
184. Evain-Brion D, et al: Growth hormone responses to thyrotropin-releasing hormone and oral glucose-loading tests in tall children and adolescents. *J Clin Endocrinol Metab* 1983; 56:429.
185. Greulich WW, Pyle SL: *Radiographic Skeletal Development of the Hand and Wrist*, 2d ed. Stanford, Calif, Stanford University Press, 1959.
186. Bayley N, et al: Attempt to suppress excessive growth in girls by estrogen treatment: Statistical evaluation. *J Clin Endocrinol Metab* 1962; 22:1127.
187. Whitelaw MJ, Foster TN, Graham WH: Estradiol valerate: Its effects on anabolism and skeletal age in the prepubertal girl. *J Clin Endocrinol Metab* 1963; 23:1125.
188. Frasier SD, Smith FG, Jr: Effect of estrogens on mature height in tall girls: A controlled study. *J Clin Endocrinol Metab* 1966; 28:416.
189. Wettenhall HNB, Cahill C, Roche AF: Tall girls: A survey of 15 years of management and treatment. *J Pediatr* 1975; 86:602.

190. Blomback M, Hall K, Ritzen EM: Estrogen treatment of tall girls: Risk of thrombosis? *Pediatrics* 1983; 72:416.
191. Evain-Brion D, et al: Studies in constitutionally tall adolescents: II. Effects of bromocriptine on growth hormone secretion and adult height prediction. *J Clin Endocrinol Metab* 1984; 58:1022.
192. Sotelo-Avila C, Gonzalez-Crussi F, Fowler JW: Complete and incomplete forms of Beckwith-Wiedemann syndrome: Their oncogenic potential. *J Pediatr* 1980; 96:47.
193. LaFranchi SH, Lippe BM, Kaplan SA: Hypoglycemia during testing for growth hormone deficiency. *J Pediatr* 1977; 90:244.
194. Penny R, Blizzard RM, Davis WT: Sequential arginine and insulin tolerance tests on the same day. *J Clin Endocrinol Metab* 1969; 29:1499.
195. Weldon VV, et al: Evaluation of growth hormone release in children using arginine and L-dopa in combination. *J Pediatr* 1975; 87:540.
196. Bacon GE, Lowrey GH, Knoller M: Comparison of arginine infusion and diethylstilbestrol as a means of provoking growth hormone secretion. *J Pediatr* 1969; 75:385.
197. Lippe B, Wong S-LR, Kaplan S: Simultaneous assessment of growth hormone and ACTH reserve in children pretreated with diethylstilbestrol. *J Clin Endocrinol Metab* 1971; 33:949.
198. Maclaren NK, Taylor GE, Raiti S: Propranolol-augmented, exercise-induced human growth hormone release. *Pediatrics* 1975; 56:804.
199. Shanis BS, Moshang T: Propranolol and exercise as a screening test for growth hormone deficiency. *Pediatrics* 1976; 57:712.
200. Collu R, et al: Stimulation of growth hormone secretion by Levodopa-Propranolol in children and adolescents. *Pediatrics* 1975; 56:262.
201. Collu R, et al: Reevaluation of Levodopa-Propranolol as a test of growth hormone reserve in children. *Pediatrics* 1978; 61:242.
202. Rowe DW, Sare Z, Kelley VC: Possible complications of the Levodopa-Propranolol test. *Pediatrics* 1977; 60:132.
203. Zadik Z, et al: The influence of age on the 24-hour integrated concentration of growth hormone in normal individuals. *J Clin Endocrinol Metab* 1985; 60:513.
204. Frasier SD: Human pituitary growth hormone (hGH) therapy in growth hormone deficiency. *Endocrine Rev* 1983; 4:155.
205. Frasier SD: A review of growth hormone stimulation tests in children. *Pediatrics* 1974; 53:929.
206. Rimoin DL, Horton WA: Short stature. Part II. *J Pediatr* 1978; 92:697.
207. Brown P: Human growth hormone therapy and Creutzfeldt-Jakob disease: A drama in three acts. *Pediatrics* 1988; 81:85.
208. Bercu BB: Growth hormone treatment and the short child: To treat or not to treat? *J Pediatr* 1987; 110:991.

4

Failure to Thrive

Failure to thrive (FTT) is a descriptive term for a syndrome of growth failure that may occur during infancy and early childhood. It is not a diagnosis, but a symptom of suboptimal development that may have many different causes. Commonly, the term FTT has been applied to the nonambulatory child, usually less than 2 years of age, who is underweight for length, and in whom no obvious organic etiology is suggested. Theoretically, however, the term could be applied to any infant or child who is making suboptimal physical or developmental progress.

Some authors have found organic illness to be the cause of the poor growth in as many as 50% of hospitalized infants with FTT (Table 4–1).[1-3] Our experience, however, more nearly parallels that of Sills,[4] who found organic disease to be the cause of poor thriving in less than 25% of cases in which a specific diagnosis was not suspected initially. Nevertheless, over 50% of FTT infants are found to have some physical abnormalities on physical examination,[2] and may have intercurrent illnesses that are not the cause of the poor thriving, but make evaluation of the infant more complex.

The evaluation of infants and toddlers who are failing to thrive is seldom easy. Both organic and nonorganic (environmental) factors may contribute to growth failure and developmental deviations, and are often interrelated. It is important, therefore, that the evaluation of the child be directed to assess these factors simultaneously. Environmental factors such as inadequate nutrition, inappropriate stimulation, and inconsistent parenting may result in an infant or child who is usually underweight for length; frequently, length, weight, and head circumference are all below the third percentile. Developmental lags and impaired social relationships are often prominent. Even when there is an organic explanation for the child's growth failure, environment may also be a contributing factor. Guidelines for the evaluation of the nonambulatory child with FTT have

TABLE 4–1.
Causes of Failure to Thrive

Illness	Riley[1]	Hannaway[2]	English[3]	Sills[4]
(No. patients)	(83)	(100)	(77)	(185)
Organic	48%	49%	54%	18%
Central nervous system	12	18	14	4
Gastrointestinal	13	12	17	8
Cardiovascular	2	4	6	1
Pulmonary	11	. . .	3	1
Urinary tract	5	5	4	0
Endocrine	0	5	4	1
Metabolic	0	0	0	1
Other	5	5	6	2
Nonorganic	31%	48%	38%	58%
Deprivation	. . .	12	. . .	50
Feeding problem	. . .	25	. . .	3
Rumination	. . .	2	. . .	3
Other	. . .	9	. . .	2
Undetermined	20%	3%	8%	24%

been developed in our hospital by a multidisciplinary team (see Appendix 4).

FAILURE TO THRIVE ASSOCIATED WITH ORGANIC DISEASE

The diagnosis of organic illness in the infant with failure to thrive is usually suggested by the history and/or physical examination.[4] Because exhaustive laboratory studies are rarely helpful,[4] and are detrimental to the optimal caloric intake of the infant under observation, screening laboratory studies should be the only organic work-up that is done initially, unless a specific diagnosis is suggested. After 10 to 14 days, if the infant has demonstrated inadequate weight gain on an adequate caloric intake, further studies are appropriate (see Appendix 4).

When an organic cause is found, it is most likely to be either neurologic or gastrointestinal disease, and is often both. Central nervous system (CNS) impairment may lead to apathy and poor responsiveness to environment, decreased appetite, malnutrition, diarrhea, infection, and further CNS disturbance—a "vicious circle."[5]

FTT associated with gastrointestinal disorders can be due to anatomic, physiologic, inflammatory, infectious, or functional abnormalities.[6] Most screening studies, such as observation of feeding patterns, caloric intake, and stools (appearance, frequency, microscopic examination, pH, Clinitest, and weight), indicate whether more extensive studies are indicated. Elevation of sweat electrolytes would suggest cystic fibrosis, but care must be taken because nonorganic FTT may occasionally show transient false positive elevations as well.[7, 8]

Failure to gain weight associated with gastroesophageal reflux in infants has received recent attention.[9] Decreased nutritional intake as a result of vomiting or anorexia, or increased energy utilization because of frequent respiratory tract infections seems to be the most likely mechanism for growth failure in these babies. Chronic vomiting in the FTT infant should suggest "infant rumination syndrome" (see the section Nonorganic Failure to Thrive). It is wise to remember that FTT infants usually have some gastrointestinal symptoms that are often intermittent, regardless of the cause of their poor thriving.

A primary neurologic disorder is not uncommonly associated with slow growth; in some instances poor weight gain may be associated with decreased caloric intake due to apathy, poor swallowing, or regurgitation. However, the neurologic examination in a child with nutritional or emotional deprivation may be markedly abnormal. Apathy, hypotonia,[10] and generalized weakness can mimic primary CNS dysfunction. Serial physical examinations and developmental testing can aid in the differentiation of nonorganic and organic neurologic abnormalities. The infant with a head circumference that is smaller than expected for length (height age) usually has primary CNS dysfunction. It is not uncommon for a nonorganic FTT infant to have a head circumference below the third percentile; however, the measurement is usually appropriate for height age.

The infant who fails to thrive because of cardiovascular disease usually has cyanosis,[11, 12] congestive heart failure,[11] and/or frequent respiratory infections. The degree of growth failure may be unrelated to the severity of the lesion.[11] Many of the children have been premature or small for dates, factors that contribute to their overall poor progress. It has been shown that many of these infants have increased metabolic rates[13-15] and decreased caloric intakes, resulting in a greater deficit in weight gain than in linear growth.

Renal disease might be suggested by the history of intermittent fevers, nausea, vomiting, poor feeding, irritability, lethargy, and decreased physical activity.[16] The failure to gain weight is probably from inadequate intake of protein and calories. Nephrogenic diabetes insipidus can produce growth failure by relative excess water intake and secondary nutritional inadequacy. Normal blood urea nitrogen (BUN), urine output, urinalysis, concentrating ability, and pH exclude most renal diseases.

Endocrine disorders are uncommon causes for FTT in infants (less than 5%). Hypothyroidism is usually evident clinically. Hypopituitarism may be suggested by the presence of frontal bossing of the skull, small hands and feet, micropenis, increased truncal adiposity, or hypoglycemia (see Chapter 3).

Failure to thrive because of acquired immune deficiency syndrome (AIDS) may be severe.[17, 18] Hepatomegaly, splenomegaly, lymphadenopathy parotitis, opportunistic infections, bacterial sepsis, lymphoid interstitial pneumonitis, and encephalopathy are common.[18] Of infants with serum positive for human immune deficiency virus (HIV [LAV/HTLV III]) observed by Blanche and associates,[18] FTT was noted only in the group with absence of antigen-induced lymphocyte proliferation. Dysmorphism consisting of growth failure, microcephaly, and craniofacial abnormalities have been associated with intrauterine HTLV III infection.[19]

Several syndromes should be considered in any infant with FTT. The *diencephalic syndrome*[20, 21] is a specific type of FTT caused by a tumor arising from the floor of the third ventricle or the optic chiasm, usually an astrocytoma. The syndrome occurs most frequently in boys in the 1st year of life. Primary clinical features are emaciation despite adequate intake, hyperactivity, and a pleasant disposition. The infant's length is usually normal or greater than average; the weight is usually considerably decreased. The diagnosis, which may be difficult to confirm, is suggested by the complete absence of subcutaneous fat on radiographic examination or by an elevated protein in the cerebrospinal fluid.[21] Elevated fasting growth hormone levels that are incompletely suppressed by hyperglycemia[22, 23] have been found in some infants with diencephalic syndrome. Because growth hormone is a stimulus to the release of free fatty acids, it is possible that this phenomenon is responsible for the malnutrition, as well as accelerated linear growth, in these patients. The diagnosis in these cases may be suggested by studies with computed axial tomography, but definitive diagnosis usually requires pneumoencephalography. The course of the disease is variable, but without therapy a fatal outcome within 2 years of onset is the rule. Longevity appears to be improved by radiation therapy. The value of surgical intervention is doubtful, since complete removal of the tumor usually is not possible.

Neurofibromatosis can produce the clinical features of the diencephalic syndrome in infants.[24] Most often a diencephalic tumor is not demonstrable; many infants, however, have a very good appetite, perhaps related to hypothalamic dysfunction. In a review of 46 children with neurofibromatosis, 63% had physical signs (café-au-lait spots) or symptoms by the age of 1 year.[25] Slow development was noted in 24%.[25] Failure to thrive is not infrequent in these infants.[26] Figure 4–1 shows the growth curve of an infant diagnosed to have neurofibromatosis at age 13 months. Note, however, that catch-up in weight occurred during his hospitalization after problems in mother-infant interaction were investigated. This case is a good example of how both organic and nonorganic factors can effect the failure to thrive pattern in the same infant.

Fetal alcohol syndrome (FAS)[27–30] is probably underdiagnosed. Infants with the syndrome have both prenatal and postnatal growth deficiency. Linear growth is usually 60% to 70% of normal, and the patients are underweight for height. All children have growth retardation, mental retardation (mean IQ = 63), and short palpebral fissures. Microcephaly, fine motor dysfunction, joint anomalies, cardiac defects, and hemangiomas are common. Upper airway obstruction has also been noted in some infants with fetal alcohol syndrome.[31] With increasing age, dysmorphic signs become less apparent.[32] Hirsutism has also been noted in early infancy, but this usually disappears by the age of 9 months. The children are usually socially uninhibited.[33] The demonstration of affection indiscriminately directed may persist into childhood. Many children demonstrate hyperactivity, distractibility, delayed gross motor milestones, poor fine motor coordination, and learning problems. Because environmental deprivation may

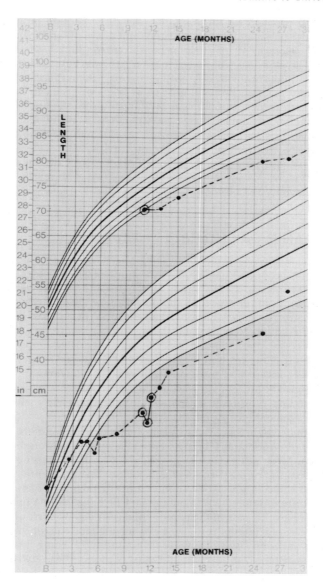

FIG 4–1.
Growth chart of infant boy with failure to thrive who was hospitalized at age 11 months. Weight loss continued despite caloric intakes of > 170 kcal/kg/day until problems in the maternal-child interaction were evaluated. Catch-up weight gain followed. He was later diagnosed to have neurofibromatosis, indicating both organic and nonorganic factors involved in his failure to thrive.

be an ongoing problem for these infants, early intervention programs are important in order to maximize their already limited growth and mental potential.

Williams' syndrome[34, 35] may also be more common than has been previously recognized. The elfin facies of these children has been associated with infantile hypercalcemia and supravalvular aortic stenosis,[36] two abnormalities that are not consistently present. Prenatal growth deficiency is mild to moderate, and postnatal growth deficiency follows in 90% of children. Mild microcephaly and mental retardation are almost always present.[35] The majority of children have a depressed nasal bridge, medial eyebrow flare, blue eyes, stellate pattern of the iris, antiverted nares, a long philtrum, prominent lips, hallux valgus, hypoplastic nails, heart murmur, and hoarse voice.[35] Only 30% of children with the elfin facies have evidence of supravalvular aortic stenosis, and few have been documented to have hypercalcemia.

NONORGANIC FAILURE TO THRIVE

The diagnosis of nonorganic FTT is not simply made by exclusion of organic causes. On the contrary, the evaluation for the presence of environmental factors is an active process and one that should be undertaken in every such case. Intervention often demands thorough psychosocial evaluation and therapy of the family in addition to behavioral therapy of the infant—an integrated approach.[37, 38]

Many young clinicians find the concept that emotional factors may be causative difficult to accept and evaluate appropriately. However, it is imperative that the physician be an active participant in this phase of the evaluation process from the start, and coordinate efforts with a multidisciplinary team in order to facilitate management (see Appendix 4).

In the family where there is obvious rejection or abandonment of the infant, the diagnosis of nonorganic FTT is seldom challenging, although the management may be. More often, however, the infant's family presents a picture of concern, interest, and initial cooperation, factors that frequently misdirect the inexperienced clinician toward evaluation for only possible organic illness.

The majority of infants with nonorganic FTT have feeding problems. Most undereat because of tension in the parent-child relationship surrounding feeding practices. Breast-fed infants can also have inadequate weight gain, and even loss, without showing signs of hunger or fussiness.[39–41] Some infants eat voraciously. In this instance the parent might think of them as "greedy" and withhold food. The mother may describe the infant's refusal of food, vomiting, or overeating in such a way as to imply that the infant is acting out of anger.

Infants may relate poorly to family and siblings, prefer to play alone, and are seldom interested in toys. Some sleep poorly, are hyperirritable, or are extremely passive and seldom cry. Diarrhea, abdominal distention, and foul-smelling stools are common. The majority of such infants are described as "different" from the siblings who preceded them.

When chronic vomiting is a prominent feature in the history of the FTT infant, the "infant rumination syndrome"[42-46] should be considered. This uncommon disorder is often difficult to distinguish from anatomic gastrointestinal disorders that cause vomiting and weight loss. The infant regurgitates previously swallowed food; the food is rechewed and reswallowed or simply vomited. There is considerable loss of calories, fluid, and electrolytes, a condition that is life-threatening if not corrected. The recognition of rumination is aided by the observation that the infants place their hands into their mouths shortly before vomiting, but this behavior is usually done when they are alone, or not at all. It has become well recognized that this syndrome is associated with a severely disturbed mother-child relationship, particularly reflecting a disturbance in feeding routines.[42-47] Lack of stimulation by the caretaker results in an adoption by the infant of self-stimulatory behavior. While behavior modification[46, 48] may improve the immediate life-threatening situation, it is rarely a cure. Intervention demands thorough psychosocial evaluation and therapy of the family. Foster care is often indicated. Figure 4–2 shows a growth curve of an infant with rumination who had catch-up growth when separated from his family by hospitalization and subsequent foster placement.

Physical examination of the nonorganic FTT infant may be normal except for decreased weight or the clinical appearance of malnutrition. Abdominal distention and hepatomegaly are common (Fig 4–3). The infant usually has decreased muscle mass and tone[10] and is often significantly delayed in both gross and fine motor development. The infant may be alert, watchful, with radar-gaze[48] and a lack of stranger anxiety, or may be passively uninterested in his environment. Many seldom cry; others are hyperirritable when approached or pull away when held. Retention of fistlike posture of the hands after the age of 4 months has been described as an early clue to sensory deprivation in some infants.[49]

Laboratory studies of these infants are usually normal. Minor and transient abnormalities may include a mildly elevated sweat sodium, BUN, aspartate aminotransferase (AST [SGOT]), and alanine aminotransferase (ALT [SGPT]). These become normal during catch-up growth. If weight gain is rapid, splitting of the cranial sutures can be demonstrated radiographically. Bone age is usually delayed appropriately for height age.

Observation of an infant feeding yields valuable information often not readily available by history.[37, 38, 50] Mothers may easily "give up" on an infant who is a particularly difficult feeder. Other mothers may have a marked aversion to letting the child self-feed because of the mess that results. Consequently the determined infant often becomes angry and refuses feedings.[50] Some caretakers may displace anger onto infants in feeding situation. Some infants give sufficient clues to help a caretaker know when a feeding is desired or when satiety has been reached. Their caretakers may likewise misinterpret the offered clues and terminate feedings prematurely. Observing feeding situations between the infant and the usual caretakers and then again between the infant and nursing personnel may also give valuable clues in the "difficult feeding" situation.

The infant with nonorganic FTT usually is the youngest in the family, after

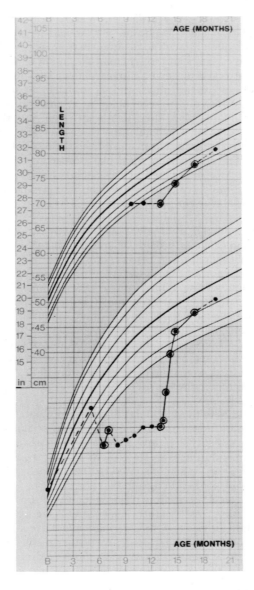

FIG 4–2.
Growth chart of an infant boy hospitalized at age 13 months after two prior hospitalizations for FTT at ages 6 and 7 months and extensive home intervention for 6 months. Rumination and vomiting were marked. This behavior ceased gradually during a 2-month hospitalization; catch-up growth continued in foster placement.

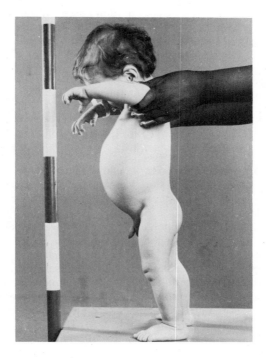

FIG 4–3.
Abdominal distention may be marked in infants with nonorganic failure to thrive.

a rapid succession of older siblings. The parents are usually not young and are usually living together; the mother seldom is employed outside the home. Financial difficulties, daily stress, and marital conflicts are frequent. Several studies have shown families of FTT infants to be psychologically ill-adapted.[51–54] Mothers of FTT infants may have limited ability to perceive and assess accurately their own needs and those of their infants, and have defective object relationships, a limited capacity for concern, and adverse affective states signifying the presence of a character disorder, which limits the potential for change.[51] Within the families of such infants, such psychopathologic entities as anxiety, depression, alcoholism, and mental retardation may also exist. The parents have usually had high stress in their own childhood, and were often abused and neglected themselves.[55, 56] The mothers have also been described as being less affectionate, relating less to their children, and using physical punishment readily.[52, 57] Expectations of the infant are often unrealistic. The family of the FTT infant can best be described as a unit that is "out-of-synchrony" in relationships. The parents are not usually adaptable and often have limited motivation and resources for change. The management of the infant with FTT and the family must be individualized and the type of intervention based on the family's potential and desire to change. Although improvement in the nurturing environment can occur in the majority of families, some infants need foster placement, based on the severity of the clinical situation, lack of potential for change, and poor progress or weight at follow-up.[58, 59]

DIFFERENTIATION BETWEEN ORGANIC AND NONORGANIC FAILURE TO THRIVE

The process by which a clinician is able to differentiate between organic and nonorganic causes of FTT is not clear-cut. Catch-up growth reflected by rapid weight gain or significant developmental gains without specific medical intervention while the child is in a different environment, such as a hospital setting, offers a valuable clue to nonorganic FTT.[60, 61] However, behavioral changes may be additional important clues that are more subtle but can be noted at the outset of the evaluation. Distinctive interactive behavioral styles have been noted by several investigators[62-64] and may help to distinguish organic FTT from nonorganic FTT by scoring social interactions of the infant with an impartial examiner. Powell and associates[64] studied the incidence of abnormal behaviors in both organic and nonorganic FTT infants and offer a valuable list of behaviors to be documented in all FTT infants (Table 4–2). The frequency and intensity of these behaviors were greater in the group of infants with nonorganic FTT. The authors point out, however, that the presence or absence of these behaviors does not rule in a nonorganic or rule out an organic etiology. However, a high frequency and intensity of these abnormal behaviors should make one suspicious of a nonorganic cause. The response to appropriate treatment is felt to be the most reliable means of confirming the correct diagnosis.[64]

TABLE 4–2.
Abnormal Behaviors Often Present in Infants With Failure to Thrive (ages 3–24 months)*

Spontaneous Behaviors	Interactive Behaviors
General inactivity	Gaze abnormality
Excessive crying	Hyperalert gaze or stare
Flexed hips	Not directed at eyes
Expressionless face	Avoidance
Infantile posture	Disinterest
Rumination	
Thumb sucking	Response to stimulus
Disproportionate hand	Lack of smile
and finger activity	Lack of motor activity
Lack of vocalization	Lack of vocalization
Crying when approached	

* From Powell GF, et al: Behavior as a diagnostic aid in failure-to-thrive. *J Dev Behav Pediatr* 1987: 8:18. Used with permission.

PSYCHOSOCIAL DWARFISM

In the child over the age of 2 years, environmental factors may continue to contribute to growth failure. The child is usually ambulatory, self-feeding, and more readily able to manifest a great variety of behavioral symptoms reflective of stress within the family. It is not surprising, therefore, that the signs and symptoms of nonorganic growth failure change as the child grows older. The majority of pediatric endocrinologists agree that nutritional factors, on the whole, are less important in the pathogenesis of stress-induced growth delay in the older child.

In the 1960s, young children were described who had severe growth retardation, developmental delay, and poor home environments.[65–70] In 1967, many of these children were found to have deficiencies of pituitary GH and adrenocorticotrophic hormone.[69] The hypopituitarism resolved with hospitalization or foster placement. Physical and emotional catch-up growth was often dramatic. This disorder has been commonly called *psychosocial dwarfism* (PSD)[71–74] to emphasize the family nature of the problem. Some authors have referred to it as maternal deprivation,[65, 75] deprivation dwarfism,[76, 77] emotional deprivation,[68, 69, 78–81] abuse dwarfism,[82, 83] or reversible hyposomatotropinism,[84–87] or they include it under the more general terminology of nonorganic failure to thrive.

Often the child has had little previous medical care and the family is unconcerned about or even denies the child's small size. When the child is brought to medical attention it is usually at the urging of the school or protective services. Sometimes the family brings the child for evaluation because of disturbing or bizarre behavior (Table 4–3) such as gorging food, stealing food, or eating bizarre nonfood items. Temper tantrums often occur in response to food restriction or rigid child-rearing practices. Developmental delays are usually prominent. Speech is immature and often indistinct, particularly in the family's presence. Regressive behaviors such as enuresis and encopresis may be present. Poor peer interaction is common; some children are reported to be withdrawn and at other times hyperactive. Poor sleeping patterns may be accompanied by night eating, wandering, drinking, or self-injury such as trichotillomania.

In a review of 35 children with PSD,[71] the pregnancy, delivery, or neonatal period were difficult in approximately 50% of the children. Developmental milestones were slow in the majority, and in more than 50% of families referral to Children's Protective Service agencies had been made previously. Six of the 35 were hospitalized for FTT in the first 2 years of life.

Physical examination of the child with PSD reveals a child at less than the 3rd percentile for height and weight. Weight age is usually less than height age. Head circumference is appropriate for height age. Appearance, behavior, and speech are immature. Dental age, however, is usually normal for chronologic age. Abdominal distention may be prominent postprandially. Hepatomegaly may become evident during rapid weight gain.

Laboratory studies may reveal mild elevations in blood eosinophils, sedimentation rate, BUN, and AST. Sweat sodium may be transiently moderately elevated. Serum protein levels are usually normal. Stools seldom reveal the

TABLE 4–3.
Diagnostic Clues to the Presence of Psychosocial Dwarfism*

Child
  Delayed growth without physical basis <3%ile height and
    weight
  Unusual eating patterns: gorging, vomiting, picky, starvation,
    or stealing food
  Unusual thirst: drinking from toilet, ditches, puddles
  Pain insensitivity
  Temper tantrums
  Shallow interpersonal relationships
  Labile age appropriateness
  Poor sleeping patterns
  Developmental delay
    Gross motor skills
    Expressive language
Family
  Multiple stresses
  Depressed, angry-hostile, or emotionally absent parents
  Abuse or deprivation in parents' background
  Poor communication or marital strife
  Rigidity, limited adaptability
  Power struggle between parent and child, may be related to
    food
  Presence of PSD in extended family
  Scapegoating of the child
  Denial of significance of child's size
  Symbiotic relationships

* From Bowden ML, Hopwood NJ: Identification of children with
psychosocial dwarfism. *Social Work Health Care* 1982; 7:15. Used
with permission.

presence of ova and parasites. Endocrine studies usually reveal low-normal levels of serum thyroxine, low 24-hour urinary 17-hydroxysteroids, and normal responses to metyrapone. Approximately 50% of these children have blunted growth hormone release to provocative stimuli if tested shortly after hospital admission.[71] Somatomedin-C levels have been shown to be low initially in some children.[88] Fasting hyperlipidemia is a frequent finding.[71] The serum may be turbid and gradually clear over the course of a week while cholesterol, triglyceride, and pre-beta lipoproteins rise, often dramatically. Whether these changes are related to nutritional or hormonal changes and/or stress is unclear. Bone maturation is delayed appropriate for height age. Growth lines in the metaphyses of the long bones may aid in distinguishing the child with PSD from the child with idiopathic hypopituitarism.[89] Skull roentgenograms show normal anatomy, splitting of cranial sutures may be seen in children with dramatic catch-up growth even though fontanelles are closed.[77] Computed tomographic scans have suggested that this phenomenon is due to increase in brain mass and not brain edema.[90] In some children gastric dilatation may also be dramatic on x-ray examination.[91] Deficit of slow-wave sleep may occur,[92] although deficiency of nocturnal growth hormone may also occur when sleep patterns are normal.[80]

Multiple stresses are present in the family of the child with PSD, but may not be readily apparent on initial interview.[71, 72] These stresses create an emotionally chaotic environment. Table 4–3 is a list of some of the most common problems. The parents tend to have fairly rigid personalities and are often controlling, particularly about food issues. In those families where only one child seems to be affected, the use of the term "scapegoating" seems appropriate. However, more than one child in the family is often affected, to varying degrees, when thorough observations of siblings are performed. Motivation and capacity for change by the parents are often limited. Some children have marked depressive symptoms, in addition to their personality disorders,[93] which are often immediately relieved by a change in environment. The precise mechanism for this change remains pathophysiologically unclear.[94]

The diagnosis of PSD requires a high index of suspicion. The evaluation requires the opportunity to demonstrate the potential reversibility of behavioral, physical, and/or hormonal abnormalities. A hospitalization in the same format as for the infant with FTT offers the best approach (see Appendix 4). A multidisciplinary team is a great asset for the observation and documentation of the changes that might occur when the child is removed from his/her stressful home environment. Decreased stranger anxiety, indiscriminate affection, and labile age appropriateness are important clues to the diagnosis of PSD (see Table 4–3). Careful calorie counts and documentation of rapid weight gain substantiate the potential reversibility of the growth delay. In a few children whose weight age is greater than height age initially, rapid weight gain may be absent; linear growth would be expected to begin to accelerate, but might not show a measurable difference during several weeks hospitalization. Psychological testing usually reveals greater delay in performance compared to verbal IQ, with overall scores in the mildly impaired intellectual range. During the hospital stay, repeated endocrine testing may reveal complete reversal of hormonal deficiencies. When this can be documented it offers indisputable evidence of the diagnosis of PSD. In lieu of such data, significant changes in weight, personality, or developmental milestones confirm the diagnosis.

The posthospitalization management of the child with PSD is complex. Usually, in the child over the age of 4 years, foster placement is indicated to give the child the opportunity for catch-up growth.[71] Foster placement is usually associated with dramatic changes in linear growth and weight gain, as shown in Figure 4–4. Prognosis for normal progress within the natural home is poor.

ANOREXIA NERVOSA AND BULIMIA

The typical patient with anorexia nervosa is a pubertal girl or young woman who has initially started to diet, either as a result of perceived obesity or because of a desire to be very thin. The constellation of symptoms includes weight loss

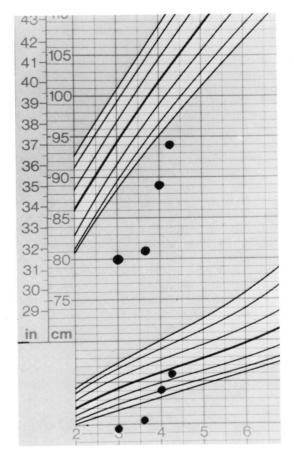

FIG 4–4.
Growth chart of a 3½-year-old girl who, on hospitalization for evaluation of growth failure and developmental delay, began to have catch-up growth. Reversible hypopituitarism was documented. Catch-up growth in a foster home further substantiated the diagnosis of psychosocial dwarfism.

of 25% to 50% of preanorexic body weight, amenorrhea, bradycardia, low blood pressure, hypothermia, constipation, and cold sensitivity. Amenorrhea precedes the weight loss in 25% of instances, but usually it is associated with the occurrence of significant weight reduction. The patient is usually from a middle or upper socioeconomic background, an overachiever, and a perfectionist. Preoccupation with food is universal and accompanied by intense rigidity concerning food and meals. There may be ritualistic eating habits and an interest in food preparation and recipes, with the individual seldom eating the prepared food.

Sometimes a pattern of gorging alternating with starvation is present. Several excellent clinical descriptions of the condition point out the similarities between these young women.[95-98]

The cause of this syndrome is poorly understood. Psychological factors are prominent, but the pathogenesis of the condition remains largely unknown. Hypothalamic dysfunction can be documented in the majority of affected patients and is probably secondary, as a result of starvation, rather than a primary cause of the behavioral symptoms.

The laboratory evaluation of the young patient with clinical symptoms of anorexia nervosa should be directed toward exclusion of organic disease, such as malignancy and adrenal insufficiency. In anorexia, sedimentation rate is low and urea nitrogen is often elevated. Hypovitaminosis A, leukopenia, and depressed serum iron are often noted.[95] Serum proteins are usually normal.

The hypothalamic dysfunction is compatible with a starvation state. Basal metabolic rate is low. Serum free and total thyroxine levels are usually in the low normal range, with low serum tri-iodothyronine levels[99] and normal serum thyroid-stimulating hormone. Response to thyrotropin-releasing hormone may be delayed in some patients.[100-102]

Serum cortisol levels are usually high, with a normal circadian rhythm but higher than normal 24-hour mean values.[99] Cortisol production rate is normal, but cortisol half-life is prolonged.[99] Urinary cortisol is normal or increased.[99] Growth hormone levels in the fasting state are usually normal or elevated;[102, 103] in some patients growth hormone may fail to respond to insulin-induced hypoglycemia[102] or may show higher rebound after glucose loading.[103]

In patients with severe forms of anorexia nervosa, gonadotrophin secretion patterns are similar to those of a prepubertal child.[104, 105] Gonadotrophin responses to gonadotrophin-releasing hormone may be absent or diminished in patients at low body weights, and return to normal as weight is regained.[7, 105, 106] Amenorrhea may persist for months or longer after weight has returned to normal.

A significant number of patients have evidence of impaired ability to maximally concentrate their urine when in the starvation state;[97] this may reflect a partial insensitivity of the renal tubule to antidiuretic hormone[107] or nitrogen depletion in patients with protein malnutrition.[108]

In anorexia nervosa, there is often a sense of urgency for correction of the abnormal weight; case fatality rates have been cited from as low as 2% to as high as 18%,[109, 110] which may be due to suicide, starvation, or electrolyte imbalance. Less commonly, a role is cited from infection, gastrointestinal catastrophe, or cardiac insufficiency.[109]

Efforts to reverse a patient's stubborn determination to starve herself are frustrating. Patients do not feel identified with their bodies and therefore attempt to control them rigidly.[111] They feel helpless, ineffective, and lack awareness of their body needs, particularly in the interpretation of hunger.[111] As a result of these attitudes, behavior modification programs have been advocated, initially to assume total care for the patient in a protective, nonpunitive environment.[95, 112] Limited contact of the child with her parents is permitted, and decision-making conflicts are avoided with regard to food. Privileges are earned, as well as personal possessions (e.g., clothing) with weight gain. Psychiatric evaluation parallels the inpatient weight regaining program. This type of behavior modification is usually helpful in achieving weight gain; however, the long-term benefit may or may not persist. The weight gain itself is not a cure for the patient with anorexia nervosa. Too-rapid gain without psychological improvement has been implicated as a partial cause for the serious depression, psychosis, or suicide attempts that sometimes occur following this approach.[111] On the other hand, persistent marginal weight fosters the continuation of the distorting effect of weight on the psychological functioning of these patients, so that only minimal emotional improvement may be evident until some gain occurs.[111] In severe conditions, if behavior modification does not succeed, temporary tube feedings or hyperalimentation may be necessary.

Perhaps even more common is bulimia, which may or may not be associated with anorexia nervosa.[113] The primary problem is not the vomiting or purging but the intense binge eating.[113] When bulimia occurs without anorexia, seldom are there overt signs of malnutrition. Group therapy is usually more successful than individual psychotherapy.[113] Currently there is no widely accepted pharmacotherapy for anorexia or bulimia, but in individual cases adjunctive therapy may be indicated.[114]

APPENDIX 4

Guidelines for Evaluation and Management of Hospitalized Infants and Toddlers With Failure to Thrive*

Both organic and nonorganic (environmental) factors may be contributing to growth failure and developmental deviations. It is important to the evaluation of a child that these factors be assessed simultaneously.

Steps for Evaluation and Management

1. *Hospitalize the infant.* Any baby with failure to thrive (FTT) who does not respond to a 1-month trial of increased calories on a prescribed diet and public health nurse visits in the home should be hospitalized immediately. These children cannot be fully assessed and are difficult to follow adequately as outpatients. It is important to delineate for the parent at the outset of hospitalization that the child's failure to grow may be a result of an organic illness or an adverse reaction to a stressful environment.

2. *Obtain a complete history* (standard pediatric format). The review of symptoms by systems should be obtained for *both* past and present time periods.

3. *Elicit a detailed diet history and feeding history in the initial interview.*
   a. Is there a schedule for feeding? What is the child's usual feeding schedule? How often is the schedule followed? For an older child: are

*Prepared by a multidisciplinary team, C. S. Mott Children's Hospital, 1978.

meals served formally or informally?

b. What types of foods are offered at each meal and what are the usual amounts taken?

c. What is the parent's opinion of the adequacy of the amounts taken?

d. What are the feeding arrangements: who gives feedings, what aids or implements are used, where is the child fed? With the family or just with children?

e. Also observe and record baby's and parent's feeding behavior on day of admission, noting interactions, quantities of food, feelings exhibited, frustrations, and time taken.

Clues to problems parents are having with their baby can sometimes be detected early through a good feeding and diet history. Vagueness and inconsistency can be an indication of difficulties the parents are having feeding their baby. Although parents frequently give a history of adequate or more than adequate caloric intake, the history may be unreliable because they are presenting what they want to believe or what they want the hospital staff to believe. Occasionally a baby is reported to be on a bizarre diet or to exhibit bizarre behavior around food or to be uninterested in food. Some parents report problems with vomiting and diarrhea. This information should be recorded as the parents describe it. Documenting this history in the medical record is important so that it can be compared with the baby's observed eating behavior in the hospital and so that the parents' experience and perceptions of their baby can be dealt with during the baby's hospitalization.

The dietitian may be consulted to obtain the detailed history and to assess the nutrient value and appropriateness of the diet as described by the parent.

4. *Perform a thorough physical examination.* The physical examination should reveal an underweight but not acutely ill child. Muscular hypotonia, decreased muscle mass and strength, abdominal distention, and mild hepatomegaly are characteristic features of both organic and nonorganic failure to thrive. On occasion, however, physical findings may suggest overt chronic disease such as cystic fibrosis, cardiac disease, or malabsorption. Dysmorphic features such as clinodactyly, low set ears, and single palmar crease should suggest congenital defects associated with growth retardation, a possible intrauterine growth retarding syndrome, or chromosomal abnormality. A good ophthalmalogic examination is essential to search for clues to metabolic disease or intrauterine infection. Note the presence of flat feet, lack of stranger anxiety, or indiscriminate affection which may suggest emotional neglect. Signs of poor hygiene or inflicted injuries may suggest physical abuse or neglect.

Obtain careful measurements of the child upon admission. It is helpful then to relate the child's measurements to the 50% age level on a growth grid. For example, Chronological age (CA) 32 months, Height age (HA) 21 months, Weight age (WA) 15 months, Occipital-Frontal Circumference (OFC) 30 months. A child who has a weight age significantly below that of HA would be more likely to have decreased caloric utilization (hypermetabolism, vomiting, diarrhea) or decreased caloric intake (primary malnutrition). A child whose head circumference is significantly below HA and WA probably has central nervous system disease.

Although the head circumference is relatively spared in emotional or caloric deprivation, this is not universal.

5. *Construct an accurate growth chart.* It is essential to obtain as much of the child's "track record" as possible (i.e., past heights and weights). A good growth chart can save thousands of dollars in nonessential medical work-up. Intermittent periods of slowing, or accelerated growth after a slowing of growth is strong evidence for environmental (nonorganic) failure to thrive. Records can often be obtained from physicians, well-child clinics, or schools. Obtain releases to seek this information on the day of admission, or prior to admission if possible.

6. *Obtain a developmental assessment on the day of admission.* Over 90% of the children who fail to thrive on a deprivation basis also manifest delays in development. A Denver Developmental Screening Test (DDST) should be obtained on the day of admission so that it can be compared to a later DDST after the child has received appropriate stimulation and nutrition. In order to have more consistent results, a clinical nursing specialist, an occupational therapist, or a physician familiar with performing DDSTs should administer these tests.

Any bizarre behavior exhibited by the child on admission should be carefully recorded in the medical chart. Discrepancies in developmental performance should also be noted (e.g., child talks with staff but not with parent). A referral to psychiatry and/or psychology and/or speech therapy for further testing and for establishing baseline capabilities should be considered.

7. *Order limited laboratory tests.* A child with failure to thrive but with a normal physical examination should undergo initial screening for organic disease, but this screening should not interfere with nutrition or regular feedings. Screening studies should include a complete blood cell count with differential erythrocyte sedimentation rate, urinalysis (with attention to ability to concentrate and produce an acid urine), stool pH, weight, Clinitest and Hematest, serum electrolytes, pH, blood urea nitrogen, fasting glucose, urine metabolic screen, tuberculin test, thyroxine, bone age and skull roentgenograms, and sweat sodium. More elaborate studies should not be ordered initially until there is a *strong suspicion* of a specific organic disease.

Such elaborate tests as malabsorption tests, intravenous pyelogram, and gastrointestinal x-ray studies may be deferred unless the infant or young child fails to gain weight after 2 or 3 weeks of documented adequate caloric intake. Both before and during the dietary trial, diagnostic tests that require fasting should be avoided in young children, unless such a test is strongly indicated. Special tests for alleged vomiting or diarrhea should not be ordered unless these symptoms are verified in the hospital setting.

8. *Order bone survey roentgenograms in selected children.* In any case of suspected emotional or physical abuse or neglect, a bone survey should be performed to search for prior fractures. Any child with limited range of motion of joints should have these done initially. The metaphyses of the long bones may show "growth" lines in infants and children who have intermittent growth patterns.

9. *Identify environmental factors.* In families of babies who are not thriving and there is no organic cause, family stress and disorganization can be identified as major problems that interfere with the parent-child attachment process. The

stress may be ongoing, such as marital problems or illness, or it may have occurred in the past during the pregnancy or postpartum periods. Stressful events in the parents' own childhood may interact with present events to revive old feelings. Some families do not recognize their own feelings and problems and focus on their "sick" baby as the only source of family disruption.

Signs of difficulties in the parent-child attachment process may be visible in parent-child interactions as "out-of-synchrony" behavior. A mother who is anxious may bounce and jostle her baby right after a feeding. A baby's behavior gives clues to how he has been parented (e.g., avoiding eye contact or being intensely watchful or stiffening when held). It is important to note any such behaviors in the chart and to take them into consideration in the treatment plan.

If environmental growth retardation is likely, social work referral is essential to assist in the family assessment and for assistance in developing a discharge and follow-up plan.

10. *Form a primary care team.* A "care team" of the various disciplines involved (physician, nurse, social worker) should be formed to coordinate an evaluation and care plan for the child and family. Parents should be considered as ad hoc members of the team. This group should meet on a regular basis to share information about the progress of the evaluation and to develop a coordinated intervention plan. The intervention should include appropriate stimulation and attention, consistent sleep and feeding management, and positive reinforcement of favorable attachment behavior between parent and child.

While these families need extra attention, reinforcement, and education during the hospitalization of the child, care should be taken to avoid overstimulation of the child and inconsistent input through multiple caretakers. Assignment of the same staff on each shift to provide care should help avoid this.

Progress or lack of progress toward established goals should be recorded in the medical chart every two to three days to keep all informed.

11. *Treat the baby's failure to thrive with unlimited feedings of a regular diet for age.* For infants less than 6 months of age, only formula and vitamins should be given during the feeding trial. This step is essential for reaching a definitive diagnosis. Avoid a formula change unless there is a strong medical indication. The formula should be identical to the one provided at home. Rapid weight gain on a special formula free of cow's milk, protein, or lactose would not prove that the child was underfed in the home setting. The daily intake should be 150 to 200 calories per kilogram (present weight) per day. The baby should be fed at regular intervals plus on demand at other times. The child who is not fed a formula should also be provided with supplemental vitamins. The dietitian should be consulted to: (1) set up a feeding plan for the child (appropriate meals and supplementary snacks), (2) document the daily hospital intake (caloric count), and (3) calculate the calories per kilo per day consumed.

12. *Involve the parents in the child's hospital care.* Because appropriate disposition may depend on the parents' involvement with the child on the ward, every effort should be made to encourage initial parental visiting and rooming-in. At a minimum this rooming-in will be required during the last 2 or 3 days of hospitalization. During this time, the medical and nursing staff should provide

emotional support as well as education to strengthen the parents' confidence in themselves and understanding of their baby. Criticism should be avoided, and when advice must be given, it should focus on behavior aspects that the parent and child can change (e.g., "He seems to eat better when held like this").

In some cases it is advantageous not to have the parents present in the hospital, especially when there is strong suspicion of an abnormal parent-child relationship. Their absence will permit the staff to assess the child's growth and behavior outside the family setting. Many infants with stress-associated failure to thrive do not gain weight in the hospital in their parents' presence in spite of good caloric intake.

13. *Confirm the diagnosis of environmental failure to thrive by documentation of a rapid weight gain.* While in the hospital, the baby should be weighed at the same time each day. Some babies with failure to thrive due to nutritional or emotional deprivation are seen to eat readily and gain rapidly. Others may be poor feeders and take 3 to 4 weeks to demonstrate weight gain and improved feeding patterns.

Average weight gains for healthy children vary according to age: 25 g/day in the first 3 months of life, 24 g/day from 3 to 6 months, 17 g/day from 6 to 9 months, and 11 g/day from 9 to 12 months of age. A rapid weight gain can be defined as a gain of over 57 g/day sustained for a 1-week period, a gain of greater than 43 g/day sustained for 2 weeks, or a gain that is strikingly greater than seen during a similar interval at home.

14. *If you suspect a failure-to-thrive infant as having been abused or neglected, seek consultation from the Suspected Child Abuse and Neglect (SCAN) Team.* Under Michigan's Child Protection Act, child abuse means "harm or threatened harm to a child's health or welfare by a person responsible for the child's health or welfare which occurs through nonaccidental physical or mental injury, sexual abuse, or maltreatment." Child neglect means "harm to a child's health or welfare by a person responsible for the child's health or welfare which occurs through negligent treatment, including the failure to provide adequate food, clothing, shelter, or medical care." If you question whether a child meets these requirements, consult the SCAN Team.

Indications for the SCAN Team referral:

a. If a parent's actions or inactions with the child resulted in a life-threatening situation, or if continued actions or inactions will result in a life-threatening situation.

b. If a parent's actions or inaction with the child result in significant developmental delays.

c. If you suspect that the child's parents did not provide adequately for the child as evidenced by: (1) history, (2) rapid weight gain, and (3) a pattern of failure to gain weight in the parents' care alternating with a pattern of weight gain in the care of others, such as foster parents and hospital staff.

d. Parental inability or unwillingness to take necessary steps to engage in necessary actions to reverse the process of physical FTT and/or developmental delay.

e. If history, physical examination, or medical work-up raises the suspicion of physical abuse.

15. *Initiate a more extensive organic work-up for the babies who fail to gain adequately in the hospital setting.* Some babies with organic failure to thrive who are given unlimited feedings for 2 to 3 weeks may gain weight. Some of them will gain 30 g/day with great effort on the part of the nursing staff, but will then level off after the initial week (e.g., those with dysphagia or cardiochalasia). Most of them do not make any substantial gain. Babies who have an organic basis for failure to thrive generally fall into five groups: (1) *inadequate intake* as a result of mechanical feeding problems (cleft palate, nasal obstruction, chalasia); (2) *failure to assimilate calories ingested* (cystic fibrosis, celiac disease, milk allergy, parasites, postdiarrheal recovery phase, portal hypertension); (3) *increased metabolism* which results in negative net caloric availability (chronic infection, malignancy, collagen disease, hyperthyroidism, diencephalic syndrome); (4) *failure to utilize available calories* ("sick cells") (rickets, hypokalemia, renal insufficiency, hypercalcemia, hepatic insufficiency, diabetes, storage diseases, amino acidopathies, and hypoxemia); and (5) *failure of stimulation* (hypothyroidism, intrauterine growth retardation, gonadal dysgenesis, mental retardation, hypopituitarism, central nervous system anomalies, neurofibromatosis). Consultation is often in order at this point.

During initiation of an organic work-up, keep in mind that both physical and emotional factors may be contributing to the poor growth. Babies with cleft palates, intrauterine growth retardation, and other physical anomalies may also be victims of their environment. Identifying the existence of both factors allows for adequate intervention and planning for the baby. It has also been our experience that some of these families need help in finding a method of feeding and caring for the baby that will enable the baby to thrive to his/her potential. Providing parents with the expertise of a staff who can help them develop a more appropriate feeding regime, or support their program and help them feel successful with the gains they have made, can be crucial in maintaining a good parent-child relationship.

16. *Provide adequate discharge planning.* Discharge the child when:

a. The members of the team are in agreement that the maximum benefit has been achieved from the child's hospitalization.

b. The child has responded to interventions.

c. The team has a clear idea of what changes have to be made and these changes have been transferred to the family or caretakers of the child or to the community through the involvement of community agencies. Team conferences and planning sessions are necessary for such arrangements.

Since full nutritional catch-up gains may take several weeks, months, or even years, arrangements must be made for adequate medical follow-up. Public Health nurses, local physicians, and community agencies must be utilized for the weekly monitoring of patients who live long distances from the hospital. In addition to the local follow-up, return clinic visits are arranged so that a consistent observer can monitor progress and assess need for changes within 3 to 4 weeks after discharge. One visit is insufficient. Catch-up growth achieved in the hospital may not be completely manifest until the first clinic visit. A second return visit is necessary to fully evaluate the gains within the home.

Expected Outcomes for Discharge From Hospital

1. If the reason for developmental lag is identified as environmental, the child shows progress toward achievement of developmental milestones within his/her identified abilities by discharge. Parents demonstrate activities to promote development.

2. Organic causes are ruled out or identified and treated.

3. Inappropriate or unusual behavioral responses of the child are diminished or absent by the time of discharge and are replaced by more appropriate behaviors (overcoming such behavioral responses as avoidance of eye contact, lack of smiling or vocalization, rigidity, flaccidness, unusual posturing, irritability, apathy, clinging or avoidance of body contact, self-stimulating behaviors).

4. Evidence of parent-child attachment is present and negative parent-child interactions have diminished by the time of discharge.

5. The parent understands and the child eats a diet appropriate in type and amount for his/her age.

6. The child demonstrates appropriate eating and self-feeding skills for age. The parent demonstrates appropriate feeding skills.

7. Weight shows an increasing trend by discharge.

Failure to Progress in the Home After Discharge

1. Readmit to hospital. Reevaluate management.

2. Refer to Children's Protective Services if failure to thrive is due to non-organic factors.

3. Arrange team meetings to make new management plan.

4. Strongly consider foster placement.

REFERENCES

1. Riley RL, et al: Failure to thrive: An analysis of 83 cases. *Calif Med* 1968; 108:32.
2. Hannaway PJ: Failure to thrive: A study of 100 infants and children. *Clin Pediatr* 1970; 9:96.
3. English PC: Failure to thrive without organic reason. *Pediatr Ann* 1978; 7:774.
4. Sills RH: Failure to thrive: The role of clinical and laboratory evaluation. *Am J Dis Child* 1978; 132:967.
5. Nelson JD: Infantile diarrhea and neurologic deficit. *Hosp Pract* 1967; 2:42.
6. Lavy V, Bauer CH: Pathophysiology of failure to thrive in gastrointestinal disorders. *Pediatr Ann* 1978; 7:743.
7. Christoffel KS, et al: Environmental deprivation and transient elevation of sweat electrolytes. *J Pediatr* 1985; 107:231.
8. Ruddy RM, Scanlin TF: Abnormal sweat electrolytes in a case of celiac disease and a case of psychosocial failure to thrive. Review of other reported cases. *Clin Pediatr* 1987; 26:83.
9. St Cyr JA, et al: Nissen fundoplication for gastroesophageal reflux in infants. *J Thorac Cardiovasc Surg* 1986; 92:661.
10. Buda FB, et al: Hypotonia and the maternal-child relationship. *Am J Dis Child* 1972; 124:906.

11. Ehlers KH: Growth failure in association with congenital heart disease. *Pediatr Ann* 1978; 7:750.
12. Strangway A, et al: Diet and growth in congenital heart disease. *Pediatrics* 1976; 57:75.
13. Krieger I: Growth failure and congenital heart disease: Energy and nitrogen balance in infants. *Am J Dis Child* 1970; 120:497.
14. Krieger I, Chen YC: Caloric requirements for weight in infants with growth failure due to maternal deprivation, undernutrition, and congenital heart disease. *Pediatrics* 1969; 44:647.
15. Stocker FP, et al: Oxygen consumption in infants with heart disease. *J Pediatr* 1972; 80:43.
16. Friedman J, Lewy JE: Failure to thrive associated with renal disease. *Pediatr Ann* 1978; 7:767.
17. Elias-Jones AC, et al: AIDS in an infant causing severe failure to thrive. *J Infect* 1987; 15:69.
18. Blanche S, et al: Longitudinal study of 18 children with perinatal LAV/HTLV III infection: Attempt at prognostic evaluation. *J Pediatr* 1986; 109:965.
19. Marion RW, et al: Human T-Cell lymphotropic virus type III (HTLV-III) embryopathy. *Am J Dis Child* 1986; 140:638.
20. Addy DP, Hudson FP: Diencephalic syndrome of infantile emaciation: Analysis of literature and report of further 3 cases. *Arch Dis Child* 1972; 47:338.
21. Burr IM, et al: Diencephalic syndrome revisited. *J Pediatr* 1976; 88:439.
22. Fisherman MA, Peake GT: Paradoxical growth in a patient with diencephalic syndrome. *Pediatrics* 1970; 45:973.
23. Hager A, Thorell JI: Studies on growth hormone secretion in a patient with the diencephalic syndrome of infancy. *Acta Paediatr Scand* 1973; 62:231.
24. Adornato B, Berg B: Diencephalic syndrome and von Recklinghausen's disease. *Ann Neurol* 1977; 2:159.
25. Fienman NL, Yakovac WC: Neurofibromatosis in childhood. *J Pediatr* 1970; 76:339.
26. Pollnitz R: Neurofibromatosis in childhood: A review of 25 cases. *Med J Aust* 1976; 2:49.
27. Jones KL, et al: Pattern of malformation in offspring of chronic alcoholic mothers. *Lancet* 1973; 1:1267.
28. Jones KL, Smith DW: Recognition of the fetal alcohol syndrome in early infancy. *Lancet* 1973; 2:999.
29. Mulvihill JJ, et al: Fetal alcohol syndrome: Seven new cases. *Am J Obstet Gynecol* 1976; 125:937.
30. Clarren SK, Smith DW: The fetal alcohol syndrome. *N Engl J Med* 1978; 298:1063.
31. Usowicz AG, et al: Upper airway obstruction in infants with fetal alcohol syndrome. *Am J Dis Child* 1986; 140:1039.
32. Spohr HL: Follow-up studies of children with fetal alcohol syndrome. *Neuropediatr* 1987; 18:131.
33. Streissguth AP, et al: Intelligence behavior, and dysmorphogenesis in the fetal alcohol syndrome: A report on 20 patients. *J Pediatr* 1978; 92:363.
34. Williams JCP, et al: Supravalvular aortic stenosis. *Circulation* 1961; 24:1311.
35. Jones KL, Smith DW: The Williams elfin facies syndrome. *J Pediatr* 1975; 86:718.
36. Smith DW: *Recognizable Patterns of Human Malformation.* Philadelphia, WB Saunders Co, 1970.
37. Chatoor I, et al: Non-organic failure to thrive: A developmental perspective. *Pediatr Ann* 1984; 13:829.

38. Chatoor I, et al: Pediatric assessment of non-organic failure to thrive. *Pediatr Ann* 1984; 13:844.

39. O'Connor PA: Failure to thrive with breast feeding. *Clin Pediatr* 1978; 17:833.

40. Habbick BF, Gerrard JW: Failure to thrive in the contented breast fed baby. *Can Med Assoc J* 1984; 131:765.

41. Weston JA, et al: Prolonged breast feeding and non-organic failure to thrive. *Am J Dis Child* 1987; 141:242.

42. Richmond JB, et al: Rumination: A psychosomatic syndrome of infancy. *Pediatrics* 1958; 22:49.

43. Menking M, et al: Rumination—a near fatal psychiatric disease of infancy. *N Engl J Med* 1969; 280:802.

44. Rothney WB: Rumination and spasmus nutans. *Hosp Pract* 1969; 6:102.

45. Fleisher DR: Infant rumination syndrome: Report of a case and review of the literature. *Am J Dis Child* 1979; 133:266.

46. Chatoor I, et al: Rumination: Etiology and treatment. *Pediatr Ann* 1984; 13:924.

47. Stein ML, et al: Psychotherapy of an infant with rumination. *JAMA* 1959; 171:2309.

48. Murray ME, et al: Behavioral treatment of ruminations. A case study. *Clin Pediatr* 1976; 15:591.

49. Krieger I, Sargent DA: Postural sign in sensory deprivation syndrome in infants. *J Pediatr* 1967; 70:332.

50. Fossen A, Wilson J: Family interactions surrounding feedings of infants with non-organic failure to thrive. *Clin Pediatr* 1987; 26:518.

51. Fischhoff J, et al: A psychiatric study of mothers of infants with growth failure secondary to maternal deprivation. *J Pediatr* 1971; 79:209.

52. Pollitt E, et al: Psychosocial development and behavior of mothers of failure-to-thrive children. *Am J Orthopsychiat* 1975; 45:525.

53. Evans SL, et al: Failure to thrive: A study of 45 children and their families. *J Am Acad Child Psych* 1972; 11:440.

54. Altemeier WA, et al: Prospective study of antecedents for non-organic failure to thrive. *J Pediatr* 1985; 106:360.

55. Leonard MF, et al: Failure to thrive in infants: A family problem. *Am J Dis Child* 1966; 111:600.

56. Barbero G, Shaheen E: Environmental failure to thrive: A clinical view. *J Pediatr* 1967; 71:639.

57. Pollitt E, Eichler A: Behavioral disturbances among failure-to-thrive children. *Am J Dis Child* 1976; 130:24.

58. Hufton IW, Oates RK: Nonorganic failure to thrive: A long-term follow-up. *Pediatrics* 1977; 59:73.

59. Glaser H, Heagarty M: Physical and psychological development of children with early failure to thrive. *J Pediatr* 1968; 73:690.

60. Hopwood NJ: Failure to thrive. Investigating the non-organic causes. *Consultant* June 1984.

61. Casey PH, Arnold WC: Compensatory growth in infants with severe failure to thrive. *Med J* 1985; 78:1057.

62. Rosenn EW, et al: Differentiation of organic from nonorganic failure to thrive in infancy. *Pediatrics* 1980; 66:698.

63. Powell GF, Low JL: Behavior in non-organic failure to thrive. *J Dev Behav Pediatr* 1983; 4:26.

64. Powell GF, et al: Behavior as a diagnostic aid in failure-to-thrive. *J Dev Behav Pediatr* 1987; 8:18.

65. Elmer E, et al: Late results of the "failure-to-thrive" syndrome. *Clin Pediatr* 1969; 8:584.
66. Patton RG, Gardner LI: Influence of family environment on growth: The syndrome of "maternal deprivation." *Pediatrics* 1962; 30:957.
67. Silver HK, Finkelstein M: Deprivation dwarfism. *J Pediatr* 1967; 70:317.
68. Powell GF, et al: Emotional deprivation and growth retardation simulating idiopathic hypopituitarism. I. Clinical evaluation of the syndrome. *N Engl J Med* 1967; 276:1271.
69. Powell GF, et al: Emotional deprivation and growth retardation simulating idiopathic hypopituitarism: II. Endocrinologic evaluation of the syndrome. *N Engl J Med* 1967; 276:1279.
70. MacCarthy D, Booth EM: Parental rejection and stunting of growth. *J Psychosome Res* 1970; 14:259.
71. Hopwood NJ, Becker DJ: Psychosocial dwarfism: Detection, evaluation, and management. *Child Abuse and Neglect* 1979; 3:439.
72. Bowden ML, Hopwood NJ: Identification of children with psychosocial dwarfism. *Social Work Health Care* 1982; 7:15.
73. Krieger I: Food restriction as a form of child abuse in ten cases of psychosocial deprivation dwarfism. *Clin Pediatr* 1974; 13:127.
74. Reinhart JB, Drash AL: Psychosocial dwarfism: Environmentally induced recovery. *Psychosom Med* 1969; 31:165.
75. Whitten CF, et al: Evidence that growth failure from maternal deprivation is secondary to undereating. *JAMA* 1969; 209:1675.
76. Gardner LI: Deprivation dwarfism. *Sci Am* 1972; 227:76.
77. Tibbles JAR, et al: Pseudotumor cerebri and deprivation dwarfism. *Dev Med Child Neurol* 1972; 14:322.
78. Frasier SD, Rallison ML: Growth retardation and emotional deprivation: Relative resistance to treatment with human growth hormone. *J Pediatr* 1972; 80:603.
79. Rayner PHW, Rudd BT: Emotional deprivation in three siblings associated with functional pituitary growth hormone deficiency. *Aust Paediatr J* 1973; 9:79.
80. Powell GF, et al: Growth hormone studies before and during catch-up growth in a child with emotional deprivation and short stature. *J Clin Endocrinol Metab* 1973; 37:674.
81. Hopwood NJ, Powell GF: Emotional deprivation: Report of a case with features of leprechaunism. *Am J Dis Child* 1974; 127:892.
82. Money J: The syndrome of abuse dwarfism (psychosocial dwarfism or reversible hyposomatotropism). *Am J Dis Child* 1977; 131:508.
84. Gardner LI: The endocrinology of abuse dwarfism. *Am J Dis Child* 1977; 131:505.
84. Wolff G, Money J: Relationship between sleep and growth in patients with reversible somatotropin deficiency (psychosocial dwarfism). *Psychol Med* 1973; 3:18.
85. Money J, Wolff G: Late puberty, retarded growth and reversible hyposomatotropinism (psychosocial dwarfism). *Adolescence* 1974; 9:121.
86. Money J, et al: Hormonal and behavioral reversals in hyposomatotropic dwarfism, in Sachar EJ (ed): *Hormones, Behavior and Psychopathology.* New York, Raven Press, 1976.
87. Money J, et al: Pain agnosia and self injury in the syndrome of reversible somatotropin deficiency (psychosocial dwarfism). *J Autism Child Schizophr* 1972; 2:127.
88. Vanden Brande JL, DuCaju MVL: Plasma somatomedin activity in children with growth disturbances, in Raiti S (eds): *Advances in Human Growth Hormone Research.* DHEW publ No 74-612, US Printing Office, 1974.

89. Hernandez RJ, et al: Incidence of growth lines in psychosocial dwarfs and idiopathic hypopituitarism. *AJR* 1978; 131:477.
90. Marks HG, et al: Catch-up brain growth—demonstration by CAT scan. *J Pediatr* 1978; 93:254.
91. Franken EA, et al: Acute gastric dilatation in neglected children. *AJR* 1978; 130:297.
92. Guilhaume A, et al: Relationship between sleep stage IV deficit and reversible HGH deficiency in psychosocial dwarfism. *Pediatr Res* 1982; 16:299.
93. Ferholt JB, et al: A psychodynamic study of psychosocial dwarfism: A syndrome of depression, personality disorder, and impaired growth. *J Am Acad Child Psych* 1985; 24:49.
94. Green WH, et al: Psychosocial dwarfism: A critical review of the evidence. *J Am Acad Child Psych* 1984; 23:39.
95. Silverman JA: Anorexia nervosa: Clinical observations in successful treatment plan. *J Pediatr* 1974; 84:68.
96. Bruch H: *The Golden Cage: The Enigma of Anorexia Nervosa.* New York, Vintage Books, 1979.
97. VandeWiele RL: Anorexia nervosa and the hypothalamus. *Hosp Pract* 1977; 12:45.
98. Vigersky R: *Anorexia Nervosa.* New York, Raven Press, 1977.
99. Boyar RM, et al: Cortisol secretion and metabolism in anorexia nervosa. *N Engl J Med* 1977; 296:190.
100. Vigersky RA, et al: Delayed pituitary hormone response to LRF and TRF in patients with anorexia nervosa with secondary amenorrhea associated with simple weight loss. *J Clin Endocrinol Metab* 1976; 43:893.
101. Vigersky RA, et al: Hypothalamic dysfunction in secondary amenorrhea associated with simple weight loss. *N Engl J Med* 1977; 297:1141.
102. Aro A, et al: Hypothalamic endocrine dysfunction in anorexia nervosa. *Acta Endocrinol* 1977; 85:673.
103. Garfinkel PE, et al: Hypothalamic-pituitary function in anorexia nervosa. *Arch Gen Psychiatry* 1975; 32:739.
104. Boyar RM, et al: Anorexia nervosa: Immaturity of the 24-hour luteinizing hormone secretory pattern. *N Engl J Med* 1974; 291:862.
105. Sherman BM, et al: LH and FSH response to gonadotropin-releasing hormone in anorexia nervosa: Effect of nutritional rehabilitation. *J Clin Endocrinol Metab* 1975; 41:135.
106. Marshall JC, Kelch RP: Low dose pulsatile gonadotropin-releasing hormone in anorexia nervosa: A model of human pubertal development. *J Clin Endocrinol Metab* 1979; 49:712.
107. Macaron C, et al: The starved kidney: A defect in renal concentrating ability. *Metabolism* 1975; 24:457.
108. Klahs S, et al: On the nature of the renal concentrating defect in malnutrition. *Am J Med* 1967; 43:84.
109. Silber T: Anorexia nervosa. Morbidity and mortality. *Pediatr Ann* 1984; 13:851.
110. Langford WS, in Barnett HL, Einhorn AH (eds): *Pediatrics,* ed 15. New York, Appleton-Century-Crofts, 1972.
111. Bruch H: Treatment of eating disorders. *Mayo Clin Proc* 1978; 51:266.
112. Delaney DW, Silber TJ: Treatment of anorexia nervosa in a pediatric program. *Pediatr Ann* 1984; 13:860.
113. DuPont RL: Bulimia: A modern epidemic among adolescents. *Pediatr Ann* 1984; 13:908.
114. Herzog DB: Pharmacotherapy of anorexia nervosa and bulimia. *Pediatr Ann* 1984; 13:915.

5

Thyrotoxicosis and Nontoxic Goiters

Knowledge of the normal feedback system that regulates the production of thyroid hormones is required to understand the pathogenesis and proposed therapy of both toxic and nontoxic goiters. Although a detailed discussion is beyond the scope of this text,[1-4] Figure 5–1 illustrates the major interrelationships in the hypothalamic-pituitary-thyroid axis.

The isolation, structural identification, and synthesis of the hypothalamic thyrotrophin-releasing hormone (TRH) (pryo-glu-his-pro-amide) greatly increased our understanding of this system and also gave clinicians a useful diagnostic tool for the assessment of pituitary thyroid-stimulating hormone (TSH) reserve.[5-10] TRH, secreted by hypothalamic neurons into the hypophysial-portal circulation, stimulates the synthesis and secretion of TSH and prolactin.[11] Although chronic administration of TRH causes hyperplasia of pituitary thyrotropes, the major role of TRH in thyroid physiology is to regulate TSH secretion. This point is emphasized best by the observation that children with hypothalamic hypopituitarism and "tertiary hypothyroidism" secondary to TRH deficiency have normal or slightly increased responses to synthetic TRH.[10]

Somatostatin and dopamine, two other hypothalamic hormones not shown in Figure 5–1, function as TSH-inhibiting factors and appear to have physiologic roles in the regulation of TSH secretion.[4] Thyroid hormones exert their principal regulatory effects by means of the thyrotroph cell T_3-nuclear receptor complex, but they also affect TSH secretion by altering the number and/or affinity of pituitary receptors for TRH and somatostatin and by direct stimulation of somatostatin and possibly dopamine by the hypothalamus.

Because of the rapid degradation of TRH in both tissue extracts and serum, the wide distribution of TRH throughout the central nervous system and gastrointestinal tract, and the technical difficulties in the measurement of TRH, the net effect of thyroid hormones on TRH secretion by the hypothalamus has not been clarified. Perhaps the most important point illustrated in Figure 5–1 is that

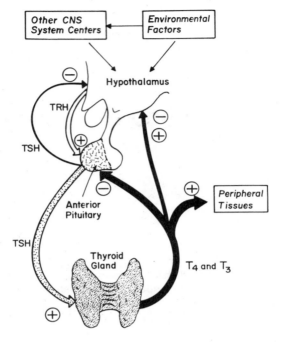

FIG 5–1.
Schematic diagram of current knowledge about the control of thyroid function. Abbreviations:
TRH = thyrotropin-releasing hormone; *TSH* = thyroid-stimulating hormone; T_3 = triiodo-
thyronine; T_4 = thyroxine.

the major site of negative feedback of thyroid hormones is the pituitary gland.[4]

Thyroid-stimulating hormone, a large glycoprotein hormone (molecular weight approximately 28,000) stimulates the production of T_4 and T_3 by the thyroid gland through binding to specific membrane receptors and activation of cyclic adenosine monophosphate. It is structurally similar to the other pituitary glycoprotein hormones—luteinizing hormone and follicle-stimulating hormone—as well as to human chorionic gonadotrophin. These hormones are composed of two noncovalently linked subunits, alpha and beta. The alpha subunits are identical, whereas the beta subunits are specific and confer biologic and immunologic specificity.

Radioimmunoassay measurements of basal serum TSH concentrations are most useful in the diagnosis of primary hypothyroidism. Until recently, differentiation of normal from low values of TSH, as occurs in hyperthyroidism, was not possible. Improvements in the TSH assay indicate that the normal range is 0.5 to 3.2 µU/mL and that hyper- and hypothyroid subjects fall below and above that range, respectively. Nonetheless, TSH assays performed in many commercial laboratories do not share this degree of sensitivity; often, the stated normal range is less than 7 µU/mL.[2]

Fortunately, serum TSH concentrations are relatively constant throughout the day. There is a modest circadian pattern, with the greatest values during the late evening or early morning hours. TSH secretion is not affected by glucose or amino acid concentrations, stress, exercise, and most drugs. However, drugs that interfere with thyroid hormone production, such as iodides and lithium carbonate, increase TSH secretion; in contrast, dopamine agonists such as L-dopa and bromergocryptine decrease TSH secretion in hypothyroid patients.[12] Hormones other than TRH, T_4, and T_3 have only slight effects on TSH secretion. Glucocorticoids suppress TSH secretion and TSH responses to TRH. Growth hormone and somatostatin also decrease TSH secretion and/or responsiveness to TRH, whereas estrogens augment TSH responses to TRH (see Appendix 5 for details of TRH test).

TSH secretion is exquisitely sensitive to the negative feedback effects of T_4 and T_3 on the pituitary gland. For example, treatment of a euthryoid individual with L-thyroxine at a dosage that maintains normal serum values for T_4 and T_3 usually results in suppression of basal TSH and TRH responsiveness. The cellular mechanisms of action of thyroid hormones are complex and involve effects on cell membranes, mitochondria, and nuclei (see reference 13 for detailed discussion). After treatment with thyroid hormones has been discontinued, at least 5 to 6—preferably 8—weeks should be allowed to elapse before evaluation of the pituitary-thyroid axis is performed. Recovery of the pituitary-thyroid axis with initial normalization of peripheral concentrations of T_4 and T_3 and, subsequently, basal TSH and TRH responsiveness, almost always occurs within 8 weeks.[14]

THYROTOXICOSIS

Thyrotoxicosis in children almost always is secondary to *Graves' disease* (also called Parry's disease, Basedow's disease, or exophthalmic goiter). The differential diagnosis of hyperthyroidism is listed in Table 5–1.[15–20]

TABLE 5–1.
Causes of Childhood Hyperthyroidism

Graves' disease
Chronic lymphocytic thyroiditis (Hashimoto's thyroiditis)
Subacute thyroiditis
Functioning adenoma(s) (Plummer's disease)
Polyostotic fibrous dysplasia (McCune-Albright syndrome)
Thyroid carcinoma
Iodide induced
Excessive TSH secretion
    Partial pituitary resistance to thyroid hormones*
    Pituitary adenoma
    Inappropriate TSH secretion (? hypothalamic hyperthyroidism)
    Factitious
* See reference 20.

Graves' disease is a multisystem disorder of unknown cause.[21–24] In adults, Graves' disease comprises three clinical entities: (1) hyperthyroidism associated with diffuse thyroid hyperplasia (with or without significant exophthalmos), (2) infiltrative ophthalmopathy ("euthyroid Graves' disease"), and (3) infiltrative dermopathy (pretibial myxedema). In practice, only the first clinical presentation is seen in children. Severe ophthalmopathy is uncommon in children, and pretibial myxedema has never been reported.

The basic defect in childhood Graves' disease is the autonomous overproduction of T_3 and T_4 by a diffusely enlarged hyperplastic thyroid gland. The thyroid gland is no longer under pituitary control; in addition to their obvious metabolic effects, excessive amounts of T_3 and T_4 suppress TSH production and block pituitary responsiveness to TRH.

Although the precise cause of the thyroid hyperfunction is still unknown, recent advances have strongly pointed toward related autoimmune defects as the cause of both Hashimoto's thyroiditis and Graves' disease.[20–25] This speculative hypothesis may explain the frequent histologic evidence of lymphocytic thyroiditis in surgically removed toxic goiters and the high degree of association of Graves' disease and Hashimoto's thyroiditis in many families. Currently, patients with Graves' disease are thought to have an inherited defect in immunologic surveillance that allows a clone of lymphoid cells to stimulate production of antibodies against the TSH receptors. These, in turn, cause thyroid hyperplasia and excess production of thyroid hormones, which produce the typical signs and symptoms of hyperthyroidism.

After the first year of life, the incidence of Graves' disease increases steadily throughout the first decade, with a peak during adolescence. Girls are affected three to six times more often than boys. Family histories frequently are positive for goiters, Graves' disease, or thyroiditis.[23, 25, 26]

The onset of the disease may be abrupt, but usually is insidious. The average duration of symptoms prior to treatment has been reported to be 1 year.[25, 26] In retrospect, most families and teachers note that school performance decreased significantly several months before thyrotoxicosis became apparent. During the initial interview, the most common complaints are nervousness, heat intolerance, excessive sweating, and increased appetite with or without weight loss. Physical examination usually reveals persistent tachycardia, systolic hypertension with markedly widened pulse pressure, mild exophthalmos, eyelid retraction and stare, tremulousness of the outstretched hands, and smooth, moist, warm skin.

Visual examination of the neck reveals an obvious goiter in nearly all patients. The thyroid gland is diffusely enlarged, with the right lobe often slightly larger than the left. Systolic bruits over the gland and venous hums in the right supraclavicular area often are present but have little prognostic value. The weight of involved thyroid glands varies between 30 and 150 g, whereas the average weight of the adult thyroid is 20 to 25 g. Blood flow to the thyrotoxic gland may be as high as 10 L/min. Thus, blood flow through the thyroid may exceed the entire cardiac output of the euthyroid individual.

Diagnosis

The diagnosis of thyrotoxicosis is seldom difficult. Usually, a thorough history and physical examination plus serum T_4 determination are all that is necessary. In questionable cases determination of the T_3 resin uptake, serum T_3, free T_4, thyroid antibody titers, or radioactive iodine (RAI) uptake may be necessary or helpful. Rarely is it necessary to show that the RAI uptake is not suppressible by administration of thyroid hormones.

A word of caution about the interpretation of thyroid function tests is necessary in view of the lack of uniformity in laboratory and reporting techniques. The single most useful thyroid function test is the serum T_4 concentration performed by competitive protein binding (Murphy-Pattee) or radioimmunoassay. Radioimmunoassay results are approximately 15% greater. These tests specifically measure the total amount of T_4. (In the past, some laboratories reported values in terms of the weight of T_4, whereas others reported values as the weight of T_4-iodine so that the normal range approximated the normal range of the serum protein-bound iodine [PBI]. As T_4 is 65% iodine by weight, the values are easily converted.) The T_3 resin uptake is an index of the amount and degree of saturation of thyroid-binding proteins (T_4-binding globulin, T_4-binding prealbumin, and serum albumin). Thus, changes in the quantity of T_4-binding proteins (genetic, hormonally induced, or secondary to disease), in addition to the amount of T_4 secreted, will affect the T_3 resin uptake value (Table 5–2). The T_3 resin uptake may be reported as normalized percentage or fraction (e.g., 86% to 114% or 0.86 to 1.14) or as an absolute percentage (e.g., 25% to 35%). When performed together, a serum T_4 and T_3 resin uptake usually will evaluate a patient's thyroid status accurately. It should be remembered, however, that the product of the

TABLE 5–2.
Factors That Affect T_3 Resin (T_3 R) Uptake Test Through Alterations in Concentration or Binding Capacity of Thyroxine-Binding Globulin*

Increased T_3 R Uptake (Decreased Binding Capacity or Concentration)	Decreased T_3 R Uptake (Increased Binding Capacity or Concentration)
Hyperandrogenic states and treatment with anabolic steroids	Pregnancy
Major illnesses and surgical stress	Hyperestrogenic states (Including oral contraceptives)
Nephrosis	Newborn period
Acromegaly, active	Perphenazine
Severe liver disease	Acute intermittent porphyria
Phenytoin	Hepatitis
Salicylates (large doses)	Genetically determined
Butazolidin	
Prednisone	
Genetically determined	

* Modified from Fisher DA, Advances in the laboratory diagnosis of thyroid disease. Part II. *J Pediatr* 1973; 82:4.

total T_4 and T_3 resin uptake provides, at best, a qualitative estimate and not a quantitative determination of free T_4.[27] For example, the calculated free T_4 index ("T_7") may be low in patients with nonthyroidal disease who have normal free T_4 but decreased serum T_4-binding capacity. Determination of free T_4 is difficult and time-consuming, but there is general agreement that free T_4 is more markedly affected than total T_4 in both hypothyroidism and hyperthyroidism. Free T_4 is measured usually by equilibration of dilute serum with isotopically labeled T_4, dialysis against a physiologic buffer to determine the ratio of bound to free hormone, and subsequent multiplication of this ratio by the total serum T_4 concentration. Serum TSH determinations are useful in differentiating among primary and secondary (hypopituitary) or "tertiary" (hypothalamic) hypothyroidism; the newer and highly sensitive TSH assays also allow for the detection of hyperthyroidism. Serum T_3 concentrations can be measured by radioimmunoassay also. The availability of this test has allowed clinicians to recognize cases of so-called T_3 toxicosis in children, as it has in adults.[28, 29] Recently, increasing numbers of clinically hyperthyroid patients have been described with normal serum T_4 concentrations but increased serum T_3 values. Furthermore, total serum T_3 determinations have been shown to be highly useful in evaluating the thyroid status of patients being treated with thionamides.[30] Serum T_3 may not be normal in such patients until serum T_4 values are low or in the low normal range. Table 5–3 is a list of the normal values for commonly used thyroid tests (see references 31 and 32 for detailed discussions).

Treatment

Treatment of Graves' disease is unsatisfactory and frustrating and probably will remain so until its cause is determined and a specific therapy is developed. Being unable to treat the cause, we are compelled to control secretion of thyroid hormones by the diseased gland. Available options include long-term treatment with thionamides, such as propylthiouracil (PTU) or methimazole. Those drugs block the formation of T_4 and T_3, and in the case of PTU, also decrease the peripheral conversion of T_4 to T_3. Subtotal thyroidectomy is also an option, but the term subtotal is now a misnomer, as nearly complete thyroidectomies are performed in children to avoid a high recurrence rate. The third option, RAI, effects control of the disease through destruction of thyroid tissue by high-energy beta rays.

Radioactive iodine (^{131}I) was established as an effective agent for the control of hyperthyroidism in the 1950s. Today it is generally accepted as the treatment of choice for hyperthyroidism in patients over age 30; indeed in many clinics, it is the preferred treatment in any patient over 20 years of age.[33] In a growing number of centers it is used routinely for the treatment of patients at any age, including children.[34–37] Advocates of this approach believe that it is safe and point out that it is safer than surgery, which has a definite, though low, mortality rate. RAI is inexpensive when compared with long-term thionamide therapy or surgery, and it is highly effective. Several concerns have limited its widespread

TABLE 5–3.
Normal Values for Commonly Used In Vitro Thyroid Function Tests

Test	Normal Range
Serum T_4 (Murphy-Pattee)	4.5–10.5 µg/100 mL
Serum T_4*	4.5–13.2 µg/100 mL
Serum T_3*	70–170 ng/100 mL
T_3 resin uptake ratio	0.86–1.14
T_4–T_3 resin uptake index ("T_7")	4.5–13.2 µg/100 mL
Serum TSH*	0.3–6.0 µU/mL†

* Determined by radioimmunoassay.
† University of Michigan Central Ligand Laboratory

acceptance. First, hypothyroidism is a common result. Indeed, most advocates of RAI recommend total thyroid ablation in children; thus hypothyroidism would be expected to be universal. Concern about the genetic risk has been expressed on numerous occasions. However, the calculated radiation dose to the gonads is equivalent to the amount of radiation one receives during either an upper gastrointestinal series or intravenous pyelography. Follow-up evaluation of the reproduction histories and health of the offspring of children and adolescents treated with large doses of ^{131}I for thyroid cancer has revealed no overt evidence of genetic damage.[37, 38] Also, there has been concern about subsequent development of malignancies. A recent report indicated that the incidence of thyroid adenomas is significantly greater when ^{131}I therapy is given before age 20.[39] It is true that developing organs or organ systems are more susceptible than adult systems to the oncogenic potential of ionizing radiation. The best example of this, of course, is the effect of radiation on the immature thyroid gland. Because RAI treatment would ablate the thyroid gland, the risk of thyroid carcinoma may be set aside. Furthermore, when the incidence of thyroid carcinoma was compared in 16,000 patients treated with RAI and 8,000 patients surgically treated, it was found that the incidence of carcinoma was significantly lower in those who had received [131]I.[39] Nonetheless, we must remain at least somewhat concerned about the effects of ionizing radiation on the malignant potential of other organ systems. Fear of the unknown has previously inhibited us from recommending RAI for the treatment of childhood thyrotoxicosis. The increased experience with the favorable outcome in children treated with RAI has lessened our concerns and has led us to offer RAI therapy as an acceptable approach for all children who have Graves' disease.[37]

Despite the trend toward greater use of RAI, a review of the pediatric endocrine literature indicates that long-term thionamide therapy remains the treatment of choice.[40–43] Most reports, however, have originated from medical centers in large metropolitan areas, and patient preference and compliance may be affected by accessibility to experienced clinicians. With long-term thionamide therapy, the sustained remission rate during the first 2 years is only 25%. The expected time of treatment to achieve a 50% remission rate is 4 to 4½ years.[43] Children are less responsive to thionamides than adults and require a longer period of time before remission is likely to occur.

In our clinics, the therapeutic options are discussed openly and thoroughly during the initial visits. Between 1972 and 1982, approximately two thirds of families at the University of Michigan chose chronic medical therapy initially; almost one third elected to have surgery performed as soon as hyperthyroidism could be controlled, and a small percentage elected RAI initially. Approximately half of the long-term PTU-treated patients experienced a remission during the first 18 to 24 months, but 50% of them had a rapid recurrence. Thirteen percent of our patients failed to respond well to medical treatment, perhaps because of poor compliance. More than half of those who initially chose medical management proceeded to have ablative therapy, usually subtotal thyroidectomy. Family and patient frustration with medical management, medical complications, and recurrent thyrotoxicosis are the common reasons for the later choice of thyroidectomy or RAI.

In prepubertal children RAI therapy was recommended when the patient was a poor surgical risk: for example, those with severe retardation, inadequately controlled thyrotoxicosis, or significant medical complications of thionamide therapy. More recently, patient and family acceptance of RAI therapy has increased modestly, but commonly held concerns about the effects of radiation still limit its acceptability.

Once the diagnosis of thyrotoxicosis has been established, treatment should be started promptly to achieve an euthyroid status. Propylthiouracil is our first drug of choice, as it also inhibits the peripheral deiodination of T_4 to T_3.[44] (Refer to reference 44 for a detailed review of antithyroid drug therapy.) The latter, however, probably has more theoretical than practical importance. Initially, PTU (150 to 300 mg total dose, 150 mg/M^2/day or 6 to 7 mg/kg/day) should be given every 6 to 8 hours to maintain fairly constant blood concentrations. Propanolol (initially 2.5 mg/kg/day orally) should be used to control symptoms, since the patient can feel better within hours rather than weeks; propranolol must be given every 6 to 8 hours for continuous effectiveness. Side effects of propranolol include bradycardia and hypoglycemia; it is contraindicated in patients with asthma or heart block. All patients should be advised to sharply control their activities and avoid physical and emotional stress. Severely toxic patients and those from unreliable families should be hospitalized until improvement has been documented; often, 10 to 14 days is required. Sedation with barbiturates may be helpful. Most patients become euthyroid in 4 to 6 weeks. The therapeutic program should be simplified as much as possible. This means tapering and discontinuing propranolol as soon as possible as well as reducing the frequency of PTU to twice a day or even once a day.[41, 44]

During the early phases of management, therapeutic options should be discussed thoroughly and frequently. This is most important as there is no specific or entirely safe mode of therapy. Both surgery and RAI trade hyperthyroidism for hypothyroidism. This concern is significant, even though the natural history of thyrotoxicosis is such that it appears to eventually result in hypothyroidism in many patients.[45]

Despite the high incidence of failures and complications with long-term thionamide therapy, that approach seems reasonable initially, as it allows the child to mature and reach an age when RAI will perhaps be safer and more acceptable (after puberty), and it does afford a 25% to 50% chance for a sustained remission. Although antithyroid drugs might have a modest suppressive effect on the intrathyroidal immune dysfunction, it should be remembered that their principal effect is the blockage of the production of thyroid hormone; this merely controls the metabolic aspects of Graves' disease and allows the disease to subside spontaneously.[44] Once the patient is euthyroid, 50 mg of PTU two to three times per day usually maintains euthyroidism. The optimal duration of therapy is unknown, but we inform families that they should expect at least 18 to 24 months of thionamide treatment. In some clinics, larger doses of PTU are used to make the patient hypothyroid. Replacement therapy with L-thyroxine is then begun, and the size of the thyroid gland is used to monitor the course of the disease. Ideally, we would like to be able to discern when (if ever) the pituitary has regained control of thyroid hormone production, as this would indicate that the disease had subsided. Suppressibility of serum T_4 or RAI uptake by T_3 (while the patient is off all medications) has been used, but this approach is expensive and time-consuming. Serial determinations of TSH or testing with TRH are also useful. Currently, we continue therapy with PTU alone for 18 to 24 months and then withdraw PTU and watch for signs of hyperthyroidism. Surgery or RAI is recommended for patients who have recurrences, but reinstitution of therapy with PTU usually controls their symptoms. Prolonged therapy with PTU for as long as 20 years has been prescribed in some pediatric endocrine clinics.[40, 42] The ability to predict which patients will have a good response to long-term thionamide therapy would be most helpful. Several findings are predictors of recurrence. If the thyroid gland is exceptionally large, that is, more than three times normal size, remission is unlikely to occur in a reasonable length of time. Likewise, severe thyrotoxicosis, failure of the thyroid gland to shrink during therapy, strongly positive microsomal antibody titer and detectable serum antibodies against the TSH receptor are poor prognostic findings. Finally, recent reports indicate that several HLA haplotypes are associated with a poor prognosis.[46, 47]

Chronic PTU therapy is not free from significant complications.[48–51] Up to 10% of children experience some complication; 8% of our patients have had a significant complication from PTU. Common complications are leukopenia and skin rash. These usually occur in the first several months of therapy and are reversible in most instances. Severe granulocytopenia secondary to PTU is uncommon. However, its onset is unpredictable, and it is sometimes difficult to distinguish from the leukopenia associated with Graves' disease itself; hence, routine white blood cell counts have limited value. We recommend blood counts during all illnesses and discontinuation of PTU in the event of significant leukopenia (white blood count less than 3,000/mm³). Rashes, fever, urticaria, arthritis, and a severe lupuslike syndrome have been caused by PTU and related drugs. These complications also dictate the discontinuance of PTU. In these cases methimazole therapy (the dose is approximately one-tenth the dose of PTU) may be tried cautiously, but it is wise to recommend surgery or RAI therapy.

Oral therapy with iodide salts (Lugol's solution or saturated solution of potassium iodide) inhibits the release of thyroid hormones and slightly impairs their synthesis. However, the beneficial effects are transient in most patients. Lithium salts also have been used, but have not been very effective.[52] Perchlorate salts were used in the past, but reports of aplastic anemia caused most clinicians to discontinue using them. Currently, they are not available through domestic pharmaceutical firms and should only be used by experienced endocrinologists.

If surgery has been agreed on, Lugol's solution (5 drops/day orally) should be given for 2 weeks before the operation. Patients must be euthyroid at the time of surgery. The preferred procedure is bilateral subtotal thyroidectomy.[53]

Subtotal thyroidectomy for the treatment of Graves' disease, when performed by highly skilled surgeons in a center well equipped for the care of children, is safe, but not without significant complications.[21, 53] In both the Mayo Clinic experience and our own, vocal cord paralysis, hypoparathyroidism, and recurrence of thyrotoxicosis have been infrequent. Contrary to our earlier experience, the incidence of postsurgical hypothyroidism is great (essentially 100%). Among the 33 patients who underwent subtotal thyroidectomy between 1972 and 1982 (approximately half of the patients seen in our clinic) there were no deaths and no vocal cord paralysis. Seven patients have had severe hypocalcemia, but in five it proved to be transient. There was one recurrence, but recently all patients have become hypothyroid. Longer follow-up and a more extensive surgical approach almost surely account for the differences between these results and our earlier report.[53]

Little is known about the natural course of untreated Graves' disease. Although there is some evidence to suggest that hypothyroidism is the natural outcome of the disease, we still should be concerned about causing hypothyroidism, especially in a growing child. It should be obvious that any child with Graves' disease deserves careful, lifelong medical observation.

Although "thyroid storm" is extremely rare in children, no discussion of Graves' disease is complete without a comment about its treatment. The best treatment, of course, is prevention. Thyroid storm can be precipitated by physical and emotional stress, infection, surgery, and RAI therapy. Treatment should consist of prompt administration of large doses of PTU, either orally or through a nasogastric tube, followed several hours later by iodides to block release of thyroid hormones. Propranolol given intravenously is useful to control adrenergic signs and symptoms. Patients may be switched to oral therapy, usually within 24 hours.[54, 55] Supportive therapy, including antipyretics, intravenous fluids, stress doses of glucocorticoids, and B vitamins, should be given.

Neonatal thyrotoxicosis is an uncommon form of Graves' disease first described in 1910. Clinically, there seem to be two forms.[24, 25, 56, 57] In some infants the disease is self-limited and has been thought to be related to the transplacental passage of thyroid-stimulating immunoglobulins.[57] In some families, neonatal Graves' disease appears to be transmitted in an autosomal dominant pattern with a predilection for female infants.[56] The disease is not transient in these infants and often is difficult to control. These infants may or may not be thyrotoxic at birth; their clinical courses cannot be attributed to the transplacental passage of thyroid-stimulating immunoglobulins. Approximately 50% of the mothers of all affected infants have had Graves' disease, either before or during the pregnancy, but only half the affected mothers have been hyperthyroid during the pregnancy.

Clinical features of neonatal Graves' disease include low birth weight; goiter; advanced bone age; increased size of thymus, liver, spleen, and lymph nodes; exophthalmus; tachycardia; irritability; congestive heart failure; jaundice; and thrombocytopenia. Although a large goiter may be present and compromise the airway, this is unusual; indeed, in many infants the thyroid may not be visibly or palpably enlarged. In contrast with the disease course in older children, there is an equal sex distribution in neonatal Graves' disease. Premature cranial synostosis, microcephaly, and minimal brain dysfunction may occur in severely affected infants. The overall mortality is between 15% and 20%.

Treatment of neonatal Graves' disease depends on the severity of symptoms. Mildly affected infants may not require treatment, but should be observed closely. Lugol's solution (1 drop orally every 8 hours), PTU (10 mg orally every 8 hours) and propranolol (2 mg/kg/day) may be used alone or in combination, along with supportive measures for treatment of congestive failure or infection.[58]

Disordered regulation of autoimmunity appears to be the cause of both classic Graves' disease and Hashimoto's thyroiditis. Moreover, recent findings strongly suggest that the clinical spectrum of autoimmune thyroid disease is much greater and, indeed, that most causes of "toxic" and "nontoxic" enlargement of the thyroid are autoimmune in nature.[23] In addition to the routinely available antithyroglobulin and antimicrosomal antibody determinations, investigators have described several other types of thyroid autoantibodies including thyroid growth stimulating immunoglobulin, thyroid growth inhibiting immunoglobulins, TSH-binding inhibiting immunoglobulins, thyroid stimulating immunoglobulins, exophthalmogenic immunoglobulin, and dermopathy associated immunoglobulin. The clinical disorders that have been associated with thyroid autoantibodies are listed in Table 5–4.

NONTOXIC GOITERS

Asymptomatic enlargement of the thyroid gland is a common reason for referral to a pediatric endocrinologist. Again, girls are affected much more frequently than boys (up to ten times more often). Although asymptomatic goiters are a common finding (7%) in grade-school girls,[59] most patients exhibit this during adolescence. A correct diagnosis can be made in most cases with the aid of laboratory studies and *without* biopsy of the thyroid gland.[31, 32]

The most common cause of a "nontoxic goiter" is Hashimoto's thyroiditis (chronic lymphocytic thyroiditis),[60–62] which accounts for 55% to 65% of patients referred to pediatric endocrine clinics for evaluation of euthyroid goiter. Simple colloid goiter is the next most common. Together, these two conditions account for the vast majority of cases. Adenomatous goiters, hyperplasia of the thyroid

TABLE 5–4.
Clinical Disorders Associated With Thyroid Autoantibodies*

Hyperthyroid conditions
  Graves' disease
  Hashitoxicosis
  Neonatal Graves' disease
  Transient thyrotoxicosis with painless thyroiditis
Euthyroid or hypothyroid conditions
  Hashimoto's thyroiditis
  Simple adolescent goiter
  Multinodular goiter
  Transient neonatal hypothyroidism
  Sporadic cretinism
  Transient (postpartum) hypothyroidism
  Focal thyroiditis
  Fibrous thyroiditis
  Primary myxedema
  Thyroid lymphoma
  Multiple endocrine deficiency disease, (e.g., diabetes
    mellitus, Addison's disease, hypoparathyroidism,
    hypogonadism)
  Associated autoimmune disorders (e.g., idiopathic
    thrombocytopenic purpura, thyroid antigen or antibody
    complex nephritis)

* Adapted from Fisher DA, Pandian MR, Carlton E: Autoimmune thyroid disease, an expanding spectrum. *Pediatr Clin North Am* 1987; 34:907.

gland, isolated thyroid nodule, and carcinoma are unusual causes, whereas goiter secondary to mild enzymatic defects in thyroid hormone production are rare.

Typically, euthyroid patients with Hashimoto's thyroiditis have a moderately enlarged, firm thyroid gland, which often has a "football pigskin-like texture." The gland is nontender and often asymptomatically enlarged and lobulated; a midline, pea-sized lymph node (so-called Delphian node) may be present above the isthmus. Despite this dramatic description, it is practically impossible to distinguish between a simple colloid goiter and thyroiditis by physical examination alone. This clinical dilemma is not surprising since most patients who have either Hashimoto's thyroiditis, a diffuse goiter, a multinodular goiter, or who merely have a single thyroid nodule have thyroid growth stimulating antibodies in their circulation.[23]

Diagnosis

The following laboratory studies and historical data allow a presumptive diagnosis of Hashimoto's thyroiditis: serum T_4, antithyroglobulin and microsomal complement-fixing antibody tests, serum TSH, thyroid scan, and family history of thyroiditis. In the past, several authors emphasized that the PBI frequently exceeds the serum T_4 (when expressed at T_4-iodine) by 2 μg/dL or more in patients with thyroiditis. More recent data indicate that this finding is not diagnostically useful. Indeed, significant PBI-T_4 differences occur in several conditions, including patients with simple colloid goiters. Antithyroglobulin titers are lower in affected children than in adults, but titers higher than 1:16 are present in many children with thyroidtitis; the thyroid microsomal complement fixation test may be positive when antithyroglobulin is undetectable. Hence, determination of both types of antibodies is helpful. When antithyroglobulin is measured by radioimmunoassay, nearly all patients with Hashimoto's thyroiditis have significant titers.[63] This determination, as well as several other types of thyroid antibody determinations, is not readily available. An elevated serum TSH or an exaggerated TSH response to TRH would suggest borderline thyroid function and point toward the diagnosis of thyroiditis. We do not find the thyroid scan as useful as others, but an irregular "patchy" uptake of RAI also suggests the presence of thyroiditis. Likewise, the perchlorate discharge test is not used routinely in our clinic. It may be useful, however, since patients with Hashimoto's thyroiditis have a partial defect in organification of iodine and hence release more than normal amounts of RAI after administration of perchlorate salts. It is not necessary to perform all of these studies, but all of them may be helpful. Indeed, if three or more of these features are present in a patient with an enlarged, firm thyroid gland, a presumptive diagnosis of Hashimoto's thyroiditis should be made. Ultrasonography and fine-needle aspiration may be helpful, but these should be reserved for unusual cases and should be performed by highly skilled personnel.[64]

Treatment

There is considerable disagreement about the correct therapeutic approach to euthyroid patients with Hashimoto's thyroiditis. A recent survey of 5,179 school children revealed a 1.2% prevalence rate for Hashimoto's thyroiditis. In that study, evaluation of affected children over 6 years of age indicated that spontaneous remission occurs in at least 50% of patients whether or not they are treated with thyroid hormones.[65] Although longer follow-up data are limited, it seems likely that many patients with thyroiditis will become hypothyroid and require lifelong treatment.[66] Furthermore, some euthyroid patients with Hashimoto's thyroiditis have elevated TSH levels.[60] These findings, plus the suggestion that chronically elevated TSH levels may be causally related to cancer of the thyroid, and the reported possible association of thyroid carcinoma and thyroiditis, support the concept of lifelong replacement therapy. We recommend full replacement therapy with synthetic L-thyroxine (average dosage: 2.5 to 3.0 μg/kg/day in adolescents) for all patients with increased TSH values and/or large or locally symptomatic goiters. All patients should be informed about the possibility of hypothyroidism in the future and should be advised about the need for long-term medical follow-up.

The natural history and course of simple colloid goiters are not known, although some evidence suggests that they may develop into large multinodular goiters later in life. In equivocal cases and in patients with suspected colloid goiters, treatment throughout adolescence, followed by attempted withdrawal after growth has ceased, is our current approach.

During the treatment of patients with Hashimoto's thyroiditis or simple colloid goiter, failure of the thyroid gland to decrease significantly while on replacement therapy should cause some concern and prompt further studies (e.g., thyroid scans and perhaps open biopsy).

Inherited defects in thyroid hormone production are rare causes of goiters in children. Patients usually are first seen at age 2 to 4 years because of thyroid enlargement. Indeed, only 20% to 25% of these patients have goiters in infancy ("goitrous cretins"). An elevated RAI uptake in a euthyroid or hypothyroid patient usually will be observed. Precise diagnoses often are difficult to arrive at, but treatment also is full replacement therapy. (See Chapter 6 for further details.)

Clinically appreciable, solitary thyroid nodules are much less common in children than in adults. In general, the presence of a solitary nodule should prompt surgical removal, because computed tomographic scanning and ultrasound have significant diagnostic limitations, and experience with fine-needle aspiration biopsy in children is limited. In studies that excluded children who had been exposed to radiation, the incidence of cancer in a thyroid nodule was approximately 15% (see Rojeski and Gharib[64] and Molitch et al.[67] for detailed discussion of nodular thyroid disease).

Despite an increasing incidence during the past 2 decades, *carcinoma of the thyroid gland* is unusual in children. The majority of affected children have received radiation therapy to the head and neck region early in life. In retrospect, such therapy was almost always inappropriate. The diagnosis usually is made after metastasis has occurred. In the University of Michigan series, cervical lymphatic metastases were present in 88% of cases of childhood thyroid carcinoma.[68]

Children with thyroid carcinoma are seldom hyperthyroid and almost never hypothyroid. They usually have persistent cervical adenopathy or a solitary thyroid nodule. The presence of a solitary nodule should always arouse a suspicion of carcinoma. The nodules usually are firm and often irregular and usually appear "cold" on a thyroid scan.

Generalized enlargement of the thyroid gland also may be found because of concomitant thyroiditis. Papillary and mixed papillary-follicular tumors account for nearly all of the pathologic diagnoses; undifferentiated carcinoma is almost unheard of in children.

Proper treatment of thyroid carcinoma consists of total thyroidectomy and removal of affected lymph nodes, followed by RAI ablation. The prognosis, despite the high incidence of metastases, is good. The overall mortality rate was 5.2% in a series of 58 consecutive children treated at the University of Michigan.[68] Although measurement of serum concentrations of thyroglobulin is not helpful in establishing a diagnosis, serial measurements may be helpful in the assessment of ablative therapies.[64]

Medullary carcinoma of the thyroid, a neoplasm of the C, or calcitonin-producing, cells of the thyroid gland, is a rare type of thyroid malignancy, accounting for 6% to 10% of thyroid cancers. In adults, it often is not recognized until the fourth or fifth decade of life, and in its sporadic form it is extremely rare in children. MCT may be familial and may be transmitted in an autosomal dominant manner. Two familial autosomal dominant forms have been well described along with other associated endocrine neoplasia, primarily pheochromocytomas and hyperparathyroidism: MEN type II (Sipple's syndrome), and MEN type III. (These were also previously known as MEN IIa and MEN IIb.) MEN type III is also known as the multiple mucosal neuroma syndrome. Because of their distinct physical appearance (Marfanoid habitus) and multiple mucosal neuromas, patients with MEN III often can be recognized early in life. Determinations of basal and pentagastrin-stimulated serum concentrations of calcitonin may be very useful in the early detection of medullary carcinoma of the thyroid in members of affected families with either MEN II or III.[69]

APPENDIX 5

Pituitary TSH Reserve Test: Intravenous TRH Test

Synthetic TRH is given intravenously over 15 to 30 seconds at time zero. Blood samples for determination of TSH and prolactin are withdrawn at the following times: -15.0, $+30$, and $+60$ minutes. Additional samples may be necessary to characterize some patients' responsiveness completely (e.g., $+90$ and $+120$ minutes). The recommended dose of TRH is 7 µg/kg, with a maximum dose of 200 µg. The test should be performed in the morning after an overnight fast, although this is not absolutely necessary. Blood pressure and pulse should be monitored often throughout the test. Side effects are minimal, but include nausea, a sensation of facial flushing, the urge to urinate, and occasionally vomiting. These effects last from several seconds to 2 minutes, but they occur in almost all patients.

The absolute values for TSH responses vary considerably between laboratories and are affected somewhat by the patient's age and sex. Although the pattern for TSH release also must be considered, a maximal rise in serum TSH of between 5 and 25 µU/mL is considered normal in most laboratories.

REFERENCES

1. Reichlin S: Regulation of the hypophysiotropic secretion of the brain. *Arch Intern Med* 1975; 135:1350.
2. Kourides IA: Pituitary thyrotropin secretion in thyroid disorders. *Thyroid Today*, vol 3, no 2, April/May 1980.
3. Harris A, et al: The physiological role of TRH in regulation of TSH and prolactin secretion in the rat. *J Clin Invest* 1978; 61:441.

4. Jackson IMD: Neuroendocrine control of pituitary TSH secretion. *Thyroid Today* vol 6, no 6, Nov/Dec 1983.

5. Haigler ED Jr, et al: : Direct evaluation of pituitary thyrotropin reserve utilizing synthetic thyrotropin releasing hormone. *J Clin Endocrinol Metab* 1971; 33:573.

6. Snyder PJ, Utiger RD: Response to thyrotropin releasing hormone (TRH) in normal man. *J Clin Endocrinol Metab* 1972; 34:380.

7. Foley TP, et al: Human prolactin and thyrotropin concentrations in the serums of normal and hypopituitary children before and after administration of synthetic thyrotropin-releasing hormone. *J Clin Invest* 1972; 51:243.

8. Faglia G, et al: Plasma thyrotropin response to thyrotropin-releasing hormone in patients with pituitary and hypothalamic disorders. *J Clin Endocrinol Metab* 1973; 37:595.

9. Schally AV, Arimura A, Kastin AJ: Hypothalamic regulatory hormones. *Science* 1973; 179:341.

10. Suter SN, et al: Plasma prolactin and thyrotropin and the response to thyrotropin-releasing factor in children with primary and hypothalamic hypothyroidism. *J Clin Endocrinol Metab* 1978; 47:1015.

11. Jacobs LS, et al: Prolactin response to thyrotropin-releasing hormone in normal subjects. *J Clin Endocrinol Metab* 1973; 36:1069.

12. Rapoport B, et al: Suppression of serum thyrotropin (TSH) by L-dopa in chronic hypothyroidism: Interrelationships in the regulation of TSH and prolactin secretion. *J Clin Endocrinol Metab* 1973; 36:256.

13. Ingbar H: The thyroid gland, in Wilson JD, Foster DW (eds): *William's Textbook of Endocrinology*, ed 7. Philadelphia, WB Saunders Co, 1985, pp 682–815.

14. Vagenakis AG, et al: Recovery of pituitary thyrotropic function after withdrawal of prolonged thyroid-suppression therapy. *N Engl J Med* 1975; 293:681.

15. McArthur RG: Hyperthyroidism in childhood. *Thyroid Today* vol 1, no 5, Jan 1978.

16. Hamilton CR, Jr, et al: Hyperthyroidism due to thyrotropin-producing pituitary chromophobe adenoma. *N Engl J Med* 1970; 283:1077.

17. Emerson CH, Utiger RD: Hyperthyroidism and excessive thyrotropin secretion. *N Engl J Med* 1972; 287:328.

18. Hopwood NJ, et al: Functioning thyroid masses in childhood and adolescence—clinical, surgical, and pathologic complications. *J Pediatr* 1976; 89:710.

19. Gorman CA, et al: Transient hyperthyroidism in patients with lymphocytic thyroiditis. *Mayo Clin Proc* 1978; 53:359.

20. Hopwood NJ, et al: Familial partial pituitary peripheral resistance to thyroid hormone. A frequently missed diagnosis. *Pediatrics* 1986; 78:114.

21. Weetman AP, McGregor AM: Autoimmune thyroid disease: Developments in our understanding. *Endocr Rev* 1984; 5:309.

22. Burman KD, Baker JR: Immune mechanisms in Graves' disease. *Endocrinol Rev* 1985; 6:183.

23. Fisher DA, Pandian MR, Carlton E: Autoimmune thyroid disease, an expanding spectrum. *Pediatr Clin North Am* 1987; 34:907.

24. Smith BR, McLachlan SM, Furmaniak J: Autoantibodies to the thyrotropin receptor. *Endocrinol Rev* 1988; 9:106.

25. Hayles AB: Problems of childhood Graves' disease. *Mayo Clin Proc* 1972; 47:850.

26. Bacon GE, Lowrey GH: Experience with surgical treatment of thyrotoxicosis in children. *J Pediatr* 1965; 67:1.

27. Schussler GC: Thyroid function tests in patients with nonthyroidal disease. *Thyroid Today* vol 3, no 3, June 1980.

28. Wahner HW: T_3 hyperthyroidism. *Mayo Clin Proc* 1972; 47:938.

29. Harland PC, McArthur RG, Fawcett DM: T_3 toxicosis in children. *Acta Paediatr Scand* 1977; 66:525.
30. Golden MP, et al: Value of simultaneous T_3, T_4, and TSH measurements for management of Graves' disease in children. *Pediatrics* 1977; 59:762.
31. Fisher DA: Advancements in the laboratory diagnosis of thyroid disease: Part I. *J Pediatr* 1973; 82:1.
32. Fisher DA: Advances in the laboratory diagnosis of thyroid disease: Part II. *J Pediatr* 1973; 82:187.
33. Becker DV: Current status of radioactive iodine treatment of hyperthyroidism. *Thyroid Today* vol 2, no 7, Nov 1979.
34. Starr P, Jaffe HL, Oettinger L, Jr: Later results of ^{131}I treatment of hyperthyroidism in 73 children and adolescents: 1967 followup. *J Nucl Med* 1969; 10:586.
35. Hayek A, Chapman EM, Crawford JD: Long-term results of treatment of thyrotoxicosis in children and adolescents with radioactive iodine. *N Engl J Med* 1970; 283:949.
36. Safa AM, Schumach OP, Rodriguez-Antunez A: Long-term follow-up results in children and adolescents treated with radioactive iodine (^{131}I) for hyperthyroidism. *N Engl J Med* 1975; 292:167.
37. Hamburger JI: Management of hyperthyroidism in children and adolescents. *J Clin Endocrinol Metab* 1985; 60:1019.
38. Sarkar SD, et al: Subsequent fertility and birth histories of children and adolescents treated with ^{131}I for thyroid cancer. *J Nucl Med* 1976; 17:460.
39. Dobyns BM, et al: Malignant and benign neoplasms of the thyroid in patients treated for hyperthyroidism: A report of the cooperative thyrotoxicosis therapy follow-up study. *J Clin Endocrinol Metab* 1974; 38:976.
40. Vaidya VA, et al: Twenty-two years' experience in the medical management of juvenile thyrotoxicosis. *Pediatrics* 1974; 54:565.
41. Barnes HV, Blizzard RM: Antithyroid drug therapy for toxic diffuse goiter (Graves' disease): Thirty years experience in children and adolescents. *J Pediatr* 1977; 91:313.
42. Shizume K: Long-term antithyroid drug therapy for intractable cases of Graves' disease. *Endocrinol Jpn* 1978; 25:377.
43. Collen RJ, et al: Remission rates of children and adolescents with thyrotoxicosis treated with antithyroid drugs. *Pediatrics* 1980; 65:550.
44. Cooper DS: Antithyroid drugs. *N Engl J Med* 1984; 311:1353.
45. Wood LC, Ingbar SH: Hypothyroidism as a late sequela in patients with Graves' disease treated with antithyroid agents. *J Clin Invest* 1979; 64:1429.
46. Ford D, et al: Histocompatibility antigens in Graves' disease. *Aust NZ J Med* 1976; 6:297.
47. Irvine WJ, et al: Correlation of HLA and thyroid antibodies with clinical course of thyrotoxicosis treated with antithyroid drugs. *Lancet* 1977; 2:898.
48. Walzer RA, Einbinder J: Immunoleukopenia as an aspect of hypersensitivity to propylthiouracil. *JAMA* 1963; 184:743.
49. Martelo OJ, Katims RB, Yunis AA: Bone marrow-aplasia following propylthiouracil therapy. *Arch Intern Med* 1967; 120:587.
50. Armheim JA, Kenny FM, Ross D: Granulocytopenia, lupus-like syndrome, and other complications of propylthiouracil therapy. *J Pediatr* 1970; 76:54.
51. Breese TJ, Solomon IL: Granulocytopenia and hemolytic anemia as complications of propylthiouracil therapy. *J Pediatr* 1975; 86:117.
52. Temple R, et al: The use of lithium in Graves' disease. *Mayo Clin Proc* 1972; 47:872.
53. Tank ES, Bacon GE, Lowrey GH: Surgical management of thyrotoxicosis in children. *J Pediatr* 1969; 4:142.

54. Mackin JF, Canary JJ, Pittman CS: Thyroid storm and its management. *N Engl J Med* 1974; 291:1396.

55. Galaburda M, Rosman NP, Haddow JE: Thyroid storm in an 11-year-old boy managed by propranolol. *Pediatrics* 1974; 53:920.

56. Hollingsworth DR, Mabry CC: Congenital Graves' disease. *Am J Dis Child* 1976; 130:148.

57. Smallridge RC, et al: Neonatal thyrotoxicosis: Alterations in serum concentrations of lats-protector, T_4, T_3, reverse T_3, and $3,3'T_2$. *J Pediatr* 1978; 93:118.

58. Smith CS, Howard NJ: Propranolol in treatment of neonatal thyrotoxicosis. *J Pediatr* 1973; 83:1046.

59. Trowbridge FL, et al: Iodine and goiter in children. *Pediatrics* 1975; 56:82.

60. Hung W, et al: Clinical, laboratory, and histologic observations in euthyroid children and adolescents with goiters. *J Pediatr* 1973; 82:10.

61. Loeb PB, Drash AL, Kenny FM: Prevalence of low titer and "negative" antithyroglobulin antibodies in biopsy-proved juvenile Hashimoto's thyroiditis. *J Pediatr* 1973; 82:17.

62. Monteleone JA, et al: Differentiation of chronic lymphocytic thyroiditis and simple goiter in pediatrics. *J Pediatr* 1973; 83:381.

63. Hopwood NJ, et al: Thyroid antibodies in children and adolescents with thyroid disorders. *J Pediatr* 1978; 93:57.

64. Rojeski MT, Gharib H: Nodular thyroid disease: Evaluation and management. *N Engl J Med* 1985; 313:428.

65. Rallison ML, et al: Occurrence and natural history of chronic lymphocytic thyroiditis in childhood. *J Pediatr* 1975; 86:675.

66. Papopetrou PD, et al: Long-term treatment of Hashimoto's thyroiditis with thyroxine. *Lancet* 1972; 1:1045.

67. Molitch ME, et al: The cold thyroid nodule: An analysis of diagnostic and therapeutic options. *Endocr Rev* 1984; 5:185.

68. Harness JK, Thompson NW, Nishiyama RN: Childhood thyroid carcinoma. *Arch Surg* 1971; 102:278.

69. Brown RS, et al: The syndrome of multiple mucosal neuromas and medullary thyroid carcinoma in childhood. *J Pediatr* 1975; 86:77.

Hypothyroidism

Hypothyroidism in children is traditionally divided into (1) congenital hypothyroidism (cretinism) and (2) acquired hypothyroidism, although the same etiologic factors may cause either type. Thyroid deficiency in cretinism is present at birth, but clinical manifestations do not always become obvious for several months and occasionally are overlooked for years. Acquired hypothyroidism usually refers to thyroid deficiency becoming apparent after the age of 2 years, although the defect may be congenital. The distinction between congenital and acquired hypothyroidism is useful because of the difference in prognosis and clinical expression, but it should be recognized that the classification is somewhat artificial and that there is no clear separation in terms of etiology or age at onset.

CONGENITAL HYPOTHYROIDISM (CRETINISM)

Incidence and Etiology

Data on the frequency of congenital hypothyroidism until recently were difficult to obtain, partly because the diagnosis rarely was made in the immediate neonatal period. With the initiation of neonatal screening programs within the past 10 years, it is now clear that the incidence of congenital hypothyroidism is one in 3,500 to 4,500 live births.[1-3]

At one time it was thought that most cases of congenital hypothyroidism reflected primary failure of the thyroid gland to develop (athyreosis). More recently, radioactive iodine or technetium 99m (^{99m}Tc) scans of many of these infants have demonstrated the presence of thyroid tissue at a high ectopic site (cryptothyroidism), especially when oblique and lateral projections are obtained.[4-5] Preliminary reports of the use of ultrasound in imagining the thyroid of neonates with hypothyroidism are beginning to appear, and may offer an alternative to radionuclide imaging in the future.[8–10]

From a population of 127 infants with congenital hypothyroidism detected by screening programs in whom scans were obtained, ectopic thyroid tissue was documented in 23%, aplastic or hypoplastic glands were present in 63%, and normal or enlarged thyroid glands in 14%.[3] Routine examination of the throat occasionally reveals a lingual thyroid at the base of the tongue. These aberrant glands are functionally inadequate and produce insufficient hormone to meet physiologic requirements.

Metabolic blocks within the thyroid gland cause clinical hypothyroidism by interfering with synthesis of hormone. At least five separate defects have been recognized (Fig 6–1), presumably the result of enzymatic deficiencies. These are relatively infrequent causes of cretinism,[11] but recognition is important because inheritance appears to be on an autosomal recessive basis, with an average of 25% of a sibship affected.[12] By contrast, most cases of athyreosis or maldescent occur sporadically, although a mild familial tendency exists.[13]

Transient hypothyroidism in the neonate may occur as a result of maternal ingestion of excessive amounts of iodide or thiourea derivatives, for example, propylthiouracil, which cross the placenta readily and block thyroid synthesis in the fetal gland, often producing goiter.[14] Adequate maternal iodine stores also are necessary for fetal thyroid production in utero. However, the fetus does not depend upon a euthyroid state in the mother for normal thyroid development or function, which occurs by the 2nd or 3rd month of gestation. Thus, a woman with hypothyroidism, if she is able to conceive and maintain the pregnancy, should be expected to deliver an infant with a normal hypothalamic-pituitary-thyroid axis. Thyroid hormones cross transplacentally to the fetus very poorly, so it is not possible to prevent congenital hypothyroidism by administration of thyroid hormone to the expectant mother.[14]

Iodide-induced transient hypothyroidism in the newborn may also be the result of iodine exposure of the mother during pregnancy or during lactation,[15] of the fetus during amniofetography,[16] or of the infant to iodine topically post-natally.[17] Other drugs administered to the pregnant mother which may cross the placenta and result in hypothyroidism in the neonate include potassium perchlorate, lithium, cobalt-containing drugs, and aminoglutethimide.[18]

Transient hypothyroidism may also result from transplacental thyrotropin-binding inhibitory immunoglobulins (TBII).[19, 20] Goiter is absent, probably because thyroid-stimulating hormone (TSH) receptor blockade during gestation may prevent compensatory hypertrophy of the infant's thyroid gland. Although perhaps an uncommon condition, this disorder might be suspected in infants whose mothers have a history of autoimmune thyroid disease, or in instances where multiple siblings have been affected. Availability of measurement of TBII is becoming more common, and with more experience, the incidence of the disorder may rise. Therapy with L-thyroxine should extend at least to 2 to 3 years, but all infants may not need lifelong replacement.

Hypothyroidism secondary to lack of TSH is rare in infancy and invariably

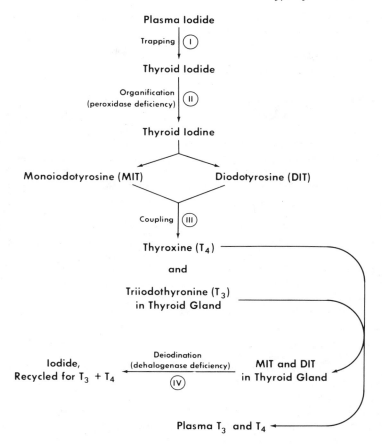

Plasma Iodide

Trapping

Thyroid Iodide

Organification
(peroxidase deficiency)

Thyroid Iodine

Monoiodotyrosine (MIT)   Diodotyrosine (DIT)

Coupling

Thyroxine (T$_4$)

and

Triiodothyronine (T$_3$)
in Thyroid Gland

Iodide,   Deiodination
Recycled for T$_3$ + T$_4$ (dehalogenase deficiency)   MIT and DIT
                                                            in Thyroid Gland

Plasma T$_3$ and T$_4$

FIG 6–1.
Enzymatic deficiencies in hypothryoidism. Sites of enzymatic defects causing hypothyroidism
are indicated by *roman numerals.* A fifth metabolic error, not illustrated, results in the formation
of abnormal iodinated proteins.

is associated with deficiency of other pituitary hormones. Of one million infants
screened for congenital hypothyroidism as of 1978, ten (incidence of one in
68,000) were suspected to have secondary hypothyroidism or TSH deficiency.[3]
As more experience with screening programs has developed, the incidence (1
in 29,000) is increasing,[21] and may be even higher because most screening programs direct their goals at detection of primary hypothyroidism. If a TSH deficiency is suspected, it is important that the infant have a thorough pituitary
evaluation because hypopituitarism in infancy can be life-threatening. The presence of micropenis, frontal bossing of the skull, and/or hypoglycemia should

make the clinician suspicious that hypopituitarism might be the cause of the infant's thyroid deficiency.

Neonatal Thyroid Screening

Because congenital hypothyroidism is one of the more common preventable causes of mental retardation if treatment is initiated early,[22] screening programs have been developed in many locations for earlier detection of affected infants. It has been determined that these programs are effective and practical when blood specimens are obtained by heel stick filter-paper blood spot at the same time phenylketonuria screening is performed.[1] Experience has shown that measurement of serum thyroxine (T_4) alone is inadequate as a screening procedure for congenital hypothyroidism, as the false positive rate of 2% to 3% is too high. Therefore, the most practical method for large screening programs at this time combines a filter paper T_4 level with a filter paper blood spot TSH where T_4 levels are low.[1] This combination aids in identification of not only infants with primary hypothyroidism, but also those infants with possible secondary hypothyroidism and thyroid-binding globulin (TBG) deficiency. Because the combination of T_4 with "backup" TSH may fail to detect infants with normal T_4 and elevated TSH (i.e., early decompensation of thyroid function), other clinics have advocated a combination of T_4 and TSH screening on a larger population of infants[3] or use of TSH screening alone when detection of primary hypothyroidism is the major goal.[23]

A high percentage of preterm and stressed infants may have lower serum T_4 and T_3 concentrations than full term healthy neonates.[24-29] The hypothyroxinemia is usually accompanied by a normal TSH level, resulting in a "positive" newborn screen. With time the majority of infants recover from this low T_4 state, although one must remember that the possibility of secondary hypothyroidism exists, necessitating careful clinical assessment of the individual infant in question. It is possible that these thyroid alterations are temporary and might even be beneficial for improved survival during this stressful period.[30] As clinical trials of L-thyroxine therapy to these sick preterm infants have not shown short-term beneficial effects,[31] and the potential that therapy might be harmful exists, treatment of these sick infants is seldom justified.[1]

Clinical Presentation

A list of clinical features found in a group of 49 hypothyroid infants by the age of 6 months at the University of Michigan is presented in Table 6–1.[32] Strabismus, another frequent sign, may persist in spite of adequate treatment; it is probably neurologic rather than muscular in origin.

These signs taken individually are relatively nonspecific, but it may be seen from Table 6–1 that they occur with considerably more frequency in infants with hypothyroidism than in healthy babies. It also is true that these features are less prominent in younger infants, but the astute observer will be able to make a

TABLE 6–1.
Features of Infants With Congenital Hypothyroidism Diagnosed Clinically and by Newborn Screening

Clinical Features	Cretinism* (n = 49)	Congenital Hypothyroidism† (n = 87)	Normal (n = 100)
Lethargy	96	31	0
Constipation	92	29	2
Feeding problems or failure to gain	83	22	5
Respiratory problems	76	NA	6
Dry skin	76	13	1
Thick tongue	67	26	0
Hoarse voice or cry	67	21	0
Umbilical hernia	67	32	8
Prolonged icterus neonatarum	12	34	0
Goiter	8	NA	0

Incidence (%) column spans Cretinism, Congenital Hypothyroidism, Normal.

NA = not available.
* Cretinism diagnosed clinically in first 6 months of life.
† Congenital hypothyroidism detected by Northwest Screening Program (Lowrey GH, et al: *Postgrad Med* 1960; 27:33).

tentative diagnosis by the age of 3 months, or earlier in some cases. For example, constipation, prolonged jaundice or cyanosis, lethargy, and failure to gain weight may be apparent within a few weeks or less.[33] Delayed closure of fontanelles is common in congenital hypothyroidism. The average size of the anterior and posterior fontanelle in affected infants is larger than in healthy infants.[34] A posterior fontanelle opening greater than 0.5 cm in diameter should arouse suspicion of hypothyroidism, as 97% of normal newborns have a smaller posterior fontanelle.[35]

From experience with hypothyroid screening programs, there is now evidence that some affected infants have subtle indications of hypothyroidism in the newborn period, before signs and symptoms become obvious clinically. Of 277 cases thus detected, only eight had been clinically suspected.[3] Such features included hypothermia, hypoactivity, edema, peripheral cyanosis, mottling of the skin, abdominal distention, lag in stooling, respiratory difficulties, and polycythemia.[33, 36–38]

In patients with athyreosis or cryptothyroidism, no thyroid tissue is felt on physical examination. (Likewise, it may be difficult to palpate the gland in healthy infants.) A goiter is present in cases of hypothyroidism resulting from maternal ingestion of goitrogens. Enzymatic defects result in thyroid enlargement, but this may not be noticeable until later infancy or childhood.

Physiologic Changes in Thyroid Function During Early Life

During the first trimester of gestation, fetal serum T_4 is present in low concentrations, which progressively rise after the 18th to 20th week of gestation until term, at which time the mean level of serum T_4 is about 11.0 $\mu g/dL$.[39, 40] Likewise, serum triiodothyronine (T_3) is undetectable by radioimmunoassay during the first two trimesters, then gradually increases to a mean level of 45 to 50 ng/dL at term.[39–41] During fetal life T_4 is predominantly metabolized to 3,3',5' triiodothyronine (reverse T_3) rather than to T_3, as is characteristic of postnatal life.[42, 43] The biologic significance of reverse T_3 remains unclear, but it has been suggested that an increase in inactive reverse T_3 may protect the body by reducing metabolic rate.[44]

At birth, there is a rapid increase in serum TSH concentration. TSH levels in cord blood are less than 20 $\mu U/mL$. Blood levels rise rapidly to peak by 30 minutes after delivery.[45] Subsequently, there is a rapid fall by 2 hours, and TSH concentrations return to near normal levels by 48 hours after delivery. Thereafter, serum TSH remains stable with age, less than 10 $\mu U/mL$.

Serum T_4 in infants at birth is higher than adult ranges;[39, 40] premature infants have lower levels.[24–29] During the 1st week of life, serum T_4 concentrations increase further to 9.8 to 16.6 $\mu g/dL$, then gradually fall to values near, but slightly higher than, adult ranges by 6 to 8 months of age.[46] Serum T_3 levels, low at birth, rise rapidly within the first 90 minutes after delivery and change little thereafter.[47] Following birth, the T_3 resin uptake also rises during the first 2 weeks of life, then subsequently declines to stable values after the child is 2 months of age.[46]

Free thyroxine and free triiodothyronine rise quickly during the first 36 hours of life then fall to parallel declines in T_4 and T_3[39, 40]; free T_4 levels in low birth weight and sick infants are lower than in term infants, but usually above 1.0 ng/dL.[28] Normal ranges of thyroid levels have not been well established for very low birth weight infants.

Laboratory Diagnosis

Assessment of thyroid function within the first few months of life must take into consideration the dynamic changes that occur in circulating hormone concentrations. It is important to be familiar with the normal values for each test at different ages, as well as with the types of assay techniques, which vary with individual laboratories.

In the approach to an infant with clinically suspected hypothyroidism, the three most useful initial laboratory procedures are a serum thyroxine (T_4) and TSH by radioimmunoassay and bone age x-ray studies. Bone age roentgenograms are useful, as bone maturity is delayed in infants with signs or symptoms of hypothyroidism. X-ray studies of the hands are not useful before the age of 3 months, since the earliest ossification of the carpal bones does not normally occur until that time. However, roentgenograms of the knees are of value; the distal femoral epiphysis is calcified in almost all term infants, but not in infants with congenital hypothyroidism.[33]

When the serum T_4 is low, it should be repeated, along with a serum TSH.

Elevation in TSH confirms the diagnosis of primary hypothyroidism, and is especially useful in evaluation of infants with suspected hypothyroidism who have marginal T_4 levels. When the serum T_4 is low and serum TSH is within the normal range, then deficiency of TBG must be differentiated from secondary hypothyroidism (TSH deficiency). An elevated resin T_3 uptake is suggestive of TBG deficiency. The diagnosis may be confirmed by direct measurement of TBG in the blood. TBG deficiency has been diagnosed in approximately one in 9,000 infants, with low serum T_4 detected by the screening programs.[3] It is important to establish the diagnosis in these infants so that inappropriate treatment for hypothyroidism can be avoided. An infant with a low T_4 and normal serum TSH and TBG must then be evaluated for hypopituitarism, particularly if there is no history to suggest stress, illness, or prematurity, which might account for a lowered T_4 level. Because infants with TSH deficiency may also have deficiencies of growth hormone and adrenocorticotrophic hormone, determination of random growth hormone, cortisol, and fasting blood glucose concentrations may be helpful. Evaluation of the hypothalamic-pituitary axis is usually difficult in young infants and should be done by individuals experienced in performing provocative tests for growth hormone release in this age group. Thyrotropin-releasing hormone (TRH) can help differentiate between hypothalamic and pituitary dysfunction.

Other studies may be obtained in doubtful or confusing cases, but usually are not necessary for diagnosis. Determination of free T_4 level is indicated if other studies appear inconsistent. Alkaline phosphatase concentrations often are low and creatine phosphokinase high in congenital hypothyroidism, but cholesterol determinations are rarely elevated until later childhood.

A thyroid scan (^{123}I or ^{99m}TC pertechnetate) detects the presence of ectopic thyroid tissue. However, this study can be technically difficult in infancy and should be performed by experienced personnel. Scan demonstration of at least some thyroid tissue has a certain prognostic value, and is valuable to obtain when possible.

Treatment

It is wise to remember that there is always a sense of urgency in establishment of the diagnosis of congenital hypothyroidism so that therapy can be started. The symptomatic infant with hypothyroidism may be lethargic, hypotonic, and poorly responsive. These signs might also mask a concomitant diagnosis of sepsis, meningitis, or pneumonia. Therefore the infant should be thoroughly evaluated with this in mind, and thyroid replacement started as soon as diagnostic tests have been obtained.

Although desiccated thyroid has been used successfully for many years, we now prefer the synthetic preparations of T_4 because of increased uniformity of the preparation,[48] and because desiccated thyroid may contain an excessive amount of T_3. Stepwise increases in dosage are seldom necessary in infancy, since it is important to quickly prevent further brain damage, and complications such as heart failure secondary to mobilization of myxedema fluid are unlikely at this age. For this reason, it may be justifiable to start therapy immediately with the predicted maintenance dose. We generally use a single daily dose of L-thyroxine: about 10 μg/kg initially, decreasing to 4 to 6 μg/kg/day from 1 to 5 years; 3 to 5 μg/kg/day from 5 to 10 years; and 2 to 3 μg/kg/day thereafter. It is important to anticipate L-thyroxine needs with weight gain and arrange repeat testing and increasing doses, so that replacement never drops below 5 μg/kg/day during the 1st year, as this is the most important time of brain growth and maturation.

Serum T_4 and TSH are monitored; adequacy of treatment is believed to be present when the serum T_4 is in the normal or high normal range and TSH is less than 7 to 10 μU/mL, depending upon the laboratory. TSH may be difficult to suppress during the first few months after diagnosis, particularly if the infant was symptomatic when therapy was initiated.[23]

In some instances, presumably because of either immaturity of feedback to the hypothalamic-pituitary axis or because of altered pituitary threshold for feedback regulation of TSH release by T_4, the infant's TSH level may be difficult to suppress into the usual adult range in spite of high T_4 levels and euthyroid clinical state. Replacement thyroxine dose must therefore take into consideration the infant's clinical picture, and one must not be guided by TSH level alone. Although the conversion of T_4 to T_3 proceeds relatively slowly during the early phases of treatment, therapy with T_3 is seldom advised.

Overdosage in a young infant with severe hypothyroidism may not always be readily detected clinically, because central nervous system function may be altered. It is therefore important to be alert to signs of excessive thyroid hormone such as tachycardia, excessive sweating, and rapid growth, and to determine levels of serum T_4. Monitoring of serum T_3 levels is usually not necessary except where clinical signs of possible toxicity are not explained by the T_4 level. Suppression of the TSH level below assay sensitivity can indicate excessive dosage. Nonreversible advancement in osseous maturation and craniosynostosis may be complications of excessive replacement therapy.[49]

Prognosis

Linear growth and skeletal maturation respond rather dramatically to treatment with thyroid hormone. However, ultimate intellectual capacity in these children is inversely proportional to the age at which adequate therapy is begun. The growing brain, at least during the first 2 years of life, is highly dependent upon thyroid hormone for normal development.[50] If treatment is delayed beyond the age of 3 to 6 months, chances for eventual attainment of normal intelligence are poor.[22, 32, 51]

Developmental testing of infants with congenital hypothyroidism detected by newborn screening where therapy was instituted before 3 months of age has shown no difference between affected infants and normal infants at 12 months of age.[52, 53] At 18 and 36 months, affected infants had significantly lower mean scores than unaffected siblings, but still over 90% of infants achieved an IQ greater than 90 by 3 to 4 years of age.[53-55] By 6 to 7 years of age, the mean quotients were not different from the accepted norm,[53] but as a group they were less advanced in speed of motor development.[54] Although outcome by etiologic classification of their hypothyroidism did not seem to be discriminatory, a bone surface area less than 0.05 cm² correlated mostly with lower IQ scores, suggesting a longer duration of severity of thyroid deficiency in utero.[53] It will still take more years of observation of these children to determine if they will have learning difficulties in the school setting.

ACQUIRED HYPOTHYROIDISM

Etiology

Hypothyroidism occurring in later childhood (after the age of 2 years) may still be due to a congenital defect, such as an ectopic gland,[10] or an enzymatic deficiency (usually autosomal recessive), which allows production of sufficient hormone to prevent the classic signs of congenital hypothyroidism during infancy. Hypothyroidism that is truly acquired is frequently a result of Hashimoto's thyroiditis (chronic lymphocytic thyroiditis; CLT) (see Chapter 5). In some cases antibodies to other endocrine target glands develop, resulting in a polyendocrine disorder (e.g., thyroid and adrenal insufficiency).

Less common causes of hypothyroidism beyond infancy include iodine deficiency (not all salt available commercially contains iodine) and hypopituitarism. Isolated TSH deficiency has been reported,[56] but lack of other pituitary hormones usually is demonstrated as well. It now seems likely that TSH deficiency in most patients actually is a result of a primary insufficiency of thyrotrophin-releasing hormone from the hypothalamus.[57]

Now that children who have been treated for cancer with head, neck, and spine irradiation are surviving long term, the incidence of primary thyroid insufficiency and hypothalamic TRH deficiency is increasing.[58] Although damage to growth hormone releasing factor and pituitary growth hormone release are the most common adverse long-term effects from radiation, primary, secondary, and tertiary hypothyroidism are not uncommon. Serial thyroid level monitoring of all children who received head and neck irradiation is very important.

Thyroid deficiency can occur in children with collagen disease[59] or during the course of subacute thyroiditis, and low T_4 and T_3 (by radioimmunoassay) also may be found in critically ill children (euthyroid sick syndrome).[60] Peripheral resistance to thyroid hormone is a rare condition, often familial, in which stigmata of hypothyroidism are occasionally found despite elevated levels of free T_4. However, these patients are usually clinically euthyroid, and even hyperthyroid if the resistance is primarily at the pituitary level.[61] Although the disease is congenital, diagnosis is often delayed beyond infancy.

Clinical Presentation

Signs and symptoms of acquired hypothyroidism may be much more subtle than those of congenital hypothyroidism. Many children have been referred to our clinic whose only complaint was short stature; additional evidence suggestive of hypothyroidism was obtained only on detailed history and physical examination. Clinical features other than slow growth may include a history of lethargy, increasing sleep requirement, poor school performance, cold intolerance, tendency to gain weight, and slow growth of nails and scalp hair.

On physical examination the thyroid gland may be small or not palpable, although an enlarged gland is consistent with an enzymatic defect, and a goiter with firm consistency is typical of CLT, particularly in the early stages.[62] These patients may also present with a solitary nodule.[63] The facies may appear dull and puffy. Hair is sometimes coarse and brittle. Skin may be dry and cool, the complexion sallow. Deep tendon reflexes often are within normal limits, with the exception of delayed return of the Achilles reflex. Although not entirely reliable,[64] this is one of the more useful physical features.

Precocious puberty occasionally occurs in association with hypothyroidism.[65] This could be caused by a nonspecific "overlap" stimulation of gonadotrophin release. Rarely, hypothyroidism is found in the presence of muscular hypertrophy (Kocher-Debré-Sémélaigne syndrome).[66, 67] The reason for this association is not clear. There also appears to be an increased incidence of hypothyroidism in children with slipped capital femoral epiphysis.[68]

Laboratory Diagnosis

The most important laboratory studies are those for T_4 (by radioimmunoassay) and TSH. TSH will be increased in primary hypothyroidism and is typically "low-normal" with hypothalamic-pituitary insufficiency,[69] although mildly elevated levels have been reported.[70] A high TSH concentration with normal T_4 suggests early or subclinical hypothyroidism, with the potential for the development of frank thyroid deficiency; therefore, although controversy exists, we agree that this group deserves thyroid treatment.

Measurement of T_3 resin uptake (RU) will help to rule out the possibility of TBG deficiency as a cause of decreased T_4, as it varies inversely with TBG concentration. Also, "free" T_4 will be normal in this situation. Measurement of this fraction rather than total T_4 is becoming more popular, since it minimizes the need for T_3RU or direct TBG determinations in patients with TBG abnormalities. Hypothyroidism may be associated with mild to moderate anemia[71] and hypercholesterolemia.[72] However, T_4 and TSH determinations are usually sufficient for confirmation of a diagnosis of primary hypothyroidism in the presence of clinical evidence of the disorder.

If serum TSH is *not* elevated in association with a low serum T_4 and there is no evidence of TBG deficiency, the possibility of associated hypofunction of the pituitary-adrenal axis must be investigated. Administration of thyroid hormone to a child with hypoadrenalism may result in adrenal crisis, although such occurrences admittedly are infrequent. Evaluation of pituitary-adrenal function usually is best accomplished on an inpatient basis. In a short child the possibility of growth hormone deficiency should also be investigated, but the patient must first be euthyroid to ensure reliable results (see Chapter 3).

Antithyroglobulin and antimicrosomal antibodies are frequently found in the serum of children with CLT,[73–76] and should probably be obtained in all patients with suspected or confirmed primary hypothyroidism even though their absence does not rule out this etiologic possibility. A "patchy" uptake of isotope also is consistent with CLT,[62, 75] and the diagnosis can be confirmed by biopsy; however, neither procedure is necessary in the usual case (see Chapter 5).

If a hypothyroid patient has an enlarged gland and there is no evidence for CLT, a 24-hour radioactive iodine uptake study is sometimes useful. Low values suggest an iodine trapping defect (see Fig 6–1). Elevated uptakes often are found in the other enzymatic deficiency states. The perchlorate discharge test is abnormal in patients with peroxidase deficiency, the most common type of metabolic block.[11] Radioactive iodine accumulates rapidly, but subsequent administration of potassium perchlorate causes the unconverted iodide to be discharged, resulting in a rapid decline of radioactivity over the gland. The association of congenital deafness with goiter also suggests an organification defect (Pendred's syndrome).[77] More precise identification of the enzymatic defects is not practical (or necessary) outside the research laboratory.

Response to TRH (thyrotrophin-releasing hormone) is useful in confirming a diagnosis of primary hypothyroidism in questionable cases, and sometimes in differentiating hypothalamic from pituitary hypothyroidism,[78–80] but is often of more academic than clinical value (see Appendix 5).

Bone age x-rays of the hand are indicated in children with hypothyroidism, and typically will reveal significant delay unless the condition is of very recent onset. Lateral skull x-ray may often show an enlarged cherry-shaped sella turcica in instances when the excess TSH secretion has been longstanding; however, we have not routinely obtained this study unless a visual field defect or other optical disturbance is present.[81] It has also been recently observed that many young hypothyroid girls have multiple small cysts present on pelvic ultrasound.[82] These appear to regress with thyroxine replacement.

Serum concentrations of T_4, TBG, T_3RU, T_3, reverse T_3, and TSH have been summarized for children 1 to 15 years of age.[83]

Treatment

Synthetic L-thyroxine is the treatment of choice. Enzymatic conversion to adequate amounts of T_3 occurs in vivo; therefore, we no longer use desiccated thyroid (which may contain excess T_3), or combination T_4 and T_3 preparations. Typical dose is 3 to 5 µg/kg/day from 5 to 10 years of age, and 2 to 3 µg/kg/day thereafter.[84, 85] The great majority of adults can be maintained on 0.1 to 0.2 mg daily.[86] When the predicted optimal dose has been given for 1 to 2 months, repeat T_4 and TSH determinations are obtained and the dose adjusted accordingly. Note that T_4 typically rises before TSH falls, probably due to delayed conversion of T_4 to T_3.[87] There is no need for haste in achieving the maximum dose, since irreversible brain damage does not appear to occur after about 2 or 3 years of age. Also, rapid increases may result in signs of thyrotoxicity and precipitate headache and pseudotumor cerebri. Congestive heart failure and psychotic behavior secondary to excessive treatment are rare in children.

Patients are monitored with periodic T_4 and TSH determinations, usually on a biannual basis once the maintenance dose has been established, but less often if the child remains clinically euthyroid and growth rate is good. Bone age roentgenograms may be obtained every 1 or 2 years until normal height is achieved and will help in determining remaining growth potential.

Prognosis

Treatment of acquired hypothyroidism is gratifying, since an increase in growth rate and reversal of the other clinical manifestations are apparent within several months, and the patient's normal height is typically reached within several years. However, in some adolescents who have been hypothyroid for several years, there appears to be lack of "catch-up" growth, with ultimate limitation of final adult stature.[88]

Permanent brain damage is not an expected consequence of this condition, and ultimate intellectual function usually is normal.[89] However, it is of interest that school performance sometimes appears to decline as a child progresses from docile hypothyroidism to a metabolic state which, although normal, is associated with more active behavior patterns, thereby reducing the attention span and irritating the teacher.

Hashimoto's thyroiditis occasionally resolves spontaneously.[90] Therefore, it may be justifiable to discontinue treatment at some point (e.g., when linear growth has ceased) and reevaluate metabolic status. In our experience, however, it has usually been necessary to reinstitute therapy. Likewise, as with other autoimmune disorders, recurrence is possible at any time. There also appears to be an increased incidence of thyroid cancer in patients with CLT, possibly related to increased antithyroid antibodies[91] or bombardment of the gland with excess TSH, although this is only speculation.

Pseudotumor cerebri has been reported during the initial phases of treatment in severely hypothyroid children,[92] and premature craniosynostosis,[49] as well as rapid advance of bone age, can result from excessively vigorous therapy, as noted in the section on congenital hypothyroidism.

REFERENCES

1. Newborn Screening for Congenital Hypothyroidism: Recommended guidelines. Committees of the American Academy of Pediatrics and American Thyroid Association. *Pediatrics* 1987; 80:745.
2. LaFranchi SH, et al: Neonatal hypothyroidism detected by the Northwest Regional Screening Program. *Pediatrics* 1979; 63:180.

3. Fisher DA, et al: Screening for congenital hypothyroidism: Results of screening one million North American infants. *J Pediatr* 1979; 94:700.
4. Wells RG, Sty JR, Duck SC: Technetium 99m pertechnetate thyroid scintigraphy: Congenital hypothyroid screening. *Pediatr Radiol* 1986; 16:368.
5. Heyman S, Crisler JF Jr, Treves S: Congenital hypothyroidism: I. Thyroidal uptake and scintigraphy. *J Pediatr* 1982; 101:571.
6. O'Connor MK, Freyne PJ, Cullen MJ: Low dose radioisotope scanning and quantitative analysis in the diagnosis of congenital hypothyroidism. *Arch Dis Child* 1982; 57:490.
7. Schoen EJ, dos Remedios LV, Backstrom M: Heterogeneity of congenital hypothyroidism: The importance of thyroid scintigraphy. *J Perinat Med* 1987; 15:137.
8. Bachrach LK, Daneman D, Daneman A, Martin DJ: Use of ultrasound in childhood thyroid disorders. *J Pediatr* 1983; 103:547.
9. Dammacco F, et al: Serum thyroglobulin and thyroid ultrasound studies in infants with congenital hypothyroidism. *J Pediatr* 1985; 106:451.
10. Miller JH: Lingual thyroid gland: Sonographic appearance. *Radiology* 1985; 156:83.
11. Carr EA, Jr, et al: The various types of thyroid malfunction in cretinism and their relative frequency. *Pediatrics* 1968; 41:113.
12. Neel JV, et al: Genetic studies on the congenitally hypothyroid. *Pediatrics* 1961; 27:269.
13. Stager J, Froesch ER: Congenital familial thyroid aplasia. *Acta Endocrinol* 1981; 96:188.
14. Cheron RG, et al: Neonatal thyroid function after propylthiouracil therapy for maternal Graves' disease. *N Engl J Med* 1981; 304:525.
15. Danziger Y, Pertzelan A, Mimouni M: Transient congenital hypothyroidism after topical iodine in pregnancy and lactation. *Arch Dis Child* 1987; 62:295.
16. Rodesh F, et al: Adverse effect of amniofetography on fetal thyroid function. *Am J Obstet Gynecol* 1976; 126:723.
17. L'Allemand D, et al: Iodine-induced alterations of thyroid function in newborn infants after prenatal and perinatal exposure to povidone iodine. *J Pediatr* 1983; 102:935.
18. McLaren EH, Alexander WD: Goitrogens. *Clin Endocrinol Metab* 1979; 8:129.
19. Connors MH, Styne DM: Transient neonatal 'athyreosis' resulting from thyrotropin-binding inhibitory immunoglobulins. *Pediatrics* 1986; 78:287.
20. Francis G, Riley W: Congenital familial transient hypothyroidism secondary to transplacental thyrotropin-blocking autoantibodies. *Am J Dis Child* 1987; 141:1081.
21. Hanna CE, et al: Detection of congenital hypopituitary hypothyroidism: Ten-year experience in The Northwest Regional Screening Program. *J Pediatr* 1986; 109:959.
22. Klein AH, Meltzer S, Kenny FM: Improved prognosis in congenital hypothyroidism treated before age three months. *J Pediatr* 1972; 81:912.
23. Foley TP, Jr, et al: Experience with primary thyrotropin (TSH) screening for congenital hypothyroidism in Pittsburgh, Pa., in Bickel, Guthrie, Hammerson (eds): *Neonatal Screening for Inborn Errors of Metabolism.* Munich Bergmann-Verlag, 1980.
24. Cuestas RA: Thyroid function in healthy premature infants. *J Pediatr* 1978; 92:963.
25. Cuestas RA, Engel RR: Thyroid function in preterm infants with respiratory distress syndrome. *J Pediatr* 1979; 94:643.
26. Uhrmann S, et al: Thyroid function in the preterm infant: A longitudinal assessment. *J Pediatr* 1978; 92:968.
27. Dussault JH, Morissette J, Laberge C: Blood thyroxine concentration is lower in low-birth-weight infants. *Clin Chem* 1979; 25:2047.
28. Wilson DM, et al: Serum free thyroxine values in term premature and sick infants. *J Pediatr* 1982; 101:113.

29. Kok JH, et al: Normal ranges of T_4 screening values in low birthweight infants. *Arch Dis Child* 1983; 58:190.
30. Klein AH, et al: Thyroid hormone and thyrotropin responses to parturition in premature infants with and without respiratory distress syndrome. *Pediatrics* 1979; 63:380.
31. Chowdhry P, et al: Results of controlled double-blind study of thyroid replacement in very low-birth-weight premature infants with hypothyroxinemia. *Pediatrics* 1987; 73:301.
32. Lowrey GH, et al: Early diagnosis and prognosis in congenital hypothyroidism. *Postgrad Med* 1960; 27:33.
33. Letarte J, LaFranchi S: Clinical features of congenital hypothyroidism, in Dussault JH, Walker P (eds): *Congenital Hypothyroidism*. New York, Marcel Dekker 1983, pp 351–383.
34. Smith DW, Popich G: Large fontanels in congenital hypothyroidism: A potential clue toward earlier recognition. *J Pediatr* 1972; 80:753.
35. Popich GA, Smith DW: Fontanels: Range of normal size. *J Pediatr* 1972; 80:749.
36. Smith DW, Klein AH, Henderson JR: Congenital hypothyroidism—Signs and symptoms in the newborn period. *J Pediatr* 1975; 87:958.
37. Klein AH, et al: Neonatal thyroid function in congenital hypothyroidism. *J Pediatr* 1976; 89:545.
38. Weinblatt ME, et al: Polycythemia in hypothyroid infants. *Am J Dis Child* 1987; 141:1121.
39. Erenberg A, et al: Total and free thyroid hormone concentrations in the neonatal period. *Pediatrics* 1974; 53:211.
40. Abuid J, et al: Total and free triiodothyronine and thyroxine in early infancy. *J Clin Endocrinol Metab* 1974; 39:263.
41. Fisher DA, et al: Serum and thyroid gland triiodothyronine in the human fetus. *J Clin Endocrinol Metab* 1973; 36:397.
42. Chopra LJ, Sack J, Fisher DA: Reverse T_3 in the fetus and newborn, in *Perinatal Thyroid Physiology and Disease*. New York, Raven Press, 1975, p 33.
43. Isaac RM, et al: Reverse triiodothyronine to triiodothyronine ratio and gestational age. *J Pediatr* 1979; 94:477.
44. Chopra IJ, et al: Reciprocal changes in serum concentrations of 3,3′,5′-triiodothyronine (reverse T_3) and 3,5′,3-triiodothyronine (T_3) in systemic illnesses. *J Clin Endocrinol Metab* 1975; 41:1043.
45. Fisher DA, Odell WD: Acute release of thyrotropin in the newborn. *J Clin Invest* 1969; 48:1670.
46. O'Halloran MT, Webster HL: Thyroid function assays in infants. *J Pediatr* 1972; 81:916.
47. Abuid J, Stinson DA, Larsen PR: Serum triiodothyronine and thyroxine in the neonate and the acute increases in these hormones following delivery. *J Clin Invest* 1973; 52:1195.
48. Stock JM, Surks MI, Oppenheimer JH: Replacement dosage of L-thyroxine in hypothyroidism: A re-evaluation. *N Engl J Med* 1974; 290:529.
49. Penfold JL, Simpson DA: Premature craniosynostosis: A complication of thyroid replacement therapy. *J Pediatr* 1975; 86:360.
50. Greenberg AH, Najjar S, Blizzard RM: Effects of thyroid hormone on growth, differentiation, and development, in *Handbook of Physiology*. Washington DC American Physiologic Society, 1974, Sect 7, Vol III.
51. Raiti S, Newns GH: Cretinism: Early diagnosis and its relation to mental prognosis. *Arch Dis Child* 1971; 46:692.

52. Gloreiux J, et al: Preliminary results on the mental development of hypothyroid infants detected by the Quebec Screening Program. *J Pediatr* 1983; 102:19.
53. Glorieux J, et al: Follow-up at ages 5 and 7 years on mental development in children with hypothyroidism detected by Quebec Screening Program. *J Pediatr* 1985; 107:913.
54. New England Congenital Hypothyroidism Collaborative. Neonatal hypothyroidism screening: Status of patients at 6 years of age. *J Pediatr* 1985; 107:915.
55. Moschini P, et al: Longitudinal assessment of children with congenital hypothyroidism detected by neonatal screening. *Helv Paediat Acta* 1986; 41:415.
56. Pittman JA: Hypopituitarism, in *The Thyroid*, ed 3. New York, Harper & Row, 1971, pp 797–806.
57. Kaplan SL, et al: Thyrotropin-releasing factor (TRF) effect on secretion of human pituitary prolactin and thyrotropin in children and in idiopathic hypopituitary dwarfism: Further evidence for hypophysiotropic hormone deficiencies. *J Clin Endocrinol Metab* 1972; 35:825.
58. Pasqualini T, et al: Long-term endocrine sequelae after surgery, radiotherapy and chemotherapy in children with medulloblastoma. *Cancer* 1987; 59:801.
59. Richards GE, Pachman LM, Green OC: Symptomatic hypothyroidism in children with collagen disease. *J Pediatr* 1975; 87:82.
60. Zucker AR, et al: Thyroid function in critically ill children. *J Pediatr* 1985; 107:552.
61. Pagliara AS, et al: Peripheral resistance to thyroid hormone in a family: Heterogeneity of clinical presentation. *J Pediatr* 1983; 103:228.
62. Fisher DA, et al: The diagnosis of Hashimoto's thyroiditis. *J Clin Endocrinol Metab* 1975; 40:795.
63. Bialas P, et al: Hashimoto's thyroiditis presenting as a solitary functioning thyroid nodule. *J Clin Endocrinol Metab* 1976; 43:1365.
64. Costin G, Kaplan SA, Ling SM: The Achilles reflex in time in thyroid disorders. *J Pediatr* 1970; 76:277.
65. Costin G, et al: Prolactin activity in juvenile hypothyroidism and precocious puberty. *Pediatrics* 1972; 50:881.
66. Najjar SS: Muscular hypertrophy in hypothyroid children: The Kocher-Debre-Semelaigne syndrome, a review of 23 cases. *J Pediatr* 1974; 85:236.
67. Spiro AJ, et al: Cretinism with muscular hypertrophy (Kocher-Debre-Semelaigne syndrome). *Arch Neurol* 1970; 23:340.
68. Hirano T, et al: Association of primary hypothyroidism and slipped capital femoral epiphysis. *J Pediatr* 1978; 93:262.
69. Hayek A, Maloof F, Crawford JD: Thyrotropin behavior in thyroid disorders of childhood. *Pediatr Res* 1973; 7:28.
70. Patel YC, Burger HG: Serum thyrotropin (TSH) in pituitary and/or hypothalamic hypothyroidism: Normal or elevated basal levels and paradoxical responses to thyrotrophin-releasing hormone. *J Clin Endocrinol Metab* 1973; 37:190.
71. Chu J, et al: Anemia in children and adolescents with hypothyroidism. *Clin Pediatr* 1981; 20:696.
72. Kutty KM, Bryant DG, and Farid NR: Serum lipids in hypothyroidism—a re-evaluation. *J Clin Endocrinol Metab* 1978; 46:55.
73. Vallotton MB, Pretell JY, Forbes AP: Distinction between idiopathic primary myxedema and secondary pituitary hypothyroidism by the presence of circulating thyroid antibodies. *J Clin Endocrinol Metab* 1967; 27:1.
74. Hopwood NJ, et al: Thyroid antibodies in children and adolescents with thyroid disorders. *J Pediatr* 1978; 93:57.

75. Rallison ML, et al: Occurrence and natural history of chronic lymphocytic thyroiditis in childhood. *J Pediatr* 1975; 86:675.

76. Hayashi Y, et al: A long term clinical, immunological, and histological follow-up study of patients with goitrous chronic lymphocytic thyroiditis. *J Clin Endocrinol Metab* 1985; 61:1172.

77. Fraser GR: The association of congenital deafness with goiter (Pendred's syndrome). A study of 207 families. *Ann Hum Genet* 1965; 28:201.

78. Haigler ED, Jr, Hershman JM, Pittman JA, Jr: Response to orally administered synthetic thyrotrophin-releasing hormone in man. *J Clin Endocrinol Metab* 1972; 35:631.

79. Hershman JM: Clinical application of thyrotrophin-releasing hormone. *N Engl J Med* 1974; 290:886.

80. Bastenie PA, Bonnyns M, Vanhaelst L: Grades of subclinical hypothyroidism in asymptomatic autoimmune thyroiditis revealed by the thyrotrophin-releasing hormone test. *J Clin Endocrinol Metab* 1980; 51:163.

81. Yamamoto K, et al: Visual field defects and pituitary enlargement in primary hypothyroidism. *J Clin Endocrinol Metab* 1983; 57:283.

82. Lindsay AN, Voorhess ML, MacGillivray MH: Multicystic ovaries detected by sonography in children with hypothyroidism. *Am J Dis Child* 1980; 134:588.

83. Fisher DA, et al: Serum T_4, TBG, T_3 uptake, T_3, reverse T_3 and TSH concentrations in children 1–15 years of age. *J Clin Endocrinol Metab* 1977; 45:191.

84. Rezvani I, DiGeorge AM: Reassessment of the daily dose of oral thyroxine for replacement therapy in hypothyroid children. *J Pediatr* 1977; 90:291.

85. Abbassi V, Aldige C: Evaluation of sodium L-thyroxine (T_4) requirement in replacement therapy of hypothyroidism. *J Pediatr* 1977; 90:298.

86. Stock JM, Surks MI, Oppenheimer JH: Replacement dosage of L-thyroxine in hypothyroidism. *N Engl J Med* 1974; 290:529.

87. Maeda M, et al: Changes in serum triiodothyronine, thyroxine, and thyrotropin during treatment with thyroxine in severe primary hypothyroidism. *J Clin Endocrinol Metab* 1976; 43:10.

88. Rivkees SA, Bode HH, Crawford JD: Long-term growth in juvenile hypothyroidism: The failure to achieve normal adult stature. *N Engl J Med* 1988; 318:599.

89. Smith DW, Blizzard RM, Wilkins L: The mental prognosis in hypothyroidism of infancy and childhood: A review of 128 cases. *Pediatrics* 1957; 19:1011.

90. Mäenpää J, et al: Natural course of juvenile autoimmune thyroiditis. *J Pediatr* 1985; 107:898.

91. Mauras N, Zimmerman D, Goellner JR: Hashimoto thyroiditis associated with thyroid cancer in adolescent patients. *J Pediatr* 1985; 106:895.

92. McVie R: Abnormal TSH regulation, pseudotumor cerebri, and empty sella after replacement therapy in juvenile hypothyroidism. *J Pediatr* 1984; 105:768.

7

Abnormal Adrenal Function

ADRENAL PHYSIOLOGY

The adrenal gland consists of the cortex and a centrally located medulla. The medulla secretes the catecholamines: epinephrine, norepinephrine, and dopamine. The cortex consists of three layers: the outermost glomerulosa, the fasciculata, and the reticularis adjacent to the medulla. Mineralocorticoids are secreted by the glomerulosa, and glucocorticoids and androgens by the inner two layers; estrogens are also formed, probably by the extra-adrenal conversion of androgens.

The secretion of glucocorticoids and androgens is under the control of adrenocorticotropin (ACTH) from the anterior pituitary, which in turn responds to a hypothalamic hormone, corticotrophin releasing factor (CRF). The CRF-ACTH system is stimulated by deficiency of cortisol (negative feedback), but also by stress. The secretion of the mineralocorticoids, on the other hand, is regulated primarily by the renin-angiotensin system, but ACTH and the serum concentrations of sodium and potassium also exert some influence.

The hypothalamic-pituitary-adrenal axis becomes functional early in intra-uterine life; there is evidence that cortisol is secreted by 10 to 18 weeks of gestation.[1, 2] The fetal adrenal gland is very large (10 to 20 times) relative to body weight, compared with the adult gland, primarily because of the extensive fetal zone.[3] This layer involutes postnatally, leaving the three distinct cortical areas found in older infants and children. It is probable that the fetal zone is responsible for the substantial secretion of adrenal androgens, reflected by increased urinary 17-ketosteroids, during the first few days after birth.

The cortisol production rate (CPR) throughout life correlates best with body

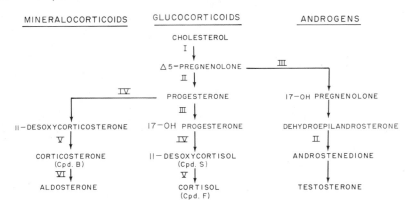

FIG 7–1.
Enzymatic deficiencies in congenital adrenal hyperplasia. Enzyme deficiency: *I* = cholesterol (20, 22) desmolase; *II* = 3-β-*ol*-dehydrogenase; *III* = 17-hydroxylase; *IV* = 21-hydroxylase; *V* = 11-hydroxylase; *VI* = 18-"oxidation" defect; *Cpd* = compound.

surface area. During the first few weeks after birth, the CPR is approximately 20 mg/M²/day; thereafter the average rate is about 12 mg/M²/day, although with some individual variation.[4] The CPR must be known when calculating replacement therapy or prescribing pharmacologic treatment with glucocorticoids.

CONGENITAL ADRENAL HYPERPLASIA

Classification and Description

Five types of congenital adrenal hyperplasia (CAH) have been recognized (Fig 7–1), each due to a specific enzymatic deficiency in the adrenal gland that prevents the synthesis of adequate amounts of cortisol.[5] A sixth type, a defect in 18-"oxidation" that does not cause cortisol deficiency, also has been described (see Hypoadrenocorticism). Sexual ambiguity is a frequent feature of this complex entity. Genetic females are typically masculinized in both 21-hydroxylase and 11-hydroxylase CAH, but in the other varieties (except 18-oxidation), it is the males who generally either have ambiguous genitalia or fail to virilize at all. The improved understanding of the pathophysiology, genetics, and spectrum of clinical and laboratory presentation in CAH that has occurred during the past decade has resulted in modification of many previously held tenets.

21-Hydroxylase deficiency (21-OHD) is by far the most common type of CAH,[6] accounting for more than 95% of all cases at our clinic. Approximately 50% of these patients have salt-losing (SL) CAH. The SL variety appears to be partly the result of a deficiency of aldosterone (21-OHD in the mineralocorticord pathway) or of relative overproduction of 18-hydroxycorticosterone as compared with aldosterone.[7] In addition, there is evidence for the secretion of an antimineralo-corticord substance,[8] possibly progesterone, 17-hydroxyprogesterone (17-OHP), or angiotensin II,[7] which might explain the apparent paradox of increased aldosterone concentrations found in some salt losers. It has generally been thought that the difference between SL and non-salt-losing (NSL) CAH is quantitative rather than qualitative and based on the severity of the metabolic block. This is consistent with the finding of increased plasma renin activity (PRA) in some clinically NSL patients with normal concentrations of serum sodium and potassium.[7] On the other hand, HLA typing has revealed a strong association of SL and NSL with different alleles, B47 and B5, respectively, consistent with a genetic difference between the two types.[9]

Lack of the 21-hydroxylase enzyme prevents the formation of adequate amounts of 11-deoxycortisol (compound S) and ultimately of cortisol (compound F). An increase in ACTH from the pituitary occurs in response to cortisol deficiency. Enhanced adrenal activity is manifested by increased production of the adrenal androgens, since this pathway is not affected by the enzymatic block. Some testosterone also is formed as a metabolite of these relatively weak adrenal androgens. Clinically, female infants are born with genitalia that are masculinized to varying degrees.[10] In mild cases, only clitoral hypertrophy is present, whereas the most severely affected infants have marked clitoromegaly simulating a male phallus with penile urethra, and the labia have a scrotal appearance.[11] Lack of palpable testes should alert the physician to the possibility that the infant may be female.

More commonly the genitalia are masculinized to an intermediate degree, manifested by a moderately enlarged clitoris, the urethral opening being at the base, and rugated labia. In many cases a urogenital sinus is present. The genitalia are sometimes hyperpigmented, but otherwise the sexual ambiguity of CAH cannot be differentiated from that of other types of hermaphroditism without laboratory studies.

Boys with 21-OHD may have slightly enlarged, hyperpigmented genitalia at birth, but the disorder is frequently undiagnosed until the child is several years of age, when excessive masculinization and increased somatic growth are obvious. Bone age (BA) at the time of diagnosis usually is advanced, thereby compromising ultimate height. The SL variety of 21-OHD is manifested in the first week or two of life by vomiting and dehydration, associated with hyponatremia and hyperkalemia. In boys this is often the first clue to the diagnosis. Frequent vomiting sometimes leads to the erroneous conclusion that the child has pyloric stenosis.

The spectrum of 21-OHD also includes two "nonclassic" types of CAH.[5, 12, 13] One, traditionally referred to as "acquired" or "attenuated,"[14, 15] is now designated as "symptomatic" nonclassic CAH. This condition is usually identified in adolescent girls, who have acne, hirsutism, and oligomenorrhea or other menstrual abnormalities, and generally is clinically indistinguishable from polycystic ovarian disease. The "cryptic" or "asymptomatic" variety, more recently described, has been identified primarily among parents and siblings of patients with confirmed CAH on the basis of hormonal abnormalities; physical appearance is normal.[16] Both the symptomatic and asymptomatic forms are strongly associated with the B14 allele and cannot be distinguished by hormonal studies (see Diagnostic Evaluation).

The frequency of occurrence of 21-OHD varies considerably depending on geographic region. The incidence of classic 21-OHD has been estimated at 1 in 5,000 to 13,000 among various white populations.[5] Probably the highest incidence occurs in western Alaska, where 1 in 490 newborn infants has the SL variety.[17] Libber et al.[18] have estimated the frequency of symptomatic, nonclassic 21-OHD in North American white women to be approximately 1 in 2,000 if there are two B14 alleles in the HLA type and 1 in 6,000 if there is only one. The frequency of asymptomatic nonclassic 21-OHD is not known, but the figures quoted above would be significantly higher if these subjects were included.

The incidence of heterozygote carriers also varies geographically, but in North America is estimated at about 5% for symptomatic nonclassic 21-OHD and 2% for the classic SL and NSL forms.[18]

Recent studies of *11-hydroxylase deficiency* (11-OHD) have emphasized the variability of this syndrome.[19] As a result of the position of the metabolic block in the mineralocorticoid pathway, these patients have traditionally been identified as hypertensive (presumably because of increased 11-desoxycorticosterone) non–salt losers, although with cortisol deficiency and virilization as in 21-OHD. It is now recognized that in some patients hypertension may not occur until adulthood, if at all.[19, 20] Therefore it seems likely that in some children 11-OHD may have been mistakenly diagnosed as the NSL form of 21-OHD, particularly before the development of the variety of steroid assays available today. Furthermore, treated patients may actually require mineralocorticord replacement because of glucocorticord-depressed 11-desoxycorticosterone superimposed on the underlying deficiency of aldosterone.[21, 22] Paradoxically, salt wasting may even occur, for unknown reasons, prior to therapy in these patients.[19]

In *17-hydroxylase deficiency* (17-OHD)[23–25] the position of the enzymatic block prevents adequate formation of androgens as well as cortisol. Girls with this syndrome have normal genitalia but do not menstruate. Boys may have ambiguous sex (male pseudohermaphroditism) or may be phenotypic females, mimicking the testicular feminization syndrome. Because only the mineralocorticoid pathway remains open in 17-OHD, increased ACTH secretion causes hypertension and hypokalemic acidosis. The diagnosis has been made in the newborn period,[26] but typically not until later in childhood or adolescence.

Early reports of *3β-hydroxysteroid dehydrogenase deficiency* described a frequently fatal condition with severe reduction of both cortisol and mineralocorticoid.[27, 28] Since then, the heterogencity of this disorder has become apparent. In the classic form, female infants are normal or only mildly masculinized, whereas males may have ambiguous genitalia because of the block in the androgen pathway. A partial form, with evidence of increasing enzymatic activity with advancing age, was described by Kenny et al. in 1971.[29] Variants now include (1) a mild enzymatic deficiency in which genetic girls do not have ambiguous genitalia and the disorder is not recognized until puberty, when there is hirsutism sometimes associated with clitoromegaly or menstrual irregularities[30, 31]; (2) an NSL form[32]; and (3) a variety in which boys have normal pubertal development, suggesting a defect in the glucocorticoid (C-21) but not in the androgen (C-19) pathway.[33]

In cholesterol desmolase deficiency[34] (also known as 20,22-desmolase deficiency or congenital lipoid adrenal hyperplasia), androgenization of genetic males does not occur, and the outcome may be fatal. However Hauffe et al.[34] described a phenotypic female who was doing well with therapy at age 18 years, when the report was published.

Diagnostic Evaluation

21-Hydroxylase Deficiency

This form should be strongly suspected in any infant with ambiguous genitalia, keeping in mind the varying degrees of expression in genetic females. Vomiting, diarrhea, or failure to gain weight should suggest the possibility of SL CAH in a male infant. Non-salt-losing males appear normal at birth except for hyperpigmentation (particularly of the nipples and genital area) or slight penile enlargement, but neither are constant features. As a result, the diagnosis in NSL boys is typically not suspected during infancy. However, neonatal screening via filter paper technique is feasible,[35] as is prenatal diagnosis[36]; both tests may become more widely used in the future.

Now that considerable experience has been gained with techniques for the measurement of appropriate steroids in serum, assay of 24-hour urinary concentrations of 17-ketosteroids or pregnanetriol is no longer necessary for detection of 21-OHD. Determination of serum 17-OHP is a dependable procedure, at least by the time the child is 2 or 3 days old.[37] Elevation of 17-OHP in cord blood may also be diagnostic,[35] but it should be noted that results must be interpreted cautiously in view of the large amount of this hormone normally produced by the fetoplacental unit. Increased levels of Δ^4-androstenedione or testosterone help to support the diagnosis in the newborn infant.

Random hormone concentrations in the nonclassic forms of CAH may be in the normal range, in which case diagnosis depends on the increase in 17-OHP after administration of synthetic ACTH (Cortrosyn); however, there is no quantitative difference between the acquired and cryptic types.[16] The increase of 17-OHP or 17-OHP-cortisol ratio is less pronounced in heterozygote carriers, and there is some overlap with the normal population.[16, 38–40]

Salt-losing 21-OHD is associated with low serum sodium and high potassium values. These abnormalities typically are present by the age of 1 week, but occasionally do not become apparent for several weeks. A more sensitive test is the estimation of PRA, which may be elevated even when serum sodium and potassium are normal.[7] Blood glucose concentration should be determined, but usually is normal. This is probably related to the discovery that patients with CAH may actually produce normal amounts of cortisol (but an excess of precursors) once the gland has hypertrophied.[41]

Infants with sexual ambiguity, including those with only mild clitoral hypertrophy, should have a chromosome count to establish the genetic sex. (A buccal smear will yield more rapid but less reliable information.) It is recommended that karyotyping also be performed in infants with laboratory evidence of CAH who appear to be males, because gross masculinization is possible in genetic females.[11] However, the presence of palpable gonads in the scrotum essentially eliminates the possibility of an XX karyotype in a patient with CAH.

Other useful studies in the infant with ambiguous genitalia include a retrograde urogram and pelvic ultrasonography to confirm the identity of the internal sexual structures (which are female in typical 21-OHD) and the presence or absence of a urogenital sinus.[42] Skeletal maturation is advanced in children with untreated CAH except in the neonatal period. Therefore BA films are of no diagnostic value at this time.

Summary of Diagnostic Procedures

Recommended studies in infants with possible 21-OHD include:
1. Serum 17-OHP and Δ^4-androstenedione.
2. Serum electrolytes and PRA.
3. Chromosome count and (?)buccal smear.
4. Retrograde urogram and pelvic ultrasonography.

Other Types of Congenital Adrenal Hyperplasia

Diagnosis of other forms of CAH may be suspected on clinical grounds, for example, hypertension (if present) in 11-OHD and 17-OHD and ambiguity of genetic males in 17-OHD and 3β-hydroxysteroid dehydrogenase deficiency. However, confirmation depends on elevation of the precursors immediately before the enzymatic blocks (e.g., increased 11-desoxycortisol in 11-OHD) or ratios of the pre- vs. postblock steroids. These studies generally are performed in specialized laboratories and require interpretation by experienced endocrinologists.

Treatment

This section on treatment of CAH, and the following section on prognosis refer primarily to 21-OHD, which has been the basis for most of the clinical studies, and to 11-OHD.

Initial Medical Management

Infants with SL CAH often are dehydrated. This is particularly true in boys, because the diagnosis may be delayed. Intravenous fluids consist primarily of normal saline solution or 0.45% saline solution with sodium bicarbonate, in the presence of hyperchloremic acidosis. Mineralocorticoid can be supplied as fludrocortisone (Florinef), 0.1 to 0.3 mg/day orally, or desoxycorticosterone acetate (Doca), 1 to 3 mg/day intramuscularly. Dose depends partly on whether supplemental sodium chloride (0.5 to 2 g/day) is used.

Treatment with glucocorticoids (which should not be initiated until blood for diagnostic laboratory studies has been drawn) serves the dual purpose of replacing cortisol and suppressing excessive ACTH production. An appropriate initial dose of hydrocortisone is 20 to 25 mg/m²/day (orally, intramuscularly, or intravenously) in three to four divided doses.

Mineralocorticoids also have some glucocorticoid activity (e.g., 0.1 mg of fludrocortisone is the equivalent of 1.5 mg of hydrocortisone). If this fact is not taken into consideration in calculating the dose of glucocorticoid, it is probable that some degree of overtreatment will occur during the first few weeks of life when the dose of mineralocorticoid may be relatively high. Elevated serum potassium levels usually can be corrected by replacement of sodium and mineralocorticoid, obviating the need for hypokalemic agents.

Children with NSL CAH do not require emergency care and are simply treated with a glucocorticoid preparation and possibly mineralocorticoid as well (see the following section).

Chronic Medical Management

High initial doses of fludrocortisone acetate in SL CAH usually can be reduced over a period of several weeks to 0.1 mg or at most 0.2 mg daily, even in the absence of salt supplements. This amount is satisfactory for patients of all ages.

It has been suggested that mineralocorticoid in CAH can be discontinued during adolescence or even earlier, on the assumption that older children are able to recognize the need for added dietary salt. Also, Limal et al. demonstrated an increased secretion of aldosterone during or near the time of puberty, and noted that this might partly explain the ability of some older children with SL CAH to remain clinically well without mineralocorticoid.[43] However, adrenal crises sometimes occurred in these circumstances. In addition, increased PRA has been reported in patients who were thought to be receiving adequate mineralocorticoid because they had normal serum concentrations of sodium and potassium.[44] Control, as judged by serum 17-hydroxyprogesterone (17-OHP) levels, improved when the dose of salt-retaining hormone was increased without any change in glucocorticoid. It was postulated that chronic sodium depletion can actually stimulate ACTH production, with a resultant increase in 17-OHP. Furthermore, as noted earlier,[7] PRA may be increased even in the NSL form of 21-OHD, and in addition the elevation of angiotensin that occurs during sodium depletion in these patients also appears to contribute to increased 17-OHP.[45] Therefore we recommend that mineralocorticoid not be discontinued in SL patients, particularly since others have now confirmed the persistence of the enzymatic block,[46] and some clinicians advocate the use of mineralocorticoids in patients who are not obvious salt losers.[7, 45]

The physiologic production rate of cortisol after the first few weeks of life is 12 mg/m²/day.[4] However, roughly twice this much given orally may be necessary to achieve adequate control of CAH. The usual replacement dose is approximately 20 to 25 mg/M²/day in at least three divided doses, but there is considerable individual variation in response to this program.[47, 48] (In fact, recommended doses of hydrocortisone have varied from 15 to 40 mg/m²/day[49, 50].) Although this requirement could be partly related to the route of administration, limited data on the intestinal absorption of steroids indicate that this process is very efficient.[51, 52] A more likely explanation might be that the hypertrophic, highly stimulatable gland disrupts the usual pituitary-adrenal feedback dynamics such that attempts at normalization of 17-OHP may result in subnormal suppression of steroidogenesis[53] and thus the inability to achieve "ideal" patterns of steroid secretion.[54]

Although hydrocortisone is traditionally administered three times a day, it is possible that this schedule does not permit effective adrenal suppression throughout a 24-hour period. We have measured serial 17-OHP concentrations in five children with CAH who were receiving hydrocortisone orally every 8 hours.[48] Simultaneous corticoid determinations provided evidence of substantial absorption of the administered hormone. In some patients, there was a definite increase in 17-OHP levels as serum corticoids declined, suggesting that this therapeutic program was not entirely adequate. In these situations, more frequent administration of the drug might permit adequate suppression with less hormone. In any case there is at least a theoretical advantage in providing the largest dose (e.g., one-half of daily amount) at bedtime in an attempt to inhibit the early morning release of ACTH,[55] although there is controversy on this point.[56]

Glucocorticoids may also be given in the form of prednisone or prednisolone, 5 to 7 mg/m²/day in two or three divided doses. These analogues afford the benefit of a relatively long half-life: about $3\frac{1}{2}$ hours for prednisolone vs. $1\frac{1}{2}$ hours for hydrocortisone[57] (prednisone is rapidly metabolized to prednisolone in vivo[58]). These preparations may be of value in selected patients not easily controlled with hydrocortisone.[59, 60] Unfortunately, there is evidence that some steroid analogues cause more growth suppression than does the naturally occurring hormone.[49, 61, 62] However, these products would be appropriate for those who have reached their final height. Even a single daily dose of dexamethasone may sometimes be satisfactory in a patient with poor compliance.

The child with CAH should be seen at intervals of 3 to 12 months, depending on age. Relatively frequent visits are appropriate during the first few years, when therapeutic errors are more likely to result in persistent abnormalities of growth, and again during adolescence. It has been our experience that steroids must often be increased rather rapidly in teenagers in order to prevent undue advancement of skeletal maturation. The efficacy of medical management is monitored by the following parameters:

1. *Measurement of height.*—Rapid linear growth and sexual maturation indicate inadequate steroid replacement. Decreased growth velocity prior to closure of epiphyses suggests excessive treatment.

2. *Skeletal maturation.*—Radiographic assessment of BA is indicated every 1 to 2 hyears, particularly in the child whose growth rate deviates from the expected pattern. Advanced skeletal maturation occurs in patients receiving insufficient steroid replacement, and retarded BA in those treated too vigorously. Ideally, BA should parallel chronological age, but discrepancies do not necessarily imply serious compromise of ultimate height, if detected early. Retarded skeletal

maturation in a short child allows the possibility of catch-up growth prior to epiphyseal fusion. Conversely, some deceleration of skeletal maturation may occur when adequate (or even excessive) treatment is instituted.[63]

3. *Measurement of serum 17-OHP and androgens.*—Steroid assays, which should be performed every 3 to 12 months, are of particular importance if growth rate and skeletal maturation suggest that therapy requires modification.

Serum 17-OHP measurements are commonly used in 21-OHD, although it must be recognized that interpretation depends partly on the interval between blood sampling and the previous steroid dose, because adrenal "escape" may occur after several hours in poorly controlled patients. However, Hughes and Winter noted a good correlation between urinary pregnanetriol, as well as other parameters of control, and the serum 17-OHP concentration at either 8:00 A.M. or noon.[44, 64] Serum Δ^4-androstenedione also appears to be an excellent index of the therapeutic response in CAH,[65] and may eventually prove to be the single most useful measurement. Adequate monitoring of 21-OHD can usually be achieved by measurement of these two steroids. We generally consider a level of 17-OHP of less than 4.0 ng/mL and a level of androstenedione of less than 3.0 ng/mL to be consistent with good control, but higher values can be accepted if linear growth and skeletal maturation are satisfactory.

Although earlier studies suggested that serum dehydroepiandrosterone sulfate concentration may be helpful in monitoring treatment (at least of the NSL form of 21-OHD) we were not able to demonstrate any elevation of this androgen in our patients, regardless of the degree of control.[60] Likewise, the relatively difficult measurement of ACTH appears to be of limited clinical value. Plasma concentrations, although characteristically elevated in 21-OHD[66] may also be normal,[53] even in untreated patients.[67]

Blood testosterone levels, however, may be a useful adjunct.[68] They are elevated in untreated and poorly controlled girls and in prepubertal boys, although the testicular contribution negates their value in pubertal males.

4. *Serum sodium and potassium.*—In children with SL 21-OHD these determinations are used to monitor the adequacy of mineralocorticoid therapy, but beyond infancy usually are needed only in patients showing clinical evidence of deficiency or excess. Maintenance of normal blood pressure is consistent with adequate replacement. The dose of fludrocortisone must be reduced if hypertension is present. Insufficient mineralocorticoid or lack of dietary salt may cause hypotension, failure to gain weight, and frequent episodes of dehydration. In the older child an increased craving for salt becomes apparent

.*Emergency Treatment*

If a child with CAH has a febrile illness, the parents are instructed to double or triple the dose of glucocorticoid and seek medical attention for treatment of the acute condition. If the patient is unable to tolerate oral medication, a physician should be contacted to administer parenteral steroids. Ideally, the parents should also be instructed in the use of an injectable preparation of hydrocortisone. A dose of 25 to 50 mg/m² may be given in emergency situations.

If an intercurrent illness is sufficiently severe to require hospitalization, or if surgery is necessary, it has been our practice to administer parenteral hydrocortisone, 50 to 100 mg/m²/day in four to six divided doses during these events, since normal individuals are able to achieve cortisol levels considerably in excess of basal concentrations during periods of maximum stress. Likewise, the following program appears satisfactory for use in preparation for surgical procedures: cortisone acetate, 100 mg/m² in three to four divided doses given at 12-hour intervals, starting 36 to 48 hours before the procedure. The last dose should be administered with the "on-call" medication. Because of the prolonged half-life of cortisone acetate, this schedule invariably provides adequate steroid coverage during operation and for at least 24 to 48 hours postoperatively.

Surgical Treatment

Boys with 21-OHD or 11-OHD require no surgical intervention. The necessity for clitorectomy in females is controversial. The enlarged clitoris may regress with adequate replacement therapy, or at least become relatively smaller in relation to general body growth. Therefore, it may be justifiable to withhold surgery in some cases, particularly in NSL patients, because a lesser degree of masculinization usually is found in these patients.[10] On the other hand, it has been our experience that the emotional trauma involved in caring for a child with an obvious genital anomaly is sufficient to warrant clitorectomy prior to discharge from the hospital or during the 1st year of life. There is evidence that sexual gratification is not compromised by this procedure,[69] but some clinics favor relocation and recession rather than amputation.[70]

Widening of the introitus in patients with a urogenital sinus is necessary to prevent urinary retention and secondary urologic problems. This can be accomplished when the clitorectomy is performed. Further revision of the vaginal orifice to allow adequate sexual function can be performed by the age of 4 to 8 years, but more appropriately after the pubertal changes have occurred. Pelvic ultrasonography can be utilized to determine when the uterus has reached adult size.[42]

Treatment of Other Types of Congenital Adrenal Hyperplasia

Glucocorticoids for replacement, and for suppression of ACTH, also constitute the basis of treatment for rarer forms of CAH. Mineralocorticoid will also be required for patients with deficiency of cholesterol desmolase or 3β-hydroxysteroid dehydrogenase. Surgical revision of genitalia is the same for children with 11-OHD as for 21-OHD. Genetic males with sexual ambiguity resulting from CAH should generally be raised as females following clitoral amputation and surgical creation of a vaginal vault.

Prognosis

Mortality

Adrenal crisis is the major threat to normal life expectancy. The risk is greatest in infancy, but it is minimal with adequate medical supervision and appropriate management during stress. The incidence of associated congenital anomalies in CAH is generally not greater than in the normal population,[71] although an apparent increase in the frequency of upper urinary tract abnormalities has been noted.[72] Also, there may be an increased incidence of testicular tumors in males; this is probably related to excess ACTH and possibly LH in these patients.[73] Likewise, the development of an adrenocortical tumor is a possible, but very unusual, complication.[74]

Growth

Significant compromise of ultimate height occurs when treatment is not instituted early in life.[75, 76] These children grow rapidly during early childhood as a result of excessive adrenal androgens and possibly because of increased growth hormone production as well.[77] However, advanced skeletal maturation leads to early epiphyseal closure. Delayed diagnosis is most likely to occur in boys with the NSL form of 21-OHD, since the abnormality in these children may not be recognized for several years.

Patients who are diagnosed and treated in infancy may be small during childhood, presumably as a result of excessive administration of steroid,[78] which appears to antagonize the action of growth hormone, primarily at the peripheral level. However, because steroids also retard skeletal maturation, significant catch-up growth is possible. The final height of most patients with CAH usually is within the low normal range if treatment is begun early and control is adequate.[75, 76, 79]

Sexual Development and Reproductivity

Masculinization without testicular hypertrophy occurs as a result of elevated adrenal androgens in male patients who are inadequately treated. These patients also tend to have early onset of true puberty, manifested by enlargement of testes and spermatogenesis. In fact, the onset of true puberty may be precipitated by steroid therapy in patients with adolescent skeletal maturation. It has been hypothesized that this is a result of suppression of adrenal androgens, which permits release of gonadotrophin inhibition.[80]

Female patients may have delayed or infrequent menses and relatively poor breast development, probably as a result of excessive production of adrenal androgens. It has been observed that the increased FSH responsiveness to gonadotrophin-releasing hormone (GnRH), noted in healthy girls when compared with boys, is preserved in CAH.[81] However, the high incidence of amenorrhea,[82] oligomenorrhea, and infertility in girls is probably at least partly related to abnormalities of gonadotrophin regulation.

It might be expected that gonadotrophins would be depressed in untreated or inadequately treated CAH, secondary to increased androgens. A lack of midcycle peaks of follicle-stimulating hormone (FSH) and luteinizing hormone (LH),[83] as well as a blunted peak LH response to GnRH,[84] have been reported. However, our data indicate that acute withdrawal of glucocorticoids for 3 days generally tends to cause a decrease in FSH, but an increase in LH, the net result being a decreased FSH/LH ratio.[48] Likewise, Boyar et al. found increased LH secretion during sleep in two males with untreated CAH.[85] It was hypothesized that chronically elevated adrenal androgens might conceivably stimulate the maturation of the hypothalamic-pituitary-gonadal axis. The cause of the differential modulation of FSH/LH following acute steroid withdrawal is not clear, but this response emphasizes the need for continuous good control to ensure regular menses and fertility.

Richards et al. postulated that the frequency of amenorrhea and oligomenorrhea (at least 25% in their experience) could be related to a local effect of androgens on the ovary,[86] as well as a suppressive effect at the hypothalamic-pituitary level. Of four patients studied in detail, all had improved menstrual regularity when their previous medication was replaced with a longer-acting glucocorticoid.

Information regarding the incidence of fertility in adequately treated CAH is now available. Klingensmith et al. reported that 10 of 18 women treated prior to age 20 years were able to conceive, but that none of four patients treated after that age were able to become pregnant.[75] It was not clear whether failure to conceive was due to prenatal or postnatal exposure to androgens. However, normal gestation has been reported in untreated women with only mild virilization.[87]

The question of sterility in males is not yet totally resolved. It has been suggested that fertility may be essentially normal, even in untreated patients,[88] or decreased.[89]

HYPOADRENOCORTICISM

Addison's disease refers to a chronic clinical state characterized by decreased production of glucocorticoids and mineralocorticoids. It is uncommon in children. Tuberculosis no longer is a frequent cause of Addison's disease. In most children the cause is idiopathic atrophy of the adrenal gland. Some cases may be due to an autoimmune mechanism, with production of adrenal antibodies. This is more likely to be the case in patients with polyhormonal disorders, for example, hypoparathyroidism associated with Addison's disease.[90, 91] A number of cases of *familial congenital hypoplasia* of the adrenal gland also have been described.[92]

Symptoms of chronic adrenal insufficiency in children consist of weakness, anorexia, and weight loss. Hyperpigmentation is due to excessive secretion of ACTH and melanocyte-stimulating hormone. Nausea, vomiting, diarrhea, and dehydration may occur, particularly during periods of physical stress. Hypoglycemia, hyponatremia, and hyperkalemia are useful diagnostic features, but are not always present. Alopecia and mucocutaneous candidiasis appear to occur in these patients with increased frequency. Associated disease of the central nervous system (cerebral sclerosis) has been reported.[93]

Many years ago, Engel and Margolin reported that 16 of 25 patients with Addison's disease had psychiatric symptoms of some type.[94] Our experience also suggests a high incidence of behavior, school, and emotional problems (as well as abdominal symptoms), which cannot be adequately explained on the basis of organic disease. It has been suggested that some of these disorders of mood and emotion may be related to increased secretion of endorphins and enkephalins.[95] These peptides are subunits of beta-lipoprotein, which is also the parent molecule of ACTH, and their secretion appears to decrease or increase in conjunction with ACTH. Interestingly, there has also been a report of achalasia, with associated vomiting, in a patient with ACTH unresponsiveness.[96]

Diagnosis of adrenal insufficiency depends upon demonstration of a blunted response to exogenous ACTH or Cortrosyn, a synthetic ACTH preparation (see Appendix 7). The latter hormone is preferable because administration of ACTH may be associated with anaphylactic reactions. The metyrapone test (see Appendix 7) also is abnormal in Addison's disease, but does not distinguish primary hypoadrenalism from ACTH deficiency.

Children with Addison's disease require treatment with both glucocorticoid and mineralocorticoid. The mineralocorticoid program described for patients with CAH (discussed earlier) is also suitable therapy for Addison's disease. However, the dose of glucocorticoid is often less, approximating the normal physiologic production rate of 12 mg/m²/day of hydrocortisone, since suppression of ACTH is not a requirement. Alternatively, the longer-acting analogues, including dexamethasone,[97] can be substituted for hydrocortisone in the fully grown patient. Also, the largest dose of glucocorticoid may be given in the morning in order to mimic diurnal variation, but there is no proof that this is of practical importance. As in CAH, glucocorticoids should be increased during periods of physical stress.

In spite of the deficiency of adrenal androgens, sexual maturation in boys with Addison's disease is generally only slightly delayed if at all, and male hormone replacement therapy is usually not necessary.[98]

Acute hypoadrenalism may occur in association with trauma or infection. Subsequently, adrenal calcification[99, 100] may be noted radiographically, but in the majority of cases, this is an incidental finding unrelated to adrenal hypofunction. Cardiovascular shock secondary to adrenal hemorrhage in the presence of meningococcemia (Waterhouse-Friderichsen syndrome) is a well-recognized entity, but an appropriate adrenal response has been noted in some patients.

Treatment of acute adrenal insufficiency in childhood consists of isotonic saline and intravenous cortisol, 2 mg/kg immediately and roughly 100 mg/m² intramuscularly each 24 hours in three or four divided doses thereafter, as needed.[101] The dose is decreased as the patient stabilizes and recovery of adrenal function occurs.

The mineralocorticoid activity in pharmacologic amounts of cortisol may preclude the necessity for specific salt-retaining hormones. However, in the presence of significant hyponatremia, desoxycorticosterone acetate, 1 to 2 mg/day intramuscularly, may be used.

Transient adrenal insufficiency in the newborn period may result from maternal Cushing's syndrome[102] or from maternal ingestion of steroids that cross the placenta,[103] but such cases are surprisingly rare.

Hypoadrenalism secondary to ACTH deficiency frequently occurs in patients with other evidence of hypopituitarism, for example, growth hormone deficiency (see Chapter 3), and also has been reported as an isolated defect in rare instances.[104, 105] These patients respond normally to ACTH (but not to metyrapone), although prolonged stimulation may be necessary. It is important not to overtreat patients who also have growth hormone deficiency, since further inhibition of growth will result.

Isolated hypoaldosteronism[106] is a rare form of adrenal disease resulting from an inherited defect of 18-"oxidation." Features of this condition are hyponatremia and hyperkalemia without hypoglycemia, susceptibility to rapid dehydration, low concentrations of aldosterone, and normal cortisol response to ACTH. Treatment is with mineralocorticoid. Differentiation from the syndrome of inappropriate secretion of antidiuretic hormone (SIADH) may be difficult, but aldosterone levels are not depressed in the latter condition. Also SIADH usually is characterized by normal or low serum potassium, good response to water restriction, and only marginal improvement following administration of mineralocorticoid (see Chapter 12).

In *hereditary adrenocortical unresponsiveness to ACTH*[107-110] cortisol production is diminished and does not increase normally following administration of ACTH. However, aldosterone is present in normal amounts, and hyponatremia does not occur. This condition appears to be transmitted as an autosomal (or X-linked in some cases) recessive trait. Replacement doses of glucocorticoid are necessary.

Iatrogenic adrenal insufficiency commonly occurs during and after prolonged therapy with corticosteroids. Gradual tapering of steroids is prudent if treatment has been given for more than 1 week. Dose may be reduced to physiologic levels in 2 or 3 weeks, although this sometimes can be accomplished more quickly without difficulty, particularly if close medical supervision is possible. Further reduction should take place over a period of about 1 month. However, more complex protocols for steroid withdrawal are available.[111]

Recovery of the pituitary-adrenal axis appears to be related to the dose and duration of treatment,[112] although there is not total agreement on this point.[113] Studies have shown that recovery may occur with 2 weeks (with stimulation)[114] to 9 months[115] following cessation of therapy. It is likely that considerable individual variation exists.

If a patient has received chronic steroid therapy during the previous year, it has been our practice to recommend pharmacologic doses of glucocorticoid during periods of physical stress.[116] This policy is admittedly conservative in view of the rapid recovery of the pituitary-adrenal axis that probably occurs in most children.[114]

Dosage schedules are the same as those suggested for CAH during acute illness. No treatment is necessary for minor forms of stress such as upper respiratory infection with little or no fever.

If there is doubt concerning the integrity of the pituitary-adrenal axis following chronic steroid therapy, the adrenal response to metyrapone or insulin-induced hypoglycemia may be tested. The latter is more physiologic but also constitutes more risk to the patient, particularly if adrenal insufficiency is present. A normal response to ACTH or Cortrosyn may be misleading, since it does not depend upon a functioning pituitary; however, recovery of the pituitary usually precedes that of the adrenal gland.[115] Unfortunately, a normal response to any artificial test does not guarantee the same result in a specific naturally occurring situation. In practice it is simpler and possibly safer to assume that adrenal insufficiency is present and to administer steroids as suggested above without relying upon test results. In contrast to chronic glucocorticoid therapy, complications are rare with short-term (less than 1 week) treatment.

Table 7–1 provides a detailed list of conditions associated with chronic adrenocortical insufficiency in childhood, not all of which have been discussed in the test.

CUSHING'S SYNDROME

Cushing's syndrome (hypercortisolism from any cause), except for the iatrogenic variety, is unusual in infancy and childhood.[117–119] Adrenal tumor, adenoma or carcinoma, is a relatively common cause up to the age of about 7 years. Thereafter, most cases are due to increased secretion of ACTH with secondary adrenal hyperplasia (Cushing's disease). In some patients, a pituitary tumor, usually a basophilic adenoma, is found. It is hypothesized that these in turn may arise as a result of increased hypothalamic secretion of CRF.[120] In addition, rare cases of hyperplasia associated with nonendocrine tumors such as bronchogenic carcinoma, ganglioneuroblastoma, and carcinoma of the thymus have been reported. It is probable that these tumors secrete a substance either identical to ACTH or having ACTH-like activity.

Increased secretion of glucocorticoid causes the physical abnormalities in most patients. However, an increase in androgen production may be present and dictates the degree of masculinization that occurs. Classic signs of Cushing's syndrome include increased weight associated with a redistribution of fat, resulting in "moon" facies, and truncal obesity with a "buffalo hump" appearance of the neck. Extremities usually are slender due to muscular wasting. Skin becomes thin, and striae develop. Hirsutism, acne, and hypertension are present to varying degrees. Decreased linear growth occurs in children[121] unless a preponderance of androgens is secreted. In fact, cases have been reported in which short stature was the only obvious clinical feature of Cushing's syndrome.[122, 123]

Fasting hyperglycemia and/or a diabetic glucose tolerance curve sometimes are present. Occasionally, the differential white blood cell count reveals leukocytosis and lymphopenia. Osteoporosis and retarded skeletal maturation are typical radiographic features if glucocorticoids predominate.

TABLE 7-1.
Chronic Adrenocortical Insufficiency in Childhood

Classification of Disorders

Enzymatic defects in steroidogenesis (autosomal recessive)
  Lipoid adrenal hyperplasia (cholesterol desmolase deficiency)
  3-β-*ol*-dehydrogenase
  21-Hydroxylase
    Salt losers
    Non-salt losers
  11-Hydroxylase
  17-Hydroxylase
  18-Dehydrogenase
Congenital adrenal hypoplasia
  X-linked recessive
  Autosomal recessive
  Sporadic
Adrenocorticotropin (ACTH)
  Isolated (sporadic)
  Multiple pituitary deficiencies (familial and sporadic)
  Anencephaly
Transient aldosterone deficiency in infancy (? delayed maturation of zona
  glomerulosa or mild 18-oxidation defect) (? autosomal recessive)
Adrenal insufficiency associated with central nervous system disease
  Diffuse cerebral sclerosis (X-linked recessive)
  Familial spastic paraplegia
Idiopathic adrenal insufficiency (Addison's Disease)
  Often familial with intrafamily similarity of syndromes; frequently
    associated with other hormonal deficiencies or antibodies against
    adrenal, thyroid, parathyroid, or gastric tissues
Acquired adrenal insufficiency
  Exogenous glucocorticoids
  Granulomatous disease
  Metastatic carcinoma
  Trauma
Hereditary ACTH unresponsiveness
  Autosomal recessive
  (?)X-linked recessive

The 24-hour excretion of urinary 17-hydroxysteroids is elevated, but this may not be apparent unless the results are expressed in terms of creatinine; the normal range is 2 to 6.5 mg/g of creatinine per day.[124] (Note that urinary 17-OH, but not serum cortisol, may be above normal in children with exogenous obesity, even when corrected for surface area.) Likewise, measurement of "free" urinary cortisol, if available, is more reliable than total 17-OH; even 1-hour samples (morning and late evening) appear to yield accurate diagnostic information.[125] An excess of urinary 17-ketosteroids or serum androgens in Cushing's syndrome favors the presence of an adrenal tumor.[126]

Serum cortisol levels usually are high, but the fluctuations that occur in healthy subjects[127] and in Cushing's syndrome as a result of adrenal hyperplasia[128] make interpretation difficult. For this reason, the expected late afternoon elevation of serum cortisol concentration cannot be depended upon to identify patients with adrenal hyperplasia. One report indicates that cortisol levels appear to be consistently high in the presence of adrenocortical adenoma,[129] but another states that the pattern of cortisol secretion does not discriminate between pituitary dependent or independent Cushing's syndrome.[130] Measurement of the integrated serum concentration of cortisol, for either 6 or 24 hours, may be the most precise test for the evaluation of Cushing's syndrome.[131] Plasma ACTH measurements may be helpful but are not definitive. Raux et al. found that plasma ACTH was increased in patients with ectopic ACTH secretion,[132] undetectable in those with adrenal tumors, but in the normal range in patients with bilateral adrenal hyperplasia, including those with pituitary tumors. Likewise, Boyar et al. reported that the mean ACTH level was higher in patients with Cushing's disease than in controls, but that the difference was not statistically significant.[133]

A dexamethasone suppression test is indicated in patients with elevated urinary 17-hydroxysteroids. This usually differentiates abnormal secretion as a result of obesity, adrenal hyperplasia, or adrenal tumor (see Appendix 7), although an occasional patient with Cushing's disease still fails to suppress under these conditions. In difficult cases, the ACTH or metyrapone tests may be helpful; in general, patients with Cushing's syndrome demonstrate an exaggerated response, whereas those with adrenal tumors show little or no change. Adrenal ultrasonography and adrenal scanning with iodocholesterol may help to distinguish adrenal tumor from hyperplasia.[42, 134]

Several treatment modalities are available for Cushing's syndrome,[135] but none is ideal. Bilateral adrenalectomy is associated with a high incidence (probably nearly 50%) of Nelson's syndrome (postoperative evidence of pituitary tumor).[136, 137] Drugs that inhibit adrenal function[138–140] or those that interfere with neurotransmitters (e.g., cyproheptadine)[141–143] tend to be unpredictable and may produce undesirable side effects. In one report, high-voltage irradiation yielded favorable results in 12 of 15 childhood cases.[144] The success rate with heavy particle irradiation could be even higher, but so is the incidence of subsequent hypopituitarism.[135] There is also considerable enthusiasm for transsphenoidal resection of pituitary microadenomas;[120, 145–147] a subtotal hypophysectomy can be performed if no tumor is identified. Cures apparently can be expected in at least two thirds of patients, and there is relatively little morbidity. However, experience with this technique in children is still limited.

A comprehensive review of the physiopathology of Cushing's disease, including a discussion of treatment modalities, has been presented by Krieger.[148]

APPENDIX 7

Oral Metyrapone Test

Baseline 24-hour urine collections are obtained for determination of 17-hydroxysteroids for 2 days. On the 3rd day the patient receives metyrapone (Metopirone), 300 mg/m^2 every 4 hours (1,800 mg/m^2/24 hr tablets are 250 mg each); 24-hour urine collections are continued on days 3 and 4.

A twofold increase in 17-hydroxysteroids on the day of or day after metyrapone indicates a normal pituitary-adrenal axis (baseline 17-hydroxysteroids must be at least 1 mg/m^2/24 hr). False negative responses may occur.

Several simplified, shorter variants of this test, all employing measurement of serum 11-desoxycortisol (11-DOCS) have been published.[149–151] A satisfactory modification consists of a fasting (8:00 AM) level of cortisol and 11-DOCS, followed by metyrapone, 15 mg/kg orally every 4 hours for six doses, and repeat cortisol and 11-DOCS at 8:00 AM. In healthy subjects, 11-DOCS will rise to at least 10 μg/dL. If the metyrapone dose has been adequate, cortisol should decrease to very low or undetectable post-test levels in both unaffected children and those with pituitary-adrenal insufficiency.

Synthetic ACTH Test

Cosyntropin (Cortrosyn) is injected IM according to the following schedule:
1. 0.10 mg, younger than 1 year.
2. 0.15 mg, 1 to 5 years.
3. 0.25 mg, older than 5 years.

Blood for serum cortisol is obtained at 0, 30, 60, 90, and 120 minutes. In our laboratory, a maximum cortisol level of 20 μg/dL or a rise of 10 μg/dL from the baseline represents a normal adrenal response. A "short" test, in which the procedure is terminated after the 30-minute sample, appears to be nearly as reliable as the complete 2-hour version.[152]

This test also may be performed intravenously. The above dose of cosyntropin is added to 250 mL of saline solution and infused over 4 hours. Cortisol is measured before and after the infusion. Interpretation is as noted for the intramuscular cosyntropin test.

Dexamethasone Suppression Test

Twenty-four hour urine collections are obtained for 17-hydroxysteroids for 8 days. (Serum cortisol concentrations may also be obtained each morning.)

Dexamethasone, 1.25 mg/100 lb (in four divided doses, every 6 hours orally) is administered on days 3, 4, and 5. The dosage is increased to 3.75 mg/100 lb/day on days 6, 7, and 8. (As an alternative, each dose of dexamethasone may be given for 2 days instead of 3, resulting in a 6-day test.)

In healthy individuals and in those who have elevated baseline 17-hydroxysteroids secondary to obesity, the 17-hydroxysteroids should decrease to less than 2 mg/24 hour by day 5. In Cushing's syndrome, as a result of bilateral adrenal hyperplasia, 17-hydroxysteroid should be less than 2 mg/24 hour by day 8. In Cushing's syndrome due to adrenal carcinoma, 17-hydroxysteroids will remain over 2 mg/24 hour during the entire test (interpretation of a 6-day test is modified accordingly).

Overnight Suppression Test

Dexamethasone, 1 mg, is given at 11:00 PM and serum for assay of cortisol is obtained between 8:00 and 9:00 AM the next morning. In healthy subjects and those with exogenous obesity, the cortisol level should fall below 10 μg/dL.

This relatively simple screening procedure may eliminate the need for in-patient investigation.

NOTE: Melby[153] has reviewed many of the laboratory procedures used to assess adrenocortical function.

REFERENCES

1. Villee DB, Engel LC, Villee CA: Steroid hydroxylation in human fetal adrenals. *Endocrinol* 1959; 65:465.
2. Kaplan SL, Grumbach MM, Aubert ML: The ontogenesis of pituitary hormones and hypothalamic factors in the human fetus: Maturation of central nervous system regulation of anterior pituitary function. *Rec Prog Hormone Res* 1976; 32:161.
3. Lanman JT: The adrenal gland in the human fetus. An interpretation of its physiology and unusual developmental pattern. *Pediatrics* 1971; 27:140.
4. Kenny FM, Richards C, Taylor FH: Reference standards for cortisol production and 17-hydroxy-corticosteroid excretion during growth: Variation in the pattern of excretion of radiolabeled cortisol metabolites. *Metabolism* 1970; 19:280.
5. Miller WL, Levine LS: Molecular and clinical advances in congenital adrenal hyperplasia. *J Pediatr* 1987; 111:1.
6. Bacon GE, Kelch RP: Congenital adrenal hyperplasia due to 21-hydroxylase deficiency: A review of current knowledge. *J Endocrinol Invest* 1979; 2:93.
7. Ulick S, et al: Evidence for an aldosterone biosynthetic defect in congenital adrenal hyperplasia. *J Clin Endocrinol Metab* 1980; 51:1346.
8. Kuhnle U, Land M, Ulick S: Evidence for the secretion of an antimineralocorticoid in congenital adrenal hyperplasia. *J Clin Endocrinol Metab* 1986; 62:934.
9. Holler W, et al: Genetic differences between the salt-wasting, simple virilizing, and nonclassical types of congenital adrenal hyperplasia. *J Clin Endocrinol Metab* 1985; 60:757.
10. Qazi QH, Thompson MW: Genital changes in congenital virilizing adrenal hyperplasia. *J Pediatr* 1972; 80:653.
11. Rosenberg B, Hendren WH, Crawford JD: Posterior urethrovaginal communication in apparent males with congenital adrenal hyperplasia. *N Engl J Med* 1969; 280:131.
12. New MI, et al: Genotyping steroid 21-hydroxylase deficiency: Hormonal reference data. *J Clin Endocrinol Metab* 1983; 57:320.

13. Lee PA, et al: Attenuated forms of congenital adrenal hyperplasia due to 21-hydroxylase deficiency. *J Clin Endocrinol Metab* 1982; 55:866.
14. Kohn B, et al: Late-onset steroid 21-hydroxylase deficiency: A variant of classical congenital adrenal hyperplasia. *J Clin Endocrinol Metab* 1982; 55:817.
15. Emans SJ, et al: Detection of late-onset 21-hydroxylase deficiency congenital adrenal hyperplasia in adolescents. *Pediatrics* 1983; 72:690.
16. Levine LS, et al: Cryptic 21-hydroxylase deficiency in families of patients with classical congenital adrenal hyperplasia. *J Clin Endocrinol Metab* 1980; 51:1316.
17. Hirschfeld JA, Feldman JK: An unusually high incidence of salt-losing congenital adrenal hyperplasia in the Alaskan Eskimo. *J Pediatr* 1969; 75:492.
18. Libber SM, Migeon CJ, Bias WB: Ascertainment of 21-hydroxylase deficiency in individuals with HLA-B14 haplotype. *J Clin Endocrinol Metab* 1985; 60:727.
19. Zachmann M, Tassinari D, Prader A: Clinical and biochemical variability of congenital adrenal hyperplasia due to 11β-hydroxylase deficiency. A study of 25 patients. *J Clin Endocrinol Metab* 1983; 56:222.
20. Cathelineau G, et al: Adrenocortical 11β-hydroxylation defect in adult women with postmenarchial onset of symptoms. *J Clin Endocrinol Metab* 1980; 51:287.
21. Zadik Z, et al: Salt loss in hypertensive form of congenital adrenal hyperplasia (11-β-hydroxylase deficiency). *J Clin Endocrinol Metab* 1984; 58:384.
22. Hochberg Z, et al: Requirement of mineralocorticoid in congenital adrenal hyperplasia due to 11β-hydroxylase deficiency. *J Clin Endocrinol Metab* 1986; 63:36.
23. Bilgieri EG, Herron MA, Brust N: 17-Hydroxylation deficiency in man. *J Clin Invest* 1966; 45:1946.
24. New MI: Male pseudohermaphroditism due to 17-α-hydroxylase deficiency. *J Clin Invest* 1970; 49:1930.
25. Kershnar AK, et al: Studies in a phenotypic female with 17-α-hydroxylase deficiency. *J Pediatr* 1976; 83:395.
26. Dean HJ, Shackleton CHL, Winter JSD: Diagnosis and natural history of 17-hydroxylase deficiency in a newborn male. *J Clin Endocrinol Metab* 1984; 59:513.
27. Bongiovanni AM: The adrenogenital syndrome with deficiency of 3-β-hydroxysteroid dehydrogenase. *J Clin Invest* 1962; 41:2086.
28. Zachmann M, et al: Unusual type of congenital adrenal hyperplasia probably due to deficiency of 3-β-hydroxysteroid dehydrogenase. Case report of a surviving girl and steroid studies. *J Clin Endocrinol Metab* 1970; 30:719.
29. Kenny FM, Reynolds JW, Green OC: Partial 3β-hydroxysteroid dehydrogenase (3β-HSD) deficiency in a family with congenital adrenal hyperplasia: Evidence for increasing 3β-HSD activity with age. *Pediatrics* 1971; 48:756.
30. Rosenfield RL, et al: Pubertal presentation of congenital 5-3β-hydroxysteroid dehydrogenase deficiency. *J Clin Endocrinol Metab* 1980; 51:345.
31. Pang S, et al: Late-onset adrenal steroid 3β-hydroxysteroid dehydrogenase deficiency. I: A cause of hirsutism in pubertal and postpubertal women. *J Clin Endocrinol Metab* 1985; 60:428.
32. Pang S, et al: Nonsalt-losing congenital adrenal hyperplasia due to 3β-hydroxysteroid dehydrogenase deficiency with normal glomerulosa function. *J Clin Endocrinol Metab* 1983; 56:808.
33. Cravioto MC, et al: A new inherited variant of the 3β-hydroxysteroid dehydrogenase-isomerase deficiency syndrome: Evidence for the existence of two isoenzymes. *J Clin Endocrinol Metab* 1986; 62:360.
34. Hauffa BP, et al: Congenital adrenal hyperplasia due to deficient side-chain cleavage activity (20,22-desmolase) in a patient treated for 18 years. *Clin Endocrinol* 1985; 23:481.

35. Pang S, et al: Microfilter paper method for 17 α-hydroxyprogesterone radioimmunoassay: Its application for rapid screening for congenital adrenal hyperplasia. *J Clin Endocrinol Metab* 1977; 45:1003.

36. Pang S, et al: Pitfalls of prenatal diagnosis of 21-hydroxylase deficiency congenital adrenal hyperplasia. *J Clin Endocrinol Metab* 1985; 61:89.

37. Lippe BM, et al: Serum 17-α-hydroxyprogesterone, progesterone, estradiol, and testosterone in the diagnosis and management of congenital adrenal hyperplasia. *J Pediatr* 1974; 85:782.

38. Gutai JP, Kowarski AA, Migeon CJ: The detection of the heterozygous carrier for congenital virilizing adrenal hyperplasia. *J Pediatr* 1977; 90:924.

39. New MI, et al: "Acquired" adrenal hyperplasia with 21-hydroxylase deficiency is not the same genetic disorder as congenital adrenal hyperplasia. *J Clin Endocrinol Metab* 1979; 48:356.

40. Lee PA, Gareis FJ: Evidence for partial 21-hydroxylase deficiency among heterozygote carriers of congenital adrenal hyperplasia. *J Clin Endocrinol Metab* 1975; 41:415.

41. Fukushima DK, et al: Pituitary-adrenal activity in untreated congenital adrenal hyperplasia. *J Clin Endocrinol Metab* 1975; 40:1.

42. Lippe BM, Sample WF: Pelvic ultrasonography in pediatric and adolescent endocrine disorders. *J Pediatr* 1978; 92:897.

43. Limal J, Rappaport R, Bayard F: Plasma aldosterone, renin activity, and 17α-hydroxyprogesterone in salt-losing congenital adrenal hyperplasia: I. Response to ACTH in hydrocortisone treated patients and effect of 9α-fluorocortisol. *J Clin Endocrinol Metab* 1977; 45:551.

44. Hughes IA, Winter JSD: The application of a serum 17 OH-progesterone radioimmunoassay to the diagnosis and management of congenital adrenal hyperplasia. *J Pediatr* 1976; 88:766.

45. Schaison G, et al: Angiotensin and adrenal steroidogenesis: Study of 21-hydroxylase-deficient congenital adrenal hyperplasia. *J Clin Endocrinol Metab* 1980; 51:1390.

46. Edwin C, et al: Persistence of the enzymatic block in adolescent patients with salt-losing congenital adrenal hyperplasia. *J Pediatr* 1979; 95:534.

47. Brook CGD, et al: Experience with long-term therapy in congenital adrenal hyperplasia. *J Pediatr* 1974; 85:12.

48. Bacon GE, Spencer ML; Kelch RP: Effect of cortisol treatment on hormonal relationships in congenital adrenal hyperplasia. *Clin Endocrinol* 1977; 6:113.

49. Laron Z, Partzelan A: The comparative effect of 6α-fluoroprednisolone, 6α-methylprednisolone, and hydrocortisone on linear growth of children with congenital adrenal virilism and Addison's disease. *J Pediatr* 1968; 73:774.

50. Rappaport R, Cornu G, Royer P: Statural growth in congenital adrenal hyperplasia treated with hydrocortisone. *J Pediatr* 1968; 73:760.

51. Hellman L, et al: Tracer studies of the absorption and fate of steroid hormones in man. *J Clin Invest* 1956; 35:1033.

52. Schedl HP: Absorption of steroid hormones from the human small intestine. *J Clin Endocrinol Metab* 1965; 25:1309.

53. Pham-Huu-Trung MT, et al: Pituitary-adrenal axis activity in treated congenital adrenal hyperplasia: Static and dynamic studies. *J Clin Endocrinol Metab* 1978; 47:422.

54. McKenna TJ, et al: Pregnenolone, 17-OH-pregnenolone, and testosterone in plasma of patients with congenital adrenal hyperplasia. *J Clin Endocrinol Metab* 1976; 42:918.

55. Nichols T, Nugent CA, Tyler FH: Diurnal variation in suppression of adrenal function by glucocorticoids. *J Clin Endocrinol Metab* 1965; 25:343.

56. Winterer J, et al: Effect of hydrocortisone dose schedule on adrenal steroid secretion in congenital adrenal hyperplasia. *J Pediatr* 1985; 106:137.

57. Sandberg AA, Slaunwhite WR, Jr: Differences in metabolism of prednisolone-C^{14} and cortisol-C^{14}. *J Clin Endocrinol Metab* 1957; 17:1040.

58. Jenkins JS, Sampson PA: Conversion of cortisone to cortisol and prednisone to prednisolone. *Br Med J* 1967; 2:205.

59. Huseman CA, et al: Treatment of congenital virilizing adrenal hyperplasia patients with single and multiple doses of prednisone. *J Pediatr* 1977; 90:538.

60. Zipf WB, et al: Hormonal and clinical responses to prednisone treatment in adolescents with congenital adrenal hyperplasia. *Hormone Res* 1980; 12:206.

61. Bailey CC, Komrower GM: Growth and skeletal maturation in congenital adrenal hyperplasia. *Arch Dis Child* 1974; 49:4.

62. Styne DM, Kaplan SL, Grumbach MM: Growth suppression in treated congenital adrenal hyperplasia (CAH) *Pediatr Res (abstract)* 1976; 10:344.

63. Bongiovanni AM, Moshang T, Parks JS: Maturational deceleration after treatment of congenital adrenal hyperplasia. *Helv Paediatr Acta* 1973; 28:127.

64. Hughes IA, Winter JSD: The relationship between serum concentrations of 170H-progesterone and other serum and urinary steroids in patients with congenital adrenal hyperplasia. *J Clin Endocrinol Metab* 1978; 46:98.

65. Korth-Schutz S, et al: Serum androgens as a continuing index of adequacy of treatment of congenital adrenal hyperplasia. *J Clin Endocrinol Metab* 1978; 46:452.

66. Cacciari E, et al: GH, ACTH, TSH, LH, and FSH reserve in prepubertal girls with congenital adrenal hyperplasia. *J Clin Endocrinol Metab* 1976; 43:1146.

67. Fukushima DK, et al: Pituitary-adrenal activity in untreated congenital adrenal hyperplasia. *J Clin Endocrinol Metab* 1975; 40:1.

68. Solomon IL, Schoen EJ: Blood testosterone values in patients with congenital virilizing adrenal hyperplasia. *J Clin Endocrinol Metab* 1975; 40:355.

69. Money J: Components of eroticism in man. II. The orgasm and genital somesthesia. *J Nerv Ment Dis* 1961; 132:389.

70. Lattimer JL: Relocation and recession of enlarged clitoris with preservation of glans: Alternative to amputation. *J Urol* 1961; 86:113.

71. Kirkland RT, et al: The incidence of associated anomalies in 105 patients with congenital adrenal hyperplasia. *Pediatrics* 1972; 49:608.

72. McMillan DE, et al: Upper urinary tract anomalies in children with adrenogenital syndrome. *J Pediatr* 1976; 89:953.

73. Kirkland RT, et al: Bilateral testicular tumors in congenital adrenal hyperplasia. *J Clin Endocrinol Metab* 1977; 44:369.

74. Pang S, et al: Adrenocortical tumor in a patient with congenital adrenal hyperplasia due to 21-hydroxylase deficiency. *Pediatrics* 1981; 68:242.

75. Klingensmith GJ, et al: Glucocorticoid treatment of girls with congenital adrenal hyperplasia: Effects on height, sexual maturation and fertility. *J Pediatr* 1977; 90:996.

76. Kirkland RT, et al: The effect of therapy on mature height in congenital adrenal hyperplasia. *J Clin Endocrinol Metab* 1978; 47:1320.

77. Finkelstein JW, et al: Growth hormone secretion in congenital adrenal hyperplasia. *J Clin Endocrinol Metab* 1973; 36:121.

78. Sperling MA, et al: Linear growth and growth hormonal responsiveness in treated congenital adrenal hyperplasia. *Am J Dis Child* 1971; 122:408.

79. Duck SC: Acceptable linear growth in congenital adrenal hyperplasia. *J Pediatr* 1980; 97:93.

80. Penny R, Olambiwonnu NO, Frasier SD: Precocious puberty following treatment in a six-year-old male with congenital adrenal hyperplasia: Studies of serum luteinizing hormone (LH), serum follicle-stimulating hormone (FSH) and plasma testosterone. *J Clin Endocrinol Metab* 1973; 36:920.

81. Reiter EO, et al: The response of pituitary gonadotropes to synthetic LRF in children with glucocorticoid-treated congenital adrenal hyperplasia: Lack of effect of intrauterine and neonatal androgen excess. *J Clin Endocrinol Metab* 1975; 40:318.

82. Jones HW, Jr, Verkauf BS: Congenital adrenal hyperplasia: Age at menarche and related events at puberty. *Am J Obstet Gynecol* 1971; 109:292.

83. Kirkland J, et al: Serum gonadotropin levels in female adolescents with congenital adrenal hyperplasia. *J Pediatr* 1974; 84:411.

84. Wentz AC, et al: Gonadotropin output and response to LRH administration in congenital virilizing adrenal hyperplasia. *J Clin Endocrinol Metab* 1976; 42:239.

85. Boyar R, et al: Twenty-four hour patterns of plasma luteinizing hormone and follicle stimulating hormone in sexual precocity. *N Engl J Med* 1973; 289:282.

86. Richards GE, et al: The effect of long acting glucocorticoids on menstrual abnormalities in patients with virilizing congenital adrenal hyperplasia. *J Clin Endocrinol Metab* 1978; 47:1208.

87. Leichter SB, Jacobs LS: Normal gestation and diminished androgen responsiveness in an untreated patient with 21-hydroxylase deficiency. *J Clin Endocrinol Metab* 1976; 42:575.

88. Urban MA, Lee PA, Migeon CJ: Adult height and fertility in men with congenital virilizing adrenal hyperplasia. *N Engl J Med* 1978; 299:1392.

89. Prader A, Zachman M, Illig R: Normal spermatogenesis in adult males with congenital adrenal hyperplasia after discontinuation of therapy, in Lee PA, Plotnick LP, Kowardski CJ (eds): *Congenital Adrenal Hyperplasia*, Baltimore, University Park Press, 1977, p 397.

90. Jackson L, Whyte WG: Addison's disease in association with idiopathic hypoparathyroidism. *J Clin Endocrinol Metab* 1967; 27:348.

91. Saenger P, et al: Progressive adrenal failure in polyglandular autoimmune disease. *J Clin Endocrinol Metab* 1982; 54:863.

92. Sperling MA, Wolfsen AR, Fisher DA: Congenital adrenal hyperplasia: An isolated defect of organogenesis. *J Pediatr* 1973; 82:44.

93. Vick NA, Morre, RY: Diffuse sclerosis with adrenal insufficiency. *Neurology* 1968; 18:1066.

94. Engel GL, Margolin SG: Neuropsychiatric disturbances in internal disease. *Arch Intern Med* 1942; 70:236.

95. Guillemin R: Beta-lipotropin and endorphins: Implications of current knowledge. *Hosp Pract* Nov 1978; 13:53–60.

96. Lanes R, et al: Glucocorticoid and partial mineralocorticoid deficiency associated with achalasia. *J Clin Endocrinol Metab* 1980; 50:268.

97. Khalid BAK, et al: Steroid replacement in Addison's disease and in subjects adrenalectomized for Cushing's disease: Comparison of various glucocorticoids. *J Clin Endocrinol Metab* 1982; 55:551.

98. Urban MD, et al: Androgens in pubertal males with Addison's disease. *J Clin Endocrinol Metab* 1980; 51:925.

99. Gardner LI: Newer knowledge of adrenal cortical disturbances. *Pediatr Clin North Am* 1957; 4:889.

100. Stevenson J, McGregor AM, Connelly P: Calcification of the adrenal glands in young children. *Arch Dis Child* 1961; 36:316.

101. Bongiovanni AM: Care of the critically ill child: Acute adrenal insufficiency. *Pediatrics* 1969; 44:109.

102. Kreines K, DeVaux WD: Neonatal adrenal insufficiency associated with maternal Cushing's syndrome. *Pediatrics* 1971; 47:516.
103. Cleveland WW: Maternal-fetal hormone relationships. *Pediatr Clin North Am* 1970; 17:273.
104. Carey DE: Isolated ACTH deficiency in childhood: Lack of response to corticotropin-releasing hormone alone and in combination with arginine vasopressin. *J Pediatr* 1985; 107:925.
105. Arky RA, Freinkel LV: The response of plasma human growth hormone to insulin and ethanol-induced hypoglycemia in two patients with "isolated adrenocorticotropin defect." *Metabolism* 1964; 13:547.
106. Visser HKA, Cost WS: A new hereditary defect in the biosynthesis of aldosterone: Urinary C 21-corticosteroid pattern in three related patients with a salt-losing syndrome, suggesting an 18-oxidation defect. *Acta Endocrinol* 1964; 47:589.
107. Migeon CJ, et al: The syndrome of congenital adrenocortical unresponsiveness to ACTH. Report of six cases. *Pediatr Res* 1968; 2:501.
108. Franks RC, Nance WE: Hereditary adrenocortical unresponsiveness to ACTH. *Pediatrics* 1970; 45:43.
109. Kelch RP, et al: Hereditary adrenocortical unresponsiveness to adrenocorticotropic hormone. *J Pediatr* 1972; 81:726.
110. Moshang T, Jr, et al: Familial glucocorticoid insufficiency. *J Pediatr* 1973; 82:821.
111. Dluhy RB, et al: Pharmacology and chemistry of adrenal glucocorticoids, in Azarnoff DL (ed): *Steroid Therapy* Philadelphia, WB Saunders Co, 1975, p 1.
112. Landen J, et al: Adrenal response to infused corticotropin in subjects receiving glucocorticoids. *J Clin Endocrinol Metab* 1965; 25:602.
113. Janches M, et al: Use of methopyrapone (SU-4885) in the study of pituitary-adrenal response in patients under corticosteroid treatment. *J Clin Endocrinol Metab* 1965; 25:534.
114. Morris GH, Jorgensen JR: Recovery of endogenous pituitary-adrenal function in corticosteroid-treated children. *J Pediatr* 1971; 79:480.
115. Graber AL, et al: Natural history of pituitary-adrenal recovery after long term suppression with corticoids. *J Clin Endocrinol Metab* 1965; 25:11.
116. Aceto T, Jr, et al: Iatrogenic ACTH-cortisol insufficiency: I. Duration of insufficiency. *Pediatr Clin North Am* 1966; 13:543.
117. Loridan L, Senior B: Cushing's syndrome in infancy. *J Pediatr* 1969; 75:349.
118. Gilbert MG, Cleveland WW: Cushing's syndrome in infancy. *Pediatrics* 1970; 46:217.
119. Schletter FE, et al: Cushing's syndrome in childhood: Report of two cases with bilateral adrenocortical hyperplasia, showing distinctive clinical features. *J Clin Endocrinol Metab* 1967; 27:22.
120. Bigso ST, et al: Cushing's disease: Management by transsphenoidal pituitary microsurgery. *J Clin Endocrinol Metab* 1980; 50:348.
121. Strickland AL, et al: Growth retardation in Cushing's syndrome. *Am J Dis Child* 1972; 123:207.
122. Lee PA, et al: Short stature as the only clinical sign of Cushing's syndrome. *J Pediatr* 1975; 86:89.
123. Solomon IL, Schoen EJ: Juvenile Cushing syndrome manifested primarily by growth failure. *Am J Dis Child* 1976; 130:200.
124. Streeten DHP, et al: Hypercortisolism in childhood: Shortcomings of conventional diagnostic criteria. *Pediatrics* 1975; 56:797.

125. Contreras LN, Hane S, Tyrrell JB: Urinary cortisol in the assessment of pituitary-adrenal function: Utility of 24-hour and spot determinations. *J Clin Endocrinol Metab* 1986; 62:965.

126. Lee PDK, Winter RJ, Green OC: Virilizing adrenocortical tumors in childhood: Eight cases and a review of the literature. *Pediatrics* 1985; 76:437.

127. Hellman L, et al: Cortisol is secreted episodically by normal man. *J Clin Endocrinol Metab* 1970; 30:411.

128. Hellman L, et al: Cortisol is secreted episodically in Cushing's syndrome. *J Clin Endocrinol Metab* 1970; 30:686.

129. Tourniaire J, Orgiazzi J, Riviere JF, Rousset H: Repeated plasma cortisol determination in Cushing's syndrome due to adrenocortical adenoma. *J Clin Endocrinol Metab* 1971; 32:666.

130. Sederberg-Olsen P, et al: Episodic variation in plasma corticosteroids in subjects with Cushing's syndrome of differing etiology. *J Clin Endocrinol Metab* 1973; 36:906.

131. Zadik Z, de LaCerda L, Kowarski AA: Evaluation of the 6-hour integrated concentration of cortisol as a diagnostic procedure for Cushing's syndrome. *J Clin Endocrinol Metab* 1982; 54:1072.

132. Raux MC, et al: Studies of ACTH secretion control in 116 cases of Cushing's syndrome. *J Clin Endocrinol Metab* 1975; 40:186.

133. Boyar RM, et al: Circadian cortisol secretory rhythms in Cushing's disease. *J Clin Endocrinol Metab* 1979; 48:760.

134. Beierwaltes WH, et al: Visualization of human adrenal glands in vivo by scintillation scanning. *JAMA* 1971; 216:175.

135. Schteingart DE: Cushing's disease: An update. *Drug Therapy*, February 1978, p 125.

136. Hopwood NJ, Kenny FM: Incidence of Nelson's syndrome after adrenalectomy for Cushing's disease in children. *Am J Dis Child* 1977; 131:1353.

137. McArthur RG, Hayles AB, Salassa RM: Childhood Cushing's disease: Results of bilateral adrenalectomy. *J Pediatr* 1979; 95:214.

138. Komanicky P, Spark RF, Melby JC: Treatment of Cushing's syndrome with trilostane (WIN 24,540), an inhibitor of adrenal steroid biosynthesis. *J Clin Endocrinol Metab* 1978; 47:1042.

139. Sonino N, et al: Prolonged treatment of Cushing's disease by ketoconazole. *J Clin Endocrinol Metab* 1985; 61:718.

140. Nieman LK, et al: Successful treatment of Cushing's syndrome with the glucocorticoid antagonist RU 486. *J Clin Endocrinol Metab* 1985; 61:536.

141. Krieger DT, Luria M: Effectiveness of cyproheptadine in decreasing plasma ACTH concentrations in Nelson's syndrome. *J Clin Endocrinol Metab* 1976; 43:1179.

142. Krieger DT, Amorosa L, Flinick F: Cyproheptadine-induced remission of Cushing's disease. *N Engl J Med* 1975; 293:893.

143. D'Ercole AJ, et al: Treatment of Cushing disease in childhood with cyproheptadine. *J Pediatr* 1977; 90:834.

144. Jennings AS, Liddle GW, Orth DN: Results of treating childhood Cushing's disease with pituitary irradiation. *N Engl J Med* 1977; 297:957.

145. Bigos ST, et al: Cure of Cushing's disease by transsphenoidal removal of a microadenoma from a pituitary gland despite a radiographically normal sella turcica. *J Clin Endocrinol Metab* 1977; 45:1251.

146. Tyrrell JB, et al: Cushing's disease: Selective trans-sphenoidal resection of pituitary microadenomas. *N Engl J Med* 1978; 298:753.

147. Kuwayama A, et al: Anterior pituitary function after transsphenoidal selective adenomectomy in patients with Cushing's disease. *J Clin Endocrinol Metab* 1981; 53:165.

148. Krieger DT: Physiopathology of Cushing's disease. *Endocrine Rev* 1983; 4:22.
149. Dickstein G, Barzilai D: Improved single-dose metyrapone test. *Isr J Med Sci* 1980; 16:365.
150. Limal JM, Basmaciogullari A, Rappaport R: Evaluation of single oral dose metyrapone tests in children with hypopituitarism. *Acta Paediatr Scand* 1976; 65:177.
151. Leisti S: Evaluation of 3 hour metyrapone test in children and adolescents. *Clin Endocrinol* 1977; 6:305.
152. Lindholm J, et al: Reliability of the 30-minute ACTH test in assessing hypothalamic-pituitary-adrenal function. *J Clin Endocrinol Metab* 1978; 47:272.
153. Melby JC: Assessment of adrenocortical function. *N Engl J Med* 1971; 285:735.

8

Sexual Ambiguity and Hermaphroditism

The newborn infant with ambiguous genitalia may present a confusing diagnostic problem,[1] but evaluation must proceed rapidly because of the necessity of determining the most appropriate sex during the neonatal period. It is possible that a change of assigned sex may be accomplished successfully up until about 2 years of age,[2] since a child's own sexual identity does not become well established until that time. However, it is obvious that the parents will want to be informed quickly of their infant's proper sex, and therefore doubts about the child's gender must be satisfactorily resolved. Investigation of such a child should be conducted efficiently with the objective of a definite sex determination prior to discharge from the hospital.

NORMAL SEXUAL DIFFERENTIATION

The mechanisms of sexual differentiation have been thoroughly reviewed by Wilson[3] and by Saenger.[4] Briefly, however, an indifferent gonad forms a fetal testis in the presence of the H-Y antigen, which resides on the Y chromosome. The testis in turn produces testosterone (under the influence of placental chorionic gonadotropin) and also anti-müllerian hormone, which causes regression of the müllerian ducts. In addition, normal male development requires conversion of testosterone to dihydrotestosterone, and appropriate androgen responsiveness of the target tissues. Errors of differentiation can occur at any point in this sequence. Normal female development occurs in the presence of intact XX chromosomes and in the absence of the androgenic factors already mentioned. The gonads become gonadotropin-dependent relatively late in embryogenesis.

Saenger[4] identifies four characteristics of sexual development, which occur at different stages: genetic sex, determined at fertilization; gonadal sex, determined by the genetic sex; phenotypic sex, regulated by differentiation of the gonads during the first half of fetal life; and psychological sex, acquired postnatally through hormonal influences plus "sociologic imprinting."

DEFINITION AND CLASSIFICATION

There is a wide spectrum of phenotypic expression in external genitalia from normal male to normal female, and it may be difficult to decide if the appearance is truly abnormal. The mean length of the stretched male phallus at full-term birth has been reported as 3.5 cm, with a normal range (3rd to 97th percentile) of 2.8 to 4.2 cm.[5] Mean clitoral *breadth* is 3.27 mm, with a range of 3.05 to 3.49 mm (± 2 SD) in white infants, and 3.66 (3.40 to 3.92) mm in black full-term babies.[6] We would estimate that the normal clitoris in a newborn should not exceed approximately 1.5 cm in *length*. These data should help to differentiate "normal" from "abnormal," but the impression of *ambiguity* (as opposed to inadequate male development, such as micropenis) also depends on other features, such as appearance of the labia (rugated or smooth), number of orifices identified, and presence or absence (and location) of palpable gonads.

Essentially all infants with ambiguous genitalia have some form of hermaphroditism, that is, discrepancy between the external genitalia and the internal gonadal structures. By strict definition, an exception might be ambiguous genitalia but no identifiable gonadal tissue of either type, only fibrous "streaks," as is sometimes found in *XY gonadal dysgenesis* (see Chapter 3).

Female pseudohermaphrodites have ambiguous genitalia, but the gonads are entirely female; karyotype is invariably XX (Fig 8–1). Male pseudohermaphrodites have only testicular tissue, and karyotype can be XY, XX, or XO/XY. True hermaphrodites have both male and female gonadal tissue, which may or may not be functional. Chromosome counts are usually XX (80%) or XY (10%; Fig 8–2).[7, 8] Some mosaic patterns, such as XX/XY (10%),[9] are also associated with true hermaphroditism.

Transverse hermaphrodites have unambiguous genitalia but discordance between gonads and external genitalia (e.g., Leydig cell hypoplasia or the complete form of androgen insensitivity); karyotype in these patients is XY. The relationship between karyotype and clinical diagnosis in children with hermaphroditism is summarized in Table 8–1.

True Hermaphroditism

True hermaphrodites[7, 8, 9] may have one ovary and one testis or elements of both structures contained in an ova-testis (often with an ovary as well), but with inadequate functioning of the testicular tissue. Internal structures often include a hypoplastic uterus that may not be contiguous with the vaginal vault.

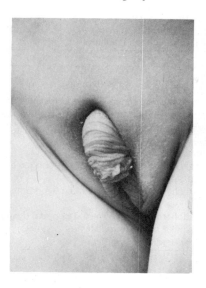

FIG 8–1.
Child with ambiguous genitalia and XX chromosome pattern (female pseudohermaphrodite) raised as a girl. Patient had enlarged clitoris with a clitoral urethra, possibly secondary to maternal ingestion of androgenic hormones. Uterus, ovaries, and small vagina were present.

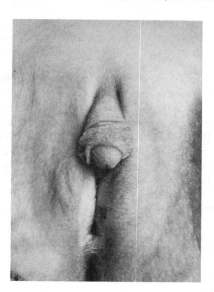

FIG 8–2.
Child with ambiguous genitalia and XY chromosome pattern, who was a true hermaphrodite. Note similarity to Fig 8–1 in appearance of external genitalia. Because of inadequacy of phallus, this patient was also raised as a girl. The phallus was amputated and intra-abdominal gonads removed.

TABLE 8–1.
Relationship of Chromosome Pattern and Clinical Diagnosis in
Children With Ambiguous Genitalia

Karyotype (and Buccal Smear)
XY (negative)
True hermaphrodite
Male pseudohermaphrodite (defect of testicular development,
testosterone synthesis/metabolism, or androgen action)
Transverse hermaphrodite
XX (positive)
True hermaphrodite
Female pseudohermaphrodite (usually congenital adrenal
hyperplasia)
Male pseudohermaphrodite (XX male syndrome)
XO/XY (negative)
Male pseudohermaphrodite (mixed gonadal dysgenesis)
XX/XY and similar mosaics (positive or negative)
True hermaphrodite

Female Pseudohermaphroditism

Exposure of the fetus to maternal androgenic hormones in utero can cause masculinization of the female infant. This may occur in the presence of a virilizing tumor[10] or congenital adrenal hyperplasia (CAH)[11] in the mother, but is more commonly a result of maternal ingestion of exogenous androgenic drugs. As expected, testosterone preparations have been implicated, but it is of interest that progestational agents[12] also may produce the same clinical picture, although the mechanism is unclear. The effect of these agents is most marked when administered during the first trimester of pregnancy.

Another type of female pseudohermaphroditism (FPH) includes the constellation of ambiguous genitalia plus müllerian duct anomalies, imperforate anus, and urinary tract malformations, probably resulting from a primary abnormality in differentiation of the genital tubercle.[13]

Congenital adrenal hyperplasia, particularly the *21-hydroxylase deficiency* (21-OHD) type, is by far the most common form of FPH; *11-hydroxylase* and *3β-hydroxysteroid dehydrogenase* (3β-HSD) deficiency can also result in masculinization of a genetic female (see Chapter 7).

Male Pseudohermaphroditism

The cause of male pseudohermaphroditism (MPH) may involve a disorder of testicular differentiation or development (karyotype XY, XX, or XO/XY), or a defect in testosterone synthesis, metabolism, or action (karyotype XY).

Defects Of Testicular Differentiation and Development

XX male syndrome[14-16] typically consists of a male phenotype and small testes in a patient with a 46,XX karyotype, but without female internal organs. These patients may also have gynecomastia and/or ambiguous genitalia,[15] and there has been at least one report in which müllerian structures were present.[16] Although several hypotheses have been proposed,[15] the discrepancy of testicular development in the absence of a Y chromosome has not been fully explained, but H-Y antigen is presumably present.

Patients with an XO/XY karyotype make up a rather diffuse group, ranging from phenotypic male to phenotypic female, sometimes with features of Turner's syndrome. However, the majority of such patients have ambiguous genitalia. A dysgenetic testis frequently is found on one side, with a fibrous streak on the other (syndrome of mixed gonadal dysgenesis).[17] It might be suspected that this streak gonad was destined to be an ovary, but since this cannot be shown histologically, these patients generally are classified as male pseudohermaphrodites rather than as true hermaphrodites.

Herniae uteri inguinale (persistent müllerian duct syndrome[18, 19]) is a form of male pseudohermaphroditism in which external genitalia are normal except for cryptorchidism and inguinal hernia, but cervix, uterus, and fallopian tubes are found internally. Testes are hypoplastic in some cases. The cause is probably a deficiency of anti-müllerian hormone from the Sertoli cells of the fetal testes, or end-organ unresponsiveness to the substance. Karyotype is XY. There also has been a report of a child with ambiguous genitalia, hypoplastic intrabdominal testes, and XY karyotype in whom the defect was thought to be reduced expression of the H-Y antigen.[20]

Defects of Testosterone Synthesis

Three defects of testosterone synthesis (deficiencies of *cholesterol desmolase*, *3β-HSD*, and *17-hydroxylase*) are forms of CAH that affect adrenal production of glucocorticoid as well as androgen synthesis (see Chapter 7; note that 3β-HSD can result in ambiguity in both genetic males or females). *17,20-Desmolase deficiency*[21] is characterized by third-degree hypospadias or, in extreme cases, female external genitalia with a vaginal pouch. Patients with *17β-hydroxysteroid dehydrogenase deficiency*[22] may not present until puberty or later when virilization occurs in a genetic male being raised as a girl. Gynecomastia may also be present, apparently secondary to peripheral conversion of estrone to estradiol.

Defects of Testosterone Metabolism

Conversion of testosterone to the more active dihydrotestosterone (DHT) is diminished in *5α-reductase deficiency*.[23] Genetic males typically demonstrate sexual ambiguity, with a large "clitoris," blind vaginal pouch, urogenital sinus, and abdominal, inguinal, or labial testes. However, some patients are phenotypic females.[24]

Defects of Androgen Action

Patients with the incomplete form of feminizing testes (androgen insensitivity) syndrome[25-27] have ambiguous genitalia and are classified as having MPH. In the complete form of this syndrome, testosterone is released by inguinal or intra-abdominal testes but, because of lack of end-organ response to male hormone,[28, 29] these patients have female secondary sexual characteristics and do not have ambiguous genitalia. It has been determined that estradiol secretion is greater than in adult men, but that the degree of feminization that occurs is also related to the estradiol-androgen ratio.[30]

In the incomplete form the external genitalia may be ambiguous, as a result of a partial response of the tissues to DHT.[25, 26, 29] In both types the uterus is rudimentary or absent, and the vagina ends in a blind pouch. This condition also is familial; statistically, half of all genetic males in a sibship would be affected. Very mild forms of androgen insensitivity, manifested only by decreased phallic length, gynecomastia, and infertility have also been reported.[31] The basic defect in these patients appears to be lack of a specific androgen receptor in skin fibroblasts,[32] although exceptions have been found, at least in subjects with the complete form.[33]

Miscellaneous Male Pseudohermaphroditism Syndromes

In the past, several forms of MPH have been categorized according to clinical features only, and a precise single cause cannot be ascribed with certainty. For example, Reifenstein's syndrome, also referred to as perineoscrotal hypospadias in neonates, may be due to 17β-hydroxysteroid dehydrogenase (17-ketosteroid reductase) deficiency,[34] 5α-reductase deficiency,[35] or partial androgen insensitivity.[25]

Transverse Hermaphroditism

Patients with Leydig cell hypoplasia[36] have an XY karyotype but lack of testicular function. These children usually are phenotypic females, without genital ambiguity, who fail to develop sexually at puberty. Patients with the complete form of androgen insensitivity also fall into this category.[28, 29]

Hermaphroditism is summarized in Table 8–2.

SCHEME OF EVALUATION

In Figure 8–3 a somewhat oversimplified scheme of evaluation is presented, which may be used in examination of an infant with ambiguous genitalia if the karyotype proves to be XX or XY. A buccal smear can also be obtained but is much less reliable, as there may be difficulties in distinguishing actual Barr bodies from artifact, and assessment of the percentage of Barr bodies present depends somewhat on individual interpretation.

TABLE 8–2.
Classification of Hermaphroditism

True hermaphroditism
Female pseudohermaphroditism
Maternal androgenic compounds
Associated with urinary tract malformations
Congenital adrenal hyperplasia (21-OHD, 11-OHD, 3β-HSD)
Male pseudohermaphroditism
Defects of testicular differentiation and development
XX male syndrome
Mixed gonadal dysgenesis
Persistent müllerian duct syndrome
Defects of testosterone synthesis
Congenital adrenal hyperplasia (17-OHD, 3β-HSD,
cholesterol desmolase deficiency)
17,20-desmolase deficiency
17-hydroxysteroid (17-ketosteroid reductase) deficiency
Defects of testosterone metabolism
5α-Reductase deficiency
Defects of androgen action
Feminizing testes (androgen insensitivity) syndrome,
incomplete form
Transverse hermaphroditism
Leydig cell hypoplasia
Feminizing testes syndrome, complete form

Additional studies that should be obtained as part of the initial work-up include pelvic ultrasound[37] and retrograde urography to evaluate the internal genitalia. More experience is also being gained with magnetic resonance imaging.

Because CAH resulting from 21-OHD is by far the most common cause of FPH, appropriate laboratory studies (serum 17-hydroxyprogesterone, androstenedione, sodium, and potassium) should be obtained in an infant with XX karyotype (see Chapter 7). In view of the frequency of this disorder, it is probably prudent to initiate these studies even before chromosome results are available. If a diagnosis of CAH is not confirmed, and there is no reason to suspect the influence of maternal androgenic hormones, laparotomy will invariably be necessary to identify the type of gonads and other internal structures present.

If the chromosome complement is XY, a diagnosis of 5α-reductase deficiency can be made on the basis of the testosterone-DHT ratio before and after human chorionic gonadotropin stimulation.[38] The types of CAH (see Chapter 7) and other defects of androgen synthesis that can cause ambiguity in a genetic male can also be defined by appropriate hormonal assays. However, if these are normal, laparotomy will probably be mandatory.

XO/XY gonadal dysgenesis can often be recognized by the clinical features, but surgery is indicated to remove the dysgenetic gonads (see Management). Patients with XX/XY or other forms of mosaicism will also invariably require

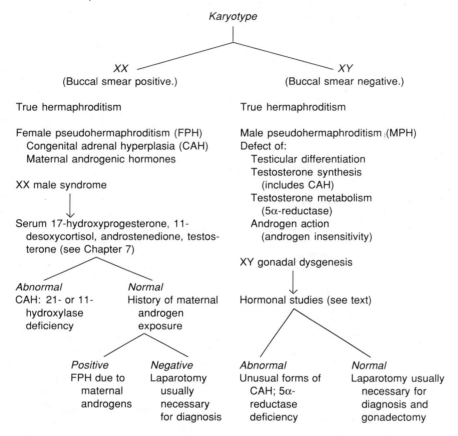

FIG 8–3.
Scheme of evaluation, somewhat oversimplified, for patients with ambiguous genitalia and XX or XY karyotype. Ultrasonagraphy is also indicated in essentially all cases.

laparotomy for diagnosis and removal of abnormal or inappropriate structures.

Because there are numerous causes of intersex problems and the diagnosis (and subsequent management) is often difficult or impossible without specialized contrast or imaging studies, hormonal assays, or surgical intervention, referral to a medical center for comprehensive evaluation is recommended.

The most important determinant of the appropriate sex of rearing is the degree to which a patient can be expected to perform in the assigned gender role. The patient whose phallus would not be sufficient for adequate function as a male should undergo the surgery necessary to simulate the external genitalia of a female, regardless of the chromatin or genetic sex. The previously outlined diagnostic procedures are thus of greater importance in the patient with an adequate phallus in whom the development of the external genitalia will permit rearing as either a boy or a girl.

MANAGEMENT

Once a definite assignment of sex has been made, appropriate surgical procedures are necessary. If the patient is to be raised as a girl, clitorectomy, dilation of the introitus, and definitive vaginoplasty are performed as described for children with CAH (see Chapter 7).

In the child to be raised as a boy, chordee can be corrected in infancy. Hypospadias is repaired during childhood, preferably prior to school age (3 to 6 years). Surgical correction of undescended testes is indicated by the age of 1 to 2 years[39] (see Chapter 9).

Suspected functional heterologous gonads should be removed prior to puberty to avoid the development of inappropriate secondary sexual characteristics. Certain types of dysgenetic gonads appear to undergo malignant degeneration with increased frequency, particularly in patients with a Y chromosome[40]; therefore gonadectomy before puberty is always recommended in this group as well. Although the exact timing is otherwise not critical, early intervention is probably prudent because malignancy in childhood, although rare, has been reported.[41] Surgical risk is probably slightly less after the age of about 1 year.

Replacement therapy in the estrogen-deficient girl is described in Chapter 3 as applied to Turner's syndrome. Androgen therapy in boys is reviewed in Chapter 3 relative to adolescents with constitutional delayed growth, and in Chapter 9 as applied to boys with delayed puberty. In general, the more potent intramuscular preparations (e.g., testosterone enanthate, 100 to 200 mg every 2 to 4 weeks) are preferable to oral androgens in patients with intersex disorders, as sexual maturation is usually a greater problem than linear growth. Priapism and fluid retention may occur if the dose is excessive. Treatment with oral or parenteral testosterone should be continued after adequate masculinization has been achieved, but the dose or frequency of administration may be reduced.

The psychological aspects of sexual ambiguity must be approached with care. Until a definite gender is assigned to the newborn infant, the problem should be presented to the parents as one of incomplete, rather than ambiguous, development. Once the more appropriate sex is determined, an effort must be made to dispel any question of alternative possibilities. If an obvious mistake of sex assignment has been made, correction may still be psychologically possible during the first 2 years of life.[2] Thereafter, any change of gender is best delayed until adulthood, when the patient is able to make a mature decision, and then only with the aid of intensive medical and psychiatric counseling.

A detailed review of the problem of abnormal sexual development has been written by Grumbach and Conte.[42] The recent review by Saenger[4] is likewise recommended.

REFERENCES

1. Donahoe PK, Hendren WH: Evaluation of the newborn with ambiguous genitalia. *Pediatr Clin North Am* 1976; 23:361.
2. Money J, Hampson JG, Hampson JL: Hermaphroditism: Recommendations concerning assignment of sex, change of sex, and psychological management. *Johns Hopkins Med J* 1955; 97:284.
3. Wilson JD: Sexual differentiation. *Annu Rev Physiol* 1978; 40:279.
4. Saenger P: Abnormal sex differentiation. *J Pediatr* 1984; 104:1.
5. Feldman KW, Smith DW: Fetal phallic growth and penile standards for newborn male infants. *J Pediatr* 1975; 86:395.
6. Riley WJ, Rosenbloom AL: Clitoral size in infancy. *J Pediatr* 1980; 96:918.
7. Miller OJ: The sex chromosome anomalies. *Am J Obstet Gynecol* 1964; 90:1078.
8. Saenger P, et al: Presence of H-Y antigen and testis in 46, XX true hermaphroditism: Evidence for Y-chromosomal function. *J Clin Endocrinol Metab* 1976; 43:1234.
9. Josso J, et al: True hermaphroditism with XX/XY mosaicism probably due to double fertilization of the ovum. *J Clin Endocrinol Metab* 1965; 23:114.
10. O'Leary TJ, et al: Virilization of two siblings by maternal androgen-secreting adrenal adenoma. *J Pediatr* 1986; 109:840.
11. Kai H, et al: Female pseudohermaphroditism caused by maternal congenital adrenal hyperplasia. *J Pediatr* 1979; 95:418.
12. Wilkins L: Masculinization of the female fetus due to the use of orally given progestins. *JAMA* 1960; 172:1028.
13. Wenstrup RJ, Pagon RA: Female pseudohermaphroditism with anorectal, müllerian duct, and urinary tract malformations: Report of four cases. *J Pediatr* 1985; 107:751.
14. Lazarus GM, Rodner RD: Probable XX male with hidden testes. *J Pediatr* 1975; 87:493.
15. Roe TF, Alfi OS: Ambiguous genitalia in XX male children: Report of two infants. *Pediatrics* 1977; 60:55.
16. Duck SC, et al: Pseudohermaphroditism with testes and a 46, XX karyotype. *J Pediatr* 1975; 87:58.
17. Davidoff F, Federman DD: Mixed gonadal dysgenesis. *Pediatrics* 1973; 52:725.
18. Stallings MW, et al: Persistent müllerian structures in a male neonate. *Pediatrics* 1976; 57:568.
19. Weiss EB, et al: Persistent müllerian duct syndrome in male identical twins. *Pediatrics* 1978; 61:797.
20. Wilson TA, et al: H-Y intermediate phenotype in male pseudohermaphroditism. *J Pediatr* 1986; 109:815.
21. Forest MG, Lecornu M, de Peretti E: Familial male pseudohermaphroditism due to 17-20-desmolase deficiency. I: In vivo endocrine studies. *J Clin Endocrinol Metab* 1980; 50:826.
22. Imperato-McGinley J, et al: Male psuedohermaphroditism secondary to 17 β-hydroxysteroid dehydrogenase deficiency: Gender role change with puberty. *J Clin Endocrinol Metab* 1979; 49:391.
23. Fisher LK, et al: Clinical, endocrinological, and enzymatic characterization of two patients with 5α-reductase deficiency: Evidence that a single enzyme is responsible for the 5α-reduction of cortisol and testosterone. *J Clin Endocrinol Metab* 1978; 47:653.
24. Johnson L, et al: Characterization of the testicular abnormality in 5α-reductase deficiency. *J Clin Endocrinol Metab* 1986; 63:1091.

25. Perez-Palacios G, et al: Familial incomplete virilization due to partial end organ insensitivity to androgens. *J Clin Endocrinol Metab* 1975; 41:946.
26. Madden JD, et al: Clinical and endocrinologic characterization of a patient with the syndrome of incomplete testicular feminization. *J Clin Endocrinol Metab* 1975; 41:751.
27. Keenan BS, et al: Male pseudohermaphroditism with partial androgen insensitivity. *Pediatrics* 1977; 59:224.
28. Rivorola MA, et al: Studies of androgens in the syndrome of male pseudohermaphroditism with testicular feminization. *J Clin Endocrinol Metab* 1967; 27:371.
29. Rosenfield RL, et al: Androgens and androgen responsiveness in the feminizing testis syndrome. Comparison of complete and "incomplete" forms. *J Clin Endocrinol Metab* 1971; 32:625.
30. MacDonald PC, et al: Origin of estrogen in normal men and in women with testicular feminization. *J Clin Endocrinol Metab* 1979; 49:905.
31. Migeon CJ, et al: A clinical syndrome of mild androgen insensitivity. *J Clin Endocrinol Metab* 1984; 59:672.
32. Griffin JE, Punyashthiti K, Wilson JD: Dihydrotestosterone binding by cultured human fibroblasts. Comparison of cells from patients with hereditary male pseudohermaphroditism due to androgen resistance. *J Clin Invest* 1976; 57:1342.
33. Brown TR, Migeon CJ: Androgen binding in nuclear matrix of human genital skin fibroblasts from patients with androgen insensitivity syndrome. *J Clin Endocrinol Metab* 1986; 62:542.
34. Knorr D, et al: Reifenstein's syndrome, a 17 β-hydroxysteroid-oxydoreductase deficiency? *Acta Endocrinol* 1973; 173 (suppl):37.
35. Walsh PC, et al: Familial incomplete male pseudohermaphroditism, type 2. Decrease dihydrotestosterone formation in pseudovaginal perineoscrotal hypospadias. *N Engl J Med* 1974; 291:944.
36. Brown DM, et al: Leydig cell hypoplasia: A cause of male pseudohermaphroditism. *J Clin Endocrinol Metab* 1978; 46:1.
37. Schneider M, Grossman H: Sonography of the female child's reproductive system. *Pediatr Ann* 1980; 9:10.
38. Sanger P, et al: Prepubertal diagnosis of steroid 5 α-reductase deficiency. *J Clin Endocrinol Metab* 1978; 46:627.
39. Kelalis P, et al: The timing of elective surgery on the genitalia of male children with particular reference to undescended testes and hypospadias. *Pediatrics* 1975; 56:479.
40. Manuel M, Katayama K, Jones HW, Jr: The age of occurrence of gonadal tumors in intersex patients with a Y chromosome. *Am J Obstet Gynecol* 1976; 124:293.
41. Frasier SD, Bashore RD, Mosier HD: Gonadoblastoma associated with pure gonadal dysgenesis in monozygotic twins. *J Pediatr* 1964; 64:740.
42. Grumbach MM, Conte FA: Disorders of sexual differentiation, in Wilson JD, Foster DW (eds): *Williams Textbook of Endocrinology*, ed 7. Philadelphia, WB Saunders Co, 1985.

9

Sexual Precocity and Delayed Development

Aberrations of the normal pattern of pubertal development are common reasons for referral to a pediatric endocrine clinic. Many of these problems do not require the expertise of a highly trained pediatric endocrinologist or sophisticated laboratory studies. The purposes of this chapter are to review briefly the endocrine and neuroendocrine changes that occur during human puberty and to outline a diagnostic apporach to abnormal sexual development.

ENDOCRINOLOGY OF ADOLESCENCE

From a physiologic perspective, the major developmental change of adolescence is maturation of the reproductive system and attainment of fertility. This complex process also results in a relatively brief growth spurt that accounts for approximately 15% to 17% of adult stature but that also results in closure of the epiphyses and cessation of linear growth. In this sense, the pubertal growth spurt is a "two-edged sword."[1, 2]

Pubertal maturation is initiated and sustained by developments in the central nervous system (CNS) that result in increased secretion of gonadotropin-releasing hormone (GnRH),* gonadotropins (follicle-stimulating hormone, FSH; and luteinizing hormone, LH), sex steroids, growth hormone, and somatomedin-C (Sm-C).[1-5] The human reproductive system undergoes many developmental changes before adolescent development becomes apparent. Indeed, maturation of the reproductive system begins during early fetal life and continues

---

* The abbreviation GnRH is used to designate the decapeptide pGlu-His-Trp-Ser-Tyr-Gly-Leu-Arg-Pro-Gly-NH$_2$, which releases both LH and FSH in many species, including human beings. This peptide also has been abbreviated LRF or LH-RH/FSH-RH.

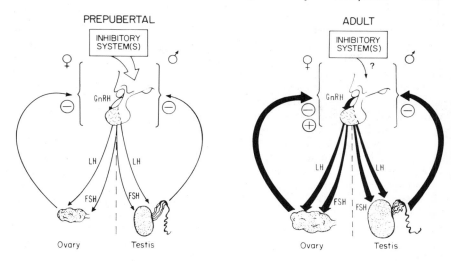

FIG 9–1.
Schematic representation of the differences in the hypothalamic-pituitary-gonadal axis between children and adults. Although a positive feedback potential has been demonstrated in adult men, this does not play a significant role in gonadotropin regulation in humans and hence is not illustrated. Abbreviations: *GnRH* = gonadotropin-releasing hormone; *LH* = luteinizing hormone; *FSH* = follicle-stimulating hormone.

into early infancy, during which time the system is remarkably active. During early infancy, plasma concentrations of FSH and LH are greater than during childhood, and these concentrations are greater in girls than in boys during most of fetal life and early infancy. Moreover, testosterone concentrations in boys and, less dramatically, estradiol concentrations in girls are higher in infancy than during childhood.[3–6] However, it appears that CNS restraint mechanisms develop in late infancy and maintain the reproductive system in a suppressed state until recrudescence occurs, usually at the beginning of the second decade of life.[3]

The major changes in the hypothalamic-pituitary-gonadal axis that occur between childhood and adulthood are illustrated schematically in Figure 9–1. During childhood this feedback system functions at a very low level.[6–11] Gonadotropin and sex steroid values are low, and there are minimal or no sex differences. The system is not completely suppressed, however.[12] Children without sex glands do have slightly greater gonadotropin concentrations than normal children do.[13, 14] In addition, pulsatile secretion of gonadotropins as well as a slight sleep-entrained increase in gonadotropin secretion have been noted in prepubertal children.[15]

From a neuroendocrine perspective, the onset of pubertal development is heralded by increased pulsatile secretion of GnRH by the hypothalamus, particularly during sleep.[16] Amplification of the preexisting, sleep-entrained increase in GnRH secretion most likely occurs slowly, about the same time as the nadir of the prepubertal growth rate. Recent studies suggest that both the amplitude and frequency of GnRH secretion increase during puberty, especially during the early hours of sleep.[17] Increased GnRH secretion leads to increased pituitary responsiveness to GnRH, increased gonadotropin secretion (particularly LH), and increased gonadal maturation and sex steroid secretion, which result in accelerated growth, physical maturation, and fertility. On average, the entire process requires 4 to 5 years. As pubertal maturation progresses the day-night difference in gonadotropin secretion decreases until it finally disappears when the reproductive system is mature.

In young adult men, LH — and presumably GnRH — is secreted episodically at approximately 90-minute intervals throughout the day. In agonadal men and women, FSH and LH are strikingly increased, and LH pulses occur approximately every 60 minutes (circhoral). In women, LH pulse frequency varies significantly throughout the menstrual cycle. During the follicular phase of the menstrual cycle, LH pulse frequency increases steadily until it appears to reach a circhoral or faster rate. Estradiol, produced by the developing follicle, increases pituitary responsiveness to GnRH and most likely increases GnRH pulse frequency as well. The rising concentrations of estradiol induce a positive feedback response that results in the midcycle LH surge and subsequent ovulation. With the formation of the corpus luteum and the resultant increase in progesterone secretion in the luteal phase, LH pulse frequency decreases remarkably and becomes irregular. With the demise of the corpus luteum, menses occurs and the cycle begins again.[3]

The estradiol-induced positive feedback potential is not present in prepubertal or early pubertal children; it is first demonstrable in midpubertal girls.[18] LH surges cannot be induced with estradiol in healthy men, but positive feedback can be demonstrated in both agonadal men and women. Although still incompletely proved, considerable data suggest that positive feedback to estradiol requires the ability of the hypothalamus to sustain pulsatile GnRH secretion at a circhoral rate throughout the day.

Secretion of GnRH in a pulsatile manner is necessary for normal functioning of the reproductive system. Indeed, continuous exposure to synthetic GnRH by way of infusions or to long-acting agonists of GnRH leads to a reduction in pituitary gonadotropin secretion, most likely by desensitization and "downregulation" of GnRH receptors.[3] As is discussed later, this finding has been put to use in clinical practice in the treatment of children with central precocious puberty.[19]

Little is known about CNS mechanism(s) that restrain or suppress the reproductive system during childhood. In adults, endogenous opiates (morphine-like neuromodulators) appear to play a role in regulating GnRH and hence gonadotropin secretion. For example, opiate drugs inhibit gonadotropin secretion and naloxone, an opiate antagonist, increases the frequency and amplitude of LH secretion in healthy men and in women during the luteal phase of the menstrual cycle. Moreover, women who have hypothalamic amenorrhea and slow LH pulse frequency frequently respond to naloxone. However, prepubertal and early pubertal children show no response to naloxone.[20] Thus, increased endogenous opiate activity does not seem to be a likely cause of the suppressed state of the reproductive system in childhood.[3]

In addition to the striking changes in gonadotropin and sex steroid secretion characteristic of puberty, secretion of androgens by the adrenal glands also increases greatly during adolescence. Similar to the development pattern of the reproductive system, the androgen-secreting inner zone of the adrenal glands, the zona reticularis, also matures in a biphasic manner. During fetal life and very early infancy, the reticularis zone of the adrenal gland is large and adrenal androgen secretion is high. Adrenal androgen secretion rapidly decreases during infancy and remains low until the child is at least 6 to 8 years of age, at which time it steadily increases until physical maturity is reached. This process is referred to as adrenarche; it is temporally related but not causally related to the onset of puberty.[5, 21] Discordant development of these two systems may be seen in several clinical situations as summarized in Table 9–1.

Adrenarche, as indicated by a rise in serum concentrations of adrenal androgens, usually occurs about 2 years before the initial pubertal rise in gonadotropins and sex steroids. Both adrenocorticotropic hormone (ACTH) and a postulated adrenal-androgen-stimulating hormone appear to be necessary for adrenarche. Dehydroepiandrosterone (DHEA), its sulfate (DHEAS), and androstenedione are the major adrenal androgens. In women, adrenal androgen secretion accounts for approximately 50% of serum testosterone, directly or by extraglandular conversion, and thus accounts for a significant proportion of sexual hair development.[22] Plasma concentrations of DHEAS, which can be measured easily and fluctuate only slightly throughout the day, are useful indices of adrenal maturation.[21] DHEAS increases progressively from about 7 to 8 years through 13 to 15 years of age in boys and girls; this increase is accompanied by a parallel increase in urinary 17-ketosteroid (17-KS) excretion. Although adrenarche usually precedes puberty, pubic hair development occurs 3 to 6 months after breast budding or early testicular enlargement in most children.

TABLE 9–1.
Pubertal (Gonadarche) and Adrenal (Adrenarche) Maturation in Clinical Disorders With Abnormal Sexual Maturation*

Diagnosis	Adrenarche	Gonadarche
Premature adrenarche	+	−
Primary adrenal insufficiency	−	+
Idiopathic precocious puberty		
Onset before 6 years	−	+
Onset after 6 years	+	+
Gonadal dysgenesis	+	−
Isolated gonadotropin deficiency	+	−
Constitutionally delayed adolescence	−	−

* Adapted from Grumbach MM: The neuroendocrinology of puberty, in Kreiger DT, Hughes JC (eds): *Neuroendocrinology.* Sunderland, Mass, Sinauer Associates, 1980.

TABLE 9–2.
Clinical Assessment of Overall Pubertal Development in Girls*

Pubertal Stage	Characteristics
P_1	No clinical signs of puberty
P_2	Breast budding; sparse labial hair; maturation of vaginal mucosa, labia majora, and labia minora
P_3	Further breast enlargement, with palpable glandular tissue; Naboth's follicles (Montgomery's follicles); sparse axillary hair; extension of pubic hair over the mons pubis; dullness of vaginal mucosa; moderate enlargement of labia majora and labia minora
P_4	Further breast enlargement, with projection of the areola to form a secondary mound; moderate axillary hair; lateral extension of pubic hair; well-developed external genitalia; no menses
P_5	Postmenarche†

* Adapted from Kelch RP, Grumbach MM, Kaplan SL: in Saxena BB, Beling CG, Gandy HM (eds): *Gonadotropins*. New York, Wiley-Interscience, 1972, p 524.
† All girls who have had menarche were classified as P_3 in this study because of the marked variability of sex hormones throughout the menstrual cycle.

Some investigators have suggested that adrenarche might account for the "midchildhood growth spurt", a slight, temporary increase in growth velocity that usually occurs in children around 7 years of age; however, the evidence in support of a significant role for adrenal androgens in either the midchildhood or pubertal growth spurt is weak at best.[2]

NORMAL SEXUAL MATURATION AND THE PUBERTAL GROWTH SPURT

The time of onset and subsequent course of hormonal and physical changes during puberty are highly variable and are influenced by genetic tendencies, chronic illnesses, nutrition, socioeconomic status, and altitude.[1, 2, 4, 23–29] Breast budding in girls and testicular enlargement, with reddening and thinning of the scrotum, in boys usually are the first signs of puberty (see Tables 9–2 and 9–3 for further classification). The appearance of secondary sex characteristics before the age of 8 years in girls and 9 years in boys should be considered precocious. On the other hand, puberty is delayed if physical changes have not developed before the age of 13 years in girls and 14 years in boys.

Indeed, fewer than 1% of healthy children develop the first signs of secondary sexual characteristics either before or after these age limits.[4] Puberty also should be considered delayed if more than 5 years elapse between the first signs of puberty and the onset of menarche or the completion of genital growth.

Pediatricians should be aware of the detailed studies of the progression of physical changes during puberty reported by Marshall and Tanner[23, 24] and by Prader.[2] Clinically there are several important facts to remember.

Except for the brief, midchildhood growth spurt, linear growth velocity decreases steadily throughout childhood.[2, 29] At approximately 10 years of age in girls and 11.5 years in boys, growth rate (velocity) reaches a nadir. This point, sometimes, referred to as minimum height or growth velocity (MHV), is the reference point for the beginning of the pubertal growth spurt. In children who exhibit constitutionally delayed growth and adolescence, the point of MHV is characteristically prolonged. As mentioned earlier, maturation of the neuroendocrine reproductive system is readily detectable before physical signs of puberty are present: that is, at and even before the age of MHV.[3]

On average, the maximal or peak growth velocity (PHV) occurs at age 12 and 14 years in girls and boys, respectively. In both sexes, the sesamoid bone of the thumb appears approximately 6 months before PHV. Peak height velocity occurs in girls when significant feminization has occurred but before menarche. The average age at menarche is between 12.5 and 13 years in the United States; and the average duration between breast budding and menarche is 2.5 years. Menstrual cycles are often irregular and anovulatory during the first 2 years. By 5 years after menarche, however, less than 20% of cycles are anovulatory. In boys, PHV occurs later in puberty when increases in LH and testosterone first occur throughout the day.

Numerous lines of evidence indicate that the principal sex steroids, estradiol (girls) and testosterone (boys), are responsible for the pubertal growth spurt.[1, 2] Large doses of estrogens suppress growth; however, very small doses of estrogens stimulate growth and most likely account for the growth spurt that occurs in early female puberty.[1] Clinical observations also support a causative role for estrogens in the pubertal growth spurt. For example, patients with testicular feminization have an entirely normal pubertal growth pattern.[2] These patients

TABLE 9–3.
Clinical Assessment of Overall Pubertal Development in Boys*

Pubertal Stage	Characteristics
P₁	No clinical signs of puberty
P₂	Early testicular enlargement and thinning and reddening of scrotum; minimal straight pubic or scrotal hair
P₃	Further testicular enlargement; definite phallic enlargement; darker, slightly curled pubic hair; early axillary and facial hair
P₄	Moderate pubic, axillary, and facial hair; acne; voice change; adult body odor
P₅	Adult body habitus, hair distribution, and genitalia

* Adapted from Kelch RP; Grumbach MM, Kaplan SL: in Saxena BB, Beling CG, Gandy HM (eds): *Gonadotropins*. New York, Wiley-Interscience, 1972, p 524.

are phenotypic females who have a 46,XY karyotype but who cannot respond to androgenic hormones. They do respond, however, to the estrogens secreted by their testes, become well feminized, and grow normally throughout childhood and adolescence.

Testosterone is a remarkably anabolic, growth-promoting hormone that undoubtedly plays a central role in the male pubertal growth spurt. However, testosterone treatment of adolescent boys who are deficient in both growth hormone and gonadotropins, does not induce a normal growth spurt.[2] Considerable evidence indicates that testosterone requires the presence of growth hormone to exert its full effect. Furthermore, it has recently been demonstrated that testosterone treatment increases the amplitude of growth hormone secretion in adolescent boys.[21] Several reports have shown that growth hormone and Sm-C production increase at puberty in both sexes almost surely as the result of increased secretion of sex steroids.[30] Available data strongly suggest that the pubertal growth spurt is caused by the combined action of testosterone and growth hormone in boys and estradiol and growth hormone in girls.[1] However, normal pubertal growth can occur only when thyroid gland function is normal and nutrition is adequate.

Although sex steroids affect the timing, magnitude, and duration of the pubertal growth spurt, they have almost no influence on adult stature unless they are given or produced at a young age. Significant exposure to sex steroids before a bone age of 10 to 12 years clearly results in a decrease in adult height; on the other hand, delayed exposure to sex steroids may increase adult height. For example, untreated agonadal or severely hypogonadal patients do not have an adolescent growth spurt, but they do grow slowly for a longer period and eventually attain entirely normal adult stature.[2] Furthermore, a recent review[1] indicates that such patients actually became taller than would have been predicted; final adult height was significantly greater (+ 4.2 cm) in men who had isolated hypogonadotrophic hypogonadism than in healthy men. Cutler and his colleagues noted, however, that all of the increased height of his population was attributable to the patients whose androgen replacement therapy had been delayed until 18 years of age or older.[1]

In adults, the average sex difference in height is approximately 5 inches (12.4 cm; ranging from 10 cm to 14 cm in various studies). Detailed longitudinal studies, as summarized recently by Prader,[2] indicate that only some of this difference may be attributable to sex steroids. Infant boys grow somewhat faster than girls, which most likely is the result of testosterone secretion in early infancy; this accounts for 1.5 cm of the difference. Why bone age does not advance more rapidly in infant boys, however, is unknown. The delayed onset of the pubertal spurt in boys accounts for 6.5 cm more of the difference, and 6 cm of the difference is caused by the higher peak velocity in boys. On the other hand, girls grow slightly more after the growth spurt, which reduces the sex difference by 1.5 cm.

ISOSEXUAL PRECOCIOUS DEVELOPMENT

Clinically it is useful to distinguish between isosexual and contrasexual (heterosexual) development. Moreover, among the causes of isosexual precocity, it is necessary to distinguish true precocious puberty from the numerous forms of incomplete isosexual precocity.

Isosexual refers to development consistent with phenotypic sex, whereas physical changes consistent with those of the opposite sex are considered contrasexual. True or central precocious puberty occurs when there is premature, sustained activation of the putative, hypothalamic GnRH pulse generator. Incomplete (pseudoprecocious or peripheral) precocity includes a large, diverse group of disorders that are not caused by premature activation of the neuroendocrine reproductive system (Tables 9–4 and 9–5).

As with most clinical conditions, a thorough history and physical examination usually point toward the correct diagnosis. Specific questions should be asked to elicit any history of recent growth acceleration, behavioral changes, body odor, vaginal discharge or bleeding, CNS trauma or infections (e.g., previous meningitis or encephalitis), similar precocious development in parent or siblings, and the use of facial creams and oral, parenteral, or topical medication. Familial precocious puberty has been reported several times, but it has been limited almost completely to boys.[31]

Physical examination must include a thorough neurologic evaluation with funduscopic and gross visual field examination. Precise measurement of height, weight, head circumference, arm span, sitting height, breast diameter, phallic length and width, and longest diameter and width of each testis (excluding epididymis) in boys must be taken and recorded. Examination of the skin for hyperpigmentation (congenital adrenal hyperplasia [CAH]), "coast of Maine" (McCune-Albright) or "coast of California" (neurofibromatosis) café-au-lait spots, carotenemia, dryness, coolness (hypothyroidism), and sebaceous gland activity (androgen effect) may be most helpful. Early signs of androgen secretion are the presence of comedones over the nose and in the external ear, and oiliness of the facial skin. Development of breasts, genitalia, and sexual hair should be assessed (see Tables 9–2 and 9–3).[26] Galactorrhea is rare, but its presence is suggestive of primary hypothyroidism or a pituitary or hypothalamic tumor.[32] Bimanual abdominal-rectal examination is helpful in the assessment of uterine development and in the detection of adnexal masses; sedation or even anesthesia may be necessary in younger patients to ensure an adequate examination.

A thorough history and physical examination along with close follow-up is often all that is required for the care of children with mild sexual precocity such as girls with premature thelarche. However, when significant sexual precocity is detected, the initial diagnostic tests should include radiographic evaluation of the skull (detailed views of the optic foramina in patients with visual defects or suspected neurofibromatosis) and hands for bone age determination, serum DHEAS or 24-hour urinary 17-KS excretion, serum thyroxine, LH and FSH, and testosterone (boys) or estradiol (girls). Single determinations of serum gonadotropins often are not useful because of the significant overlap of normal

TABLE 9–4.
Differential Diagnosis of Isosexual Precocious Development

Premature activation of GnRH (LRF) pulse generator (true or
central precocious puberty); pubertal or adult-type response
to synthetic GnRH
Idiopathic true precocious puberty
Sporadic (most common)
Familial (rare)
Other central nervous system disorders: hypothalamic
hamartoma, congenital anomalies, tumors, trauma, post
inflammation or irradiation of the CNS, neurofibromatosis,
tuberous sclerosis, Russell-Silver syndrome, septo-optic
dysplasia
True precocious puberty after late treatment of congenital
virilizing adrenal hyperplasia or other chronic exposure to
sex steroids
GnRH (LRF)–independent, "incomplete" or "peripheral"
isosexual precocity; prepubertal or severely blunted response
to synthetic GnRH
Gonadal tumors and gonadotropin-independent
hyperfunctioning disorders
Ovarian: granulosa cell tumor, granulosa-luteal cell cysts,
McCune-Albright syndrome, Peutz-Jeghers syndrome
Testicular: Leydig cell tumor, adrenal rest tumor,
"testoxicosis"
Adrenal disorders
Congenital adrenal hyperplasia (in boys)
Adenomas and carcinomas: virilizing (in boys), feminizing
(in girls)
Gonadotrophin-secreting tumors
hCG-secreting tumors (within or outside of the CNS);
chorioepithelioma, choriocarcinoma, germinoma,
hepatoblastoma, and teratoma
LH-secreting pituitary adenoma
Exogenous sex steroid or hCG administration
Severe primary hypothyroidism
Normal variants
Premature thelarche
Premature adrenarche

values between prepubertal and adult subjects.[33] Nonetheless, because of the
cross-reactivity of chorionic gonadotropin and LH, the radioimmunoassay
technique is used to detect the presence of the rare gonadotropin-producing
tumor. Sensitive urinary pregnancy tests, which detect human chorionic
gonadotropin (hCG) or its β-subunit immunologically may also be useful. Urinary
gonadotropin determinations by bioassay are not useful in most cases;
radioimmunoassay determinations of urinary LH and FSH may be helpful as
may bioassay determinations of serum gonadotropins, but these techniques are
not readily available. Further diagnostic evaluation — which may include a
synthetic GnRH test, pelvic sonography, cranial computed tomographic (CT)
scanning or magnetic resonance (MR) imaging — will depend on the degree

and rapidity of the sexual maturation, results of the preliminary tests, and the sex of the patient.

Isosexual precocity is a much more common disorder in girls (Table 9–6) than in boys.[34] The recent widespread use of high-resolution, CT brain scans has revealed a much higher than suspected incidence of hypothalamic hamartomas

TABLE 9–5.
Differential Diagnosis of Contrasexual
Development During Childhood and Adolescence

GIRLS
    Congenital adrenal hyperplasia
        21-Hydroxylase deficiency
        11-Hydroxylase deficiency
        3-β-Hydroxysteroid dehydrogenase deficiency
    Androgen-producing tumors
        Adrenal adenoma or carcinoma
        Ovarian arrhenoblastoma
        Teratoma
    Idiopathic hirsutism
    Polycystic ovarian disease
    Exogenous androgens
BOYS
    Adolescent gynecomastia
    Klinefelter's syndrome
    Estrogen-producing tumors
        Adrenal adenoma or carcinoma
        Teratoma
    Marihuana smoking
    Exogenous estrogens

TABLE 9–6.
Usual Clinical Findings in Girls With Isosexual Precocity

	Premature Thelarche	Exogenous Estrogen Exposure	Unsustained Isosexual Precocity	True Precocious Puberty
Breast development ($+ / + + + +$)	$+/+ +$	$+ / + + +$	$+ + / + + +$	$+ + / + + +$
Growth velocity	Normal	Normal	Normal or slightly increased	Accelerated
Bone age	Normal	Normal	Normal	Advanced
Serum estradiol	Prepubertal	Prepubertal	Strikingly increased or prepubertal	Pubertal
GnRH test	Prepubertal*	Suppressed	Suppressed or prepubertal	Pubertal or adult
Pelvic ultrasonography	Normal*	Normal	Small ovarian cyst(s)	Ovarian enlargement (+/- small cysts)

* Seldom, if ever indicated in evaluation.

in children with true precocious puberty. However, idiopathic precocious puberty remains as the most common final diagnosis in girls. On the other hand, CNS lesions, especially tumors, are commonly found in boys with sexual precocity. Indeed, in a recent series of 20 consecutive boys with true (central) precocious puberty referred to the National Institute of Health for treatment with GnRH (LRF)-analogue, only two had a final diagnosis of idiopathic precocious puberty.[35] Thus, despite the overall high incidence of idiopathic precocious puberty, clinicians must diligently search for evidence of other disorders outlined in Table 9–4, especially in boys.

Idiopathic true precocious puberty most commonly is sporadic but may be familial.[36] Children with idiopathic precocious puberty typically have normal skull roentgenograms, advanced bone age (often greater than height age), urinary 17-KS excretion appropriate or somewhat less than expected for the degree of pubertal development, and serum gonadotropins and sex steroid concentrations in the broad pubertal range. However, their clinical courses are highly variable. Girls usually show breast development, sexual hair, development of labia minora and majora, and in due course periodic menstruation. If untreated, ovulation occurs in some very young girls with precocious puberty, and pregnancies have been reported. Boys display phallic enlargement, testicular enlargement, and progressive signs of androgen secretion: pubic and axillary hair, acne to a variable degree, facial hair, and emission. Often, however, the rate of progression of sexual maturation is unpredictable and does not follow the normal pattern. Many children with precocious puberty have been observed for extended periods and have led normal lives as adults. Although significant manifestations of CNS disease are usually absent, there is an increased incidence of abnormal electroencephalographic tracings.[37]

Isosexual precocity in girls may also be secondary to CNS tumors or to estrogen secretion by ovarian or adrenal tumors. Testing with synthetic GnRH is helpful diagnostically.[4, 16] Recent studies indicate that patients with precocious puberty of central origin have augmented LH responsiveness, whereas girls with incomplete or GnRH-independent forms of isosexual precocity have blunted or prepubertal-type responses.[16] Radionuclide brain scans have limited usefulness, but cranial CT scanning and pelvic ultrasonography are most useful in evaluating suspected nervous system or ovarian abnormalities, respectively.[38, 39] Although there is not universal agreement on this point, it is our opinion that cranial CT scans should be obtained in all patients (boys and girls) with true precocious puberty. Because of the associated risks, pneumoencephalography or carotid arteriography should be performed only for further delineation of lesions demonstrated by CT scanning or when the clinical condition remains highly suggestive of intracranial disease despite a normal appearance on the CT scan. However, in those instances, it would be prudent to refer the patient to a center where sophisticated MR imaging could be performed first.

In patients with well-described syndromes such as McCune-Albright[40] (see below), the condition should be recognized by careful physical examination alone. Silver-Russell syndrome is characterized by intrauterine growth retardation, subnormal growth velocity, triangular facies, clinodactyly, simian creases, increased prevalence of structural abnormalities of the genitourinary tract, and in some patients skeletal asymmetry (see Chapter 3). Patients with neurofibromatosis may harbor a glioma in or around the hypothalamus, which may lead to increased, or more commonly, decreased pituitary function. Septo-optic dysplasia (deMorsier syndrome) includes abnormalities of the optic nerves and associated visual defects, absence of the septum pellucidum or corpus callosum, and hypothalamic hypopituitarism including diabetes insipidus. Despite the high incidence of hypothalamic hypopituitarism in the disorder, precocious sexual development has also been reported.[41]

Various CNS tumors, malignant and benign, may impinge on ventral hypothalamic areas and activate the centers that control gonadotropin secretion. The classic example of a benign tumor is hamartoma of the tuber cinereum. These tumors rarely damage the hypothalamus; they generally have secondary effects on other parts of the CNS and usually are asymptomatic, except for sexual precocity. With these facts in mind and especially since hypothalamic hamartomas respond nicely to GnRH-analogue therapy, attempted surgical removal of such lesions is unwise.

Analysis of a hypothalamic hamartoma revealed GnRH and neurosecretory cells, which presumably caused sexual precocity by increased or uncontrolled secretion of GnRH.[42] Nonparenchymatous tumors of the pineal gland also may cause sexual precocity in boys, whereas parenchymatous tumors are associated with delayed sexual development. Therapeutic radiation of the CNS may frequently lead to neuroendocrine dysfunction; unfortunately, both growth hormone deficiency and true precocious puberty are common sequelae.

Estrogen-producing ovarian tumors are usually palpable on bimanual abdominal-rectal examination.[37, 43–48] The average diameter of such tumors at the time of diagnosis has been approximately 11 to 12 cm. They are usually unilateral, smooth, firm, and encapsulated. Histologically they are either granulosa–theca cell tumors or cysts; at times there is luteinization of the cyst. Granulosa–theca cell tumors generally grow rapidly, but usually are benign. Approximately 30% are malignant, but accurate statistics on this are not available. It may be difficult to differentiate small ovarian tumors because of the overlap in laboratory values. For example, at times urinary and serum estrogens may be only slightly elevated, and gonadotropin determinations may be in the normal range. The GnRH test and pelvic ultrasonography would be most useful in such cases. Small ovarian cysts and the resultant isosexual precocity may regress spontaneously. Indeed, if pelvic ultrasonography reveals an ovarian mass less than 2.5 cm in diameter, a period of careful, close observation is a reasonable approach. On the other hand, treatment of large ovarian tumors is primarily surgical and often involves unilateral ovariectomy. The presence of a palpable adnexal mass requires surgical exploration by an experienced pediatric surgeon or gynecologist. Small or moderate-sized ovarian cysts are sometimes palpable in girls with idiopathic precocious puberty. These are usually bilateral and may recur after careful excision. These cysts are probably the result of the precocious release of gonadotropins; care must be taken to avoid surgical trauma to the remaining ovarian tissue.

McCune-Albright syndrome is more common in girls and is associated with polyostotic fibrous dysplasia and prominent areas of skin pigmentation, usually unilateral and generally on the same side as the osseous lesions. Recent reports indicate that the endocrine disorders associated with McCune-Albright syndrome — for example, hyperthyroidism, Cushing's syndrome, giantism, and isosexual precocity — may result from autonomous hyperfunctioning of the target glands.[40] Indeed, functioning ovarian cysts have been found to be the cause of isosexual precocity in several patients.

Isosexual precocity has also been observed in patients with Peutz-Jeghers syndrome, a familial disorder characterized by the association of mucocutaneous pigmentation and polyposis. Girls and boys may have functioning gonadal sex cord tumors which result in feminization. In girls, these tumors have a histologic appearance similar to granulosa–theca cell tumors.

"Testotoxicosis," another form of gonadal autonomy, is a sex-limited autosomal dominant disorder in which Leydig cell hyperplasia and germ cell maturation occur in the absence of gonadotropin stimulation. The precise cause of this form of gonadotropin-independent sexual precocity is unknown. On the other hand, this disorder probably accounts for most of the reports of familial precocious puberty.

Feminizing adrenal tumors are rare and often difficult to recognize. Frequently they secrete excessive amounts of androgens, hence 17-KS excretion is increased. Intravenous pyelography may be helpful when an adrenal adenoma or carcinoma is a distinct possibility. CT or ultrasonography are noninvasive and have now become the preferred diagnostic approaches. Adrenal scans performed by the administration of radioiodinated cholesterol before and after dexamethasone suppression have been helpful in selected patients. Adrenal venography or arteriography should only be performed by highly skilled personnel when the index of suspicion is great, and when absolutely necessary.

Leydig cell (interstitial cell) tumors of the testis are rare, but usually are unilateral and palpable.[49] Although many of these are benign, metastases have been reported years after removal of a primary tumor. Most boys with Leydig cell tumors have been under 6 years of age. Detailed studies of individual plasma sex steroids and urinary 17-KS have assisted in the differentiation from adrenal lesions. In instances of Leydig cell tumors, the urinary 17-KS are usually metabolites of testosterone, and the principal circulating androgen is testosterone, whereas adrenal androgen-producing lesions secrete primarily DHEA and DHEAS as well as their 16α-hydroxy derivatives.

Adrenocortical tumors, adenomas, or carcinomas can occur in either sex at any time in life. Adrenal tumors are exceedingly rare in earliest infancy and are not an important consideration in the differential diagnosis of neonatal sexual ambiguity. These tumors are usually unilateral and may be associated principally with the secretion of excessive quantities of androgens. In such instances, serum DHEAS is usually remarkably high and urinary 17-KS levels are strikingly elevated, sometimes reaching levels in excess of 50 mg/day. In some cases, the contralateral adrenal gland may be atrophic secondary to glucocorticoid secretion by the tumor. Thus when unilateral adrenalectomy is planned, the patient should receive stress doses of glucocorticoids to prevent the possibility of acute adrenal insufficiency. Surgical removal of adenomas is usually curative, but adrenal carcinomas are usually rapidly fatal.

In both boys and girls, gonadotropin-producing tumors are rare. These neoplasms arise in an extrapituitary site; gonadotropin-producing tumor of the pituitary gland is essentially unknown as a cause of sexual precocity. Chorioepitheliomas are the classic gonadotropin-producing tumors. They may occur in any part of the body, even within the cranial cavity. Generally they are highly malignant. Hepatoblastoma may produce a chorionic gonadotropin–like hormone and cause sexual precocity in boys. Testicular biopsy reveals Leydig cell hyperplasia. Hepatomegaly may be present, but without evidence of gross hepatic functional disturbance. Teratomas may occur in the gonads or retroperitoneum or anywhere along the median or paramedian line from the base of the skull to the sacrococcygeal region. They are often benign and may secrete chorionic gonadotropins.

Because the source of the androgen excess frequently is not obvious, adrenal gland suppression with oral dexamethasone (1.25 mg/m²/day in four equal doses) may be necessary. When evaluating adrenal androgen secretion through determination of 17-KS excretion, suppression should be carried out for at least 4 to 5 days because of the slow clearance rate of circulating adrenal androgens (see Appendix 9, Dexamethasone Suppression Test). Serum DHEAS, 17-hydroxyprogesterone, and possibly 17-hydroxypregnenolone should be measured before and at the end of dexamethasone suppression. If those studies are not readily available, then urinary 17-KS and pregnanetriol measurements may be substituted. Increased but suppressible values for serum DHEAS and 17-hydroxyprogesterone will usually confirm the diagnosis of CAH; additional measurements of 17-hydroxypregnenolone and 17-hydroxyprogesterone before and after ACTH stimulation may be required to differentiate mild forms of 21-hydroxylase and 3β-hydroxysteroid dehydrogenase deficiencies. Strikingly increased and nonsuppressible serum DHEAS suggests an androgen-producing tumor, most likely adrenal in origin. Measurements of serum DHEAS and 17-hydroxyprogesterone have essentially replaced urinary 17-KS and pregnanetriol determinations because of greater ease of collection and reliability. If the baseline urinary level of 17-hydroxycorticosteroids were elevated, suppression with a higher dose of dexamethasone (3.75 mg/m²/day in four equal doses) for an additional 2 days would be necessary to differentiate between an adrenal tumor and Cushing's disease. However, the effects of excess glucocorticoids should be obvious clinically.

When evaluating isosexual precocity in boys true precocious puberty must be differentiated from excessive androgen production alone. The most common cause of excessive androgen production is CAH (usually a non-salt-losing form of 21-hydroxylase deficiency). Thorough examination of the external genitalia will almost always distinguish between true precocious puberty and excess androgen production alone. Boys with true precocious puberty will have bilateral testicular enlargement (testes 2.5 to 3.0 cm or greater in longest diameter) and skeletal age and adrenal and testicular sex steroid values appropriate for the degree of pubertal development. Boys with androgen excess alone usually have small, prepubertal-sized testes despite advanced genital development, more striking advancement of skeletal age, and marked increases in adrenal sex steroid values (serum androstenedione, DHEAS, or urinary 17-KS). There are some exceptions to these general statements. Occasionally boys who have CAH also have testicular enlargement because they have entered puberty or because of bilateral hyperplasia of adrenal rests in the testes.

In all instances of sexual precocity, clinicians must diligently search for possible exposure to sex steroids. Ingestion of estrogen-contaminated pharmaceutical products, or birth control pills, as well as exposure to estrogen-containing creams, lotions, and ointments have all been associated with precocious sexual development in infants and children. In both sexes, severe primary hypothyroidism has been associated with sexual precocity.[32] Galactorrhea is a common finding in affected girls. The precocious development in primary hypothyroidism appears to be secondary to inappropriate secretion of pituitary gonadotropins, and the galactorrhea appears to be a consequence of increased secretion of prolactin in the presence of severe thyroid hormone deficiency.

The term *incomplete sexual precocity* should be limited to girls who have precocious development of breast tissue (premature thelarche) or precocious appearance of sexual hair (premature adrenarche). In the past these conditions were thought to be the result of increased end organ sensitivity to sex hormones. However, considerable evidence now indicates that the concentrations of sex hormones are increased in most of these patients, suggesting precocious, but often unsustained, secretion of ovarian or adrenal sex steroids.[37, 50]

Premature thelarche must be differentiated from neonatal hyperplasia of the breast, which can occur in either sex and generally subsides spontaneously within a few weeks or months. No treatment is necessary for this type of neonatal breast enlargement. Typically girls with premature thelarche are between 6 months and 2 years of age. Breast development is only modest and often regresses over several months to a year, but it may persist, even until the onset of normal puberty. There is no history of accelerated growth, and the bone age and 17-KS values are normal. Girls with premature adrenarche are usually older, 5 to 8 years of age. Growth velocity may be increased; 17-KS and plasma DHEAS are in the early pubertal range; bone age is slightly advanced; and comedones, axillary sweating, and hair may be present in addition to pubic hair. Urinary pregnanetriol or serum 17-hydroxyprogesterone determinations, before and after acute ACTH stimulation, usually differentiate premature adrenarche from mild forms of virilizing CAH.

Treatment

A precise diagnosis is necessary before initiation of therapy for sexual precocity. Reassurance and close follow-up only are required in the management of patients with premature thelarche or premature adrenarche. Diagnostic evaluation should be severely limited in those patients; breast biopsy should never be performed. Tumors of the gonads, adrenal glands, or CNS require a medical-surgical approach. Central nervous system tumors that are associated with true precocious puberty are seldom completely resectable, because of their proximity to vital structures. A carefully performed biopsy, followed by radiation therapy if the tumor is radiosensitive, is the preferred treatment in most instances. A typical hypothalamic hamartoma, on the other hand, should not be biopsied, but should be observed closely with serial CT scans to be certain that the lesion is not enlarging, and GnRH-analogue therapy should be considered. Patients with CAH should be given replacement doses of glucocorticoids and their adrenal steroid levels and growth should be observed closely (see Chapter 7). Usually only replacement doses of thyroid hormone are necessary for severe primary hypothyroidism associated with sexual precocity.

One of the most important aspects of the management of precocious development is detailed supportive counseling for the child and the parents. Parental anxieties and concerns must be addressed, and practical guidance should be provided. Parents should be advised to respond to their child in a manner appropriate to the chronologic age and not in relation to physical appearance; similar advice should be given to teachers and other school personnel. Affected children will require counseling and support in the maintenance of self-esteem and in their ability to handle ridicule, rejection, self doubt, and difficult encounters with other children and adults. On occasion, acceleration in school has been helpful in lessening some of the psychosocial difficulties associated with sexual precocity, but this can be accomplished only if the child is able to cope with increased academic stress. Parents, especially fathers, often have great difficulty relating to a physically precocious child, and they must be taught to accept the normal caresses and physical contact appropriate for the child's chronologic age. Many parents physically shun their child, who interprets this as frank rejection. Finally, the patient must be assisted with adaptation to the possibility of a short adult height despite having been tall as a child.

Until recently, the medical treatment of precocious puberty has been unsatisfactory and difficult to evaluate. Several steroid drugs have been used with variable success: medroxyprogesterone acetate (Provera),[51, 52] an ethinyl testosterone analogue (Danazol)*,[53, 54] cyproterone acetate,[55] and chlormadinone.[56] None of these compounds has controlled sexual precocity completely without significant side effects. Provera has been the most widely used compound; it is a progestational steroid that decreases gonadotropin secretion, but also has significant glucocorticoid activity. Adrenal suppression and even Cushing's syndrome have resulted when Provera has been given parenterally in large doses. Treatment with Provera has also been associated with the finding of chromosomal alterations in testicular germ cells.[57] Although Provera controls menses and frequently causes regression of breast tissue, it usually has not altered the rapid growth rate or bone maturation appreciably. Danazol has definite antigonadotropin activity in human beings, but its inherent androgenic activity limits its clinical usefulness. Cyproterone acetate, an antiandrogen, has not been used in the United States, but it appears to have no major advantages over Provera.

---

* 17α-Prega-2,dien-20-yno[2,3-d]isoxazol-17-ol.

All of these drugs must still be considered investigational.

The most promising therapeutic approach to patients with true precocious puberty has been the administration of potent, long-acting GnRH agonists.[18, 34, 58-60] Analogues of GnRH have been developed that have up to 200-fold greater potency, prolonged action, and apparent low toxicity. Rather than inducing chronic overstimulation of pituitary gonadotrophes, these analogues have the paradoxical effect of densensitizing the gonadotrophe, and in so doing profoundly suppress gonadotropin secretion. These agents are usually effective when given as a singly daily subcutaneous injection; intranasal administration is also effective, but much larger dosages are required.[60] Early results from several centers suggest that central precocity can be controlled in nearly all patients and that treatment results in an increase in adult height prediction. Nonetheless, until results from longer term studies are available, treatment with GnRH analogues must be considered investigational. In our opinion, the current treatment of choice for centrally mediated precocious puberty is administration of a long-acting agonist of GnRH, because it appears to offer a beneficial effect on adult height. If analogue therapy is unavailable, treatment with Provera should be considered. Medical intervention should be considered when menarche has occurred or seems imminent in a child in whom this would produce significant psychosocial trauma. Patients with rapidly progressive precocious puberty may be given Provera (5 to 10 mg once or twice per day orally). Adrenal suppression with this dosage is minimal, and menses and breast development are arrested; in general, patients who have tumors or structural abnormalities of the CNS respond poorly. In many patients with idiopathic precocious puberty, the waxing and waning course makes it difficult to assess the results of therapy. Since it has not been established that ultimate height is increased by treatment with progestational steroids, treatment is indicated only to lessen the psychosocial trauma.

Antagonists to the hypothalamic hormone GnRH have been developed and are in the earliest stage of clinical trials; at least theoretically, these compounds would provide a more specific and effective means of therapy for central precocious puberty.

Neither GnRH agonists nor progestational steroids have been effective in the treatment of gonadotropin-independent sexual precocity. Some success has been reported with the use of ketoconazole or a combination of testolactone and spironalactone in "testotoxicosis" and testolactone alone in the McCune-Albright syndrome.[61-63] These approaches also are at the investigational stage.

CONTRASEXUAL DEVELOPMENT

Contrasexual development (virilization of a girl or feminization of a boy) is uncommon after the newborn period (see Table 9–5). The diagnostic approach is similar to that outlined earlier, but special attention must be given to the possibility of CAH and sex hormone-producing tumors. Thus, selective serum measurements of DHEAS, 17-hydroxyprogesterone, 11-deoxycortisol, 17-hydroxypregnenolone, and total or free testosterone may be necessary; in addition, measurements before and after ACTH stimulation or dexamethasone suppression may be required to arrive at a final diagnosis.

Some young girls develop moderately generalized hirsutism without other signs of an endocrine disorder (idiopathic hirsutism). This is often constitutional or familial, but is distressing in some cultures. Urinary 17-KS excretion and serum androgen levels may be slightly elevated. These patients must be differentiated from those with mild forms of CAH. Medical treatment is not indicated, but reassurance should be given, and depilatory creams or electrolysis for cosmetically unacceptable facial hair can be recommended. Some of these girls may have early polycystic ovarian disease (PCO; Stein-Leventhal syndrome), although most do not develop the other features of this syndrome.

The classic signs of Stein-Leventhal syndrome were amenorrhea, hirsutism, and obesity; now it is well recognized that these findings may be seen in Cushing's syndrome, CAH, virilizing ovarian and adrenal tumors, and hyperthyroidism or hypothyroidism, as well as in typical PCO. Analysis of 100 consecutive patients with PCO revealed that menarche occurs at a normal age (mean 12.3 years), but postmenarchal menstrual irregularity is maintained; usually excessive hair growth occurs before or at about menarche; and most patients are considered "overweight" before menarche.[21] These findings suggest that the endocrine abnormalities of PCO syndrome are present before final maturation of the cyclic hypothalamic-pituitary-ovarian axis. Physicians may see such patients before ovarian enlargement is detectable by routine pelvic examination. Although the initial abnormality is not known, the pathophysiology of PCO syndrome is complex.[21] Excess androgen production by the ovaries, and to some degree by the adrenal glands, causes hirsutism and allows for increased estrogen production by means of extraglandular conversion. The latter occurs to a great degree within fat cells. The increased estrogen production results in increased LH and decreased FSH secretion, which in turn causes ovarian hyperthecosis and chronic anovulation. Typical laboratory findings include an increased serum LH-FSH ratio, normal or slightly increased levels of urinary 17-KS, increased total and to a greater degree free concentration of serum testosterone, and normal urinary pregnanetriol and serum 17-hydroxyprogesterone values.

During adolescence, most patients seek medical help because of hirsutism. There is no rational and highly effective endocrine therapy for hirsutism.[21, 64] Oral contraceptive steroids (low-dose estrogen-progestin combinations) or adrenal suppression with dexamethasone (0.5 to 1.0 mg orally at bedtime) may be effective alone or in combination. However, it is 4 to 6 months before decrease in hair growth is appreciable. Some patients fail to show any significant effect despite clear suppression of serum androgen values. Spironalactone, primarily used as a antihypertensive, also has antiandrogenic properties, and has been effective at a dose of 100 to 200 mg/day.[22] When fertility is desired, in contrast, administration of clomiphene is usually successful; this treatment should be supervised by an experienced gynecologist.

Gynecomastia is common in male adolescents. The overall incidence is estimated at approximately 40%, with a peak prevalence at 13 to 14 years of age.[26] In most cases it is mild and transitory and is noticed only during careful physical examination. Severe gynecomastia is uncommon and in many patients is accompanied by obesity. The differential diagnosis includes Klinefelter's syndrome and estrogen-producing tumors. Recently, heavy marihuana smoking has also been associated with gynecomastia and arrested or delayed sexual maturation.[65] A thorough physical examination should suggest Klinefelter's syndrome (eunuchoid body habitus, incomplete masculinization, small firm testes). Estrogen-producing tumors also cause testicular atrophy. The tumors may be palpable if they are testicular, but estrogen-producing Leydig cell tumors occur only after adolescence. Diagnostic studies in severe gynecomastia should include buccal smear or karyotype, serum gonadotropins, serum prolactin, serum estradiol, and total urinary estrogens.

An increase in prolactin may result from drug use or abuse or from a prolactin-secreting pituitary tumor. In disorders of androgen deficiency, testosterone administration may result in some regression of breast tissue, but occasionally such treatment will actually make the condition worse. Recently, percutaneous dihydrotestosterone administration has been reported to be beneficial in the treatment of idiopathic gynecomastia; clomiphene citrate has also been effective in some patients.[66] Usually weight reduction, reassurance, and time are the only necessary remedies. When the patient is especially disturbed by his appearance and the breast diameter is greater than 4 cm, a transareolar mastectomy, a relatively simple procedure, should be considered.

DELAYED ADOLESCENT DEVELOPMENT

In contrast to precocious sexual development, delayed adolescent development is much more common in boys than in girls. A similar, careful history and a physical examination with precise measurement are mandatory. However, special attention should be paid to clues suggestive of chronic illness, hypopituitarism, hypothyroidism, hyposmia or anosmia (Kallmann's syndrome), Turner's syndrome, or Klinefelter's syndrome. Table 9–7 is a list of causes of delayed adolscence based primarily on whether the serum gonadotropins are normal or increased. The basic examination should include lateral radiographs of the skull to evaluate the pituitary fossa; bone age determinations; studies of serum thyroxine, serum gonadotropins, serum testosterone, or estradiol; and urinalysis with specific gravity determination, complete blood cell count, and sedimentation rate. Significantly short girls with delayed development should be karyotyped during the first visit.

Serum gonadotropins, especially FSH, are increased significantly in children with primary hypogonadism who are 12 years or older.[13, 14] Gonadotropins also are slightly increased in younger hypogonadal children, but there may be some overlap with the normal range during the middle of the first decade. Problems arise, however, in attempting to differentiate normal from low serum gonadotropin levels.

TABLE 9–7.
Differential Diagnosis of Delayed or Incomplete Adolescent Development

Normal or low serum gonadotropin values
  Constitutional delayed adolescence
  Hypopituitarism: idiopathic or acquired
    Multiple pituitary tropic hormone deficiencies
    Isolated deficiencies: gonadotropins (Kallman's syndrome), growth hormone
  Chronic illness (e.g. anorexia nervosa, regional enteritis, sickle cell anemia)
  Hypothyroidism
  Severe exogenous obesity
  Hyperprolactinemia: drug-induced, pituitary adenoma
  Congenital anomalies: absent uterus or vagina, imperforate hymen
Increased serum gonadotropin values
  Gonadal dysgenesis (Turner's syndrome)
  Klinefelter's syndrome
  Bilateral gonadal failure: traumatic, autoimmune destruction, infectious,
    postsurgical, postirradiation or chemotherapy, galactosemia, idiopathic (empty-
    scrotum or vanishing-testes syndrome), resistant ovary syndromes
Miscellaneous conditions
  Prader-Willi syndrome
  Laurence-Moon-Biedl syndrome
  Alstrom syndrome
  Testicular feminization (complete and incomplete)
  Germinal cell aplasia
  Steroidogenic enzyme deficiencies (adrenal and gonadal): cholesterol desmolase
    complex
  3β-hydroxysteroid dehydrogenase, 17α-hydroxylase, C17,20-desmolase, 17β-
    hydroxysteroid oxidoreductase (see Chapter 8)
  Myotonic dystrophy

    The most common final diagnosis for adolescents with delayed development and "normal" serum gonadotropins is constitutional delayed growth pattern. Typically the patient is a healthy but short boy with a moderately retarded bone age and a history of short stature since late infancy or early childhood. Frequently his father or brother(s) also developed slowly and may not have achieved their full adult height until after 20 years of age. Because of the failure of many clinicians to recognize the earliest signs of puberty in boys, many referred to our clinic are really in early puberty and can be reassured that they are developing normally. Thus the physical examination is extremely important, because undue concern and laboratory evaluation only increase anxiety and hinder the patient's psychosocial development.

    Hypopituitarism is not a common cause of delayed adolescent development, but must always be kept in mind, especially in patients with severe short stature (more than 3 SD below the mean for chronologic age). The diagnostic approach to growth failure is discussed in Chapter 3. Perhaps the most difficult condition to rule out is isolated gonadotropin deficiency. The typical patient is of average height and has eunuchoid body proportions.[67] Isolated gonadotropin deficiency in association with hyposmia or anosmia is Kallmann's syndrome. However, olfaction may be normal; the condition may occur in girls as well as in boys;

and at times is associated with facial defects such as cleft lip or palate. Only time can reliably differentiate isolated gonadotropin deficiency from constitutional delayed adolescence, but recent studies indicate that a standard intravenous GnRH stimulation test (2.5 μg/kg intravenous bolus) can be of some reassurance. Patients with delayed adolescence and bone age greater than 12 years usually have LH responses within the adult range (maximum LH increment >12 mIU/ mL, Second International Reference Preparation of human menopausal gonadotropin), whereas patients with isolated gonadotropin deficiency characteristically have blunted or immature LH responses. Prolactin responses to thyrotropin-releasing hormone have also been used to aid in the differential diagnosis. It is reported that boys with isolated gonadotropin deficiency have lower prolactin responses. Responsiveness to hCG is also blunted in boys with isolated gonadotropin deficiency, but no single test is completely reliable. Thus careful follow-up is mandatory.[68, 69]

Almost any chronic illness (e.g., sickle cell disease, diabetes mellitus, cyanotic congenital heart disease, collagen diseases, anorexia nervosa, regional enteritis) can delay growth and sexual development. Although childhood obesity is commonly associated with tall stature and normal or early pubertal development, severe obesity may be associated with delayed adolescence, the appearance of small external genitalia, and blunted responses to synthetic GnRH.[69]

Hyperprolactinemia, either drug induced or the result of pituitary microadenoma, is a rare cause of primary amenorrhea or delayed adolescence. Serum prolactin should be measured in all girls with galactorrhea and should be a routine part of the evaluation of secondary amenorrhea.

Congenital anomalies of the müllerian system are usually associated with delayed onset of menses but normal progression of secondary sex characteristics. Abnormal development of the müllerian system should be suspected in any girl who has not menstruated within 5 years of the onset of breast development. When a vagina is present, a cervix should be looked for. If a cervix is present, the possibility of uterine aplasia or uterine synechiae should be considered. Normal development of the vagina and uterus may occur in the rare syndrome of congenital absence of the cervix.

If the vagina is absent or not patent, imperforate hymen, vaginal atresia, or vaginal aplasia (in order of increasing severity) should be considered. These disorders will require surgical correction. Because ovarian function in these girls is usually normal, the endometrium, if present, responds appropriately to ovarian estrogen and progestogen; but lack of egress through the vagina leads to spillage of menstrual fluid into the abdomen and pelvis, and the fluid contains viable endometrium. This ectopic endometrium is also hormonally responsive and forms endometriomas, which are commonly associated with cyclic abdominal pain and masses that can be palpated rectally.[45]

Turner's syndrome (gonadal dysgenesis) is by far the most common cause of delayed development associated with increased serum gonadotropins. Affected girls are short and have primary amenorrhea. Seldom are their physical findings as blatant as those pictured in most texts; nonetheless, careful examination commonly reveals a low hairline, high-arched palate, low posteriorly rotated ears, numerous pigmented nevi, increased carrying angle, short fourth metacarpals, lymphedema, and dystrophic fingernails and toenails. The buccal smear is chromatin negative in the majority of patients; however, in approximately 20% of girls with gonadal dysgenesis a buccal smear is positive because of the presence of mosaicism or a structurally abnormal X chromosome. Thus even if the buccal smear is positive, karyotyping should be performed in girls with increased gonadotropins and delayed adolescence.

In most boys with Klinefelter's syndrome, this relatively common disorder is not diagnosed until puberty or early adulthood, although it may be diagnosed at birth because of undescended or unusual testes, or in childhood because of borderline mental retardation, behavioral abnormalities, or relatively small external genitalia. Such patients seldom come to a pediatrician because of delayed sexual maturation. Gynecomastia, on the other hand, is often a presenting complaint in adolescence. The patients are tall and slender, with decreased upper to lower body segment ratio. Arrested testicular growth usually occurs at around midpuberty, with maximal testicular volume of 3.5 ± 1.5 mL. Late in the second decade azoospermia or oligospermia are usually found and indicate progression of testicular damage. Early in puberty, serum gonadotropins and serum testosterone as well as response to hCG may be normal, but by midpuberty basal plasma FSH is usually increased and testosterone production is subnormal. Testosterone replacement therapy may be helpful in the management of gynecomastia, but if significant gynecomastia persists, mastectomy may be necessary.

In most patients with Klinefelter's syndrome the buccal smear reveals a chromatin-positive pattern consistent with the most common karyotype, 46,XXY. All patients who are found to have hypogonadism and clinical findings consistent with Klinefelter's syndrome should have a chromosomal analysis performed. In addition to the XXY pattern, patients with Klinefelter's syndrome may have multiple X (XXXY) or Y (XXYY) chromosomal patterns or mosaic patterns (e.g., XXY/XY).

Bilateral gonadal failure has many possible causes, but is uncommon. As therapy for various childhood malignancies has become more successful, there has been an increased incidence of primary hypogonadism secondary to chemotherapy, radiation therapy, and sometimes surgical removal. Autoimmune oophoritis, a rare cause of ovarian failure, is most often associated with Addison's disease and other autoimmune endocrinopathies. Delayed puberty, lack of pubertal progression, and menstrual irregularities in girls and young women with galactosemia are believed to result from acquired ovarian failure secondary to the toxic effects of galactose or its metabolites on the ovary in utero or in the immediate neonatal period. Patients with the so-called vanishing-testes syndrome hava a normal 46,XY karyotype and masculine appearance of the external genitalia; testes, however, are not palpable, and normal male puberty does not occur. Presumably, both testes atrophied or were destroyed sometime after fetal differentiation of the external genitalia. Stimulation with chorionic gonadotropin is useful to determine whether some abdominal testicular tissue is present; however, in the face of elevated serum FSH and LH, it is unlikely that this would be so. Although the risk of surgery may equal the risk of possible malignant degeneration, we believe that these boys should undergo exploratory laparotomy to detect and remove gonadal tissue. At the same time, prosthetic testes may be placed in the scrotum.

Patients with resistant ovary syndrome usually have primary amenorrhea, sexual immaturity, chromatin-positive buccal smear (46,XX), and small ovaries that contain primordial follicles. This constellation of findings is being identified with increasing frequency; gonadal biopsy is critical for the diagnosis.

Whenever a Y chromosome is detected in a phenotypic girl, the gonadal tissue should be removed to prevent occurrence of gonadal tumors, particularly gonadoblastomas. Gonad removal or biopsy is not required when a 45,X, 46,XX, or mosaic karyotype without an XY- or Y-bearing cell line has been found.

The miscellaneous conditions listed in Table 9–7 are rare and are not discussed in detail. Most of these conditions cause incomplete or abnormal sexual development. Prader-Willi syndrome is characterized by obesity, short stature, hypogonadism, small hands and feet, mental retardation, and infantile hypotonia. Bilateral cryptorchidism and a small flat scrotum are characteristic. The phallus appears small in childhood, and as the obesity progresses the phallus seemingly disappears. The primary defect has not been defined precisely, but there is evidence to suggest abnormal hypothalamic function. There is usually a blunted response or failure to respond to intravenous administration of synthetic GnRH. Girls as well as boys can be affected, and glucose intolerance is common. Most cases have been sporadic.

Laurence-Moon-Biedl syndrome is characterized by retinitis pigmentosa, polydactyly, obesity, and hypogonadism. Hypogonadotropic hypogonadism occurs in most affected boys and in approximately half of affected girls. The condition seems to be inherited as an autosomal recessive trait, with marked intrafamily variability.

Alstrom syndrome includes hypogonadism, retinitis pigmentosa, diabetes mellitus, and neurogenic deafness. Testicular feminization and Reifenstein's syndrome are extreme variants of familial male pseudohermaphroditism secondary to end organ insensitivity to androgens.[70, 71] Defects in testosterone biosynthesis (e.g., 17α-hydroxylase and 17β-hydroxysteroid oxidoreductase deficiency) also cause male pseudohermaphroditism. In girls, 17α-hydroxylase deficiency can cause hypertension, glucocorticoid insufficiency, and sexual infantilism[72]; boys have had hypospadias along with other endocrine disorders. Patients with germinal cell aplasia, del Castillo syndrome, or Sertoli cell–only syndrome have moderately increased serum FSH, but are normally virilized. Postpubertal seminiferous tubule sclerosis and cataracts occur in boys with chronic muscular dystrophy. Finally, a wide variety of genetic disorders can be associated with gonadal dysplasia and primary hypogonadism. Among them are Bloom, leopard, Louis-Bar (ataxia-telangiectasia), Rothmund-Thomson, Smith-Lemli-Opitz, and Opitz-Soffer syndromes. One of the most common disorders of this type is Noonan syndrome, characterized by short stature, webbed neck, congenital heart disease, ptosis, and abnormal testes; the karyotype in both boys and girls is normal.

Treatment

Evaluation of typical constitutionally delayed growth and adolescence in boys should be limited to avoid further increase in patient and parental anxiety. The boy should be reassured that he is developing normally and that medical intervention will not increase adult height. However, when emotional well-being is adversely affected, there is evidence of withdrawal from age-appropriate social activities or decreased academic performance, and no evidence of significant masculinization by 14 to 15 years of age, short-term treatment with androgens may be wise. Androgens can be given orally or intramuscularly for 3 to 6 months without significant adverse effects on adult height.[73, 74] This often produces enough masculinization to alleviate anxiety and social pressures; several prospective and retrospective studies have not shown a deleterious effect on ultimate height. Our therapeutic preference is to use a long-acting salt of testosterone, such as testosterone enanthate, 50 to 100 mg/mo, for a total of six intramuscular injections.

At initiation of therapy, the patient must agree to discontinuation of therapy after 6 months and observation of his spontaneous growth during the following 6 months. Usually, spontaneous growth velocity increases, the rate of sexual maturation is satisfactory, and no further therapy is needed. Rarely, short-term therapy with low-dose estrogens, for example, conjugated estrogens 0.3 mg/day or ethinyl estradiol 5 μg/day orally, is indicated in the treatment of markedly delayed development in girls. As in boys, a 6-month treatment course followed by 6 months of observation is recommended. In most girls, reassurance, close observation, and encouragement to wear a padded brassiere, age-appropriate clothing, and cosmetics are sufficient.

Patients with gonadal failure or proved gonadotropin deficiency require replacement therapy with sex steroids. If the age of the patient permits, the dosage of sex steroids should be gradually increased to full replacement over 2 to 3 years in an attempt to mimic the normal course of pubertal changes. In girls, treatment with conjugated or semisynthetic estrogens may be initiated, then gradually increased to full replacement. When vaginal spotting occurs, cyclical therapy should begin for 21 or 25 days per month; a progestational steroid such as medroxyprogesterone (5 to 10 mg/day orally) should be added during the last week of estrogen therapy. In boys, intramuscular testosterone enanthate, 50 to 100 mg/month initially, with increases up to 300 mg every 3 to 4 weeks, is highly effective. Initially some adolescent boys will not agree to long-term intramuscular therapy, and in those patients oral medication can be used to initiate pubertal changes. Methyltestosterone (25 to 50 mg/day orally), fluoxymesterone (Halotestin, 2 to 10 mg/day orally), or testosterone proprionate (10 mg/day orally) can be used, but full masculinization is seldom achieved at reasonable and safe dosages. Gonadotropin-deficient patients should be treated with sex steroid replacement until they wish to become fertile. When fertility is desired, therapy with gonadotropins or pulsatile GnRH should be considered; experience with GnRH is limited, but initial results are highly promising in patients with hypothalamic hypogonadotropism.[75]

ADOLESCENT MENOMETRORRHAGIA

Excessive, irregular vaginal bleeding is relatively common in adolescent girls. Whether the pathophysiologic basis for this disorder is primarily at the ovarian or the hypothalamic-pituitary level is unknown. Follicular maturation that terminates in atresia rather than ovulation is associated with sufficient ovarian hormone secretion to stimulate growth of extraovarian estrogen-dependent target tissues, including the endometrium. In such instances, ovarian progesterone secretion is inconsequential because ovulation has not occurred and thus the endometrium is responding to estrogen alone. Continuous production of estrogen unopposed by cyclic progestogen frequently results in acute or chronic vaginal bleeding, which may be sufficient to cause anemia and hypovolemia. Similar problems may be encountered during initiation of estrogen replacement therapy in girls with primary ovarian failure or gonadal dysgenesis. Once local causes of bleeding, such as polyps or vaginal lesions, have been excluded, bleeding usually can be controlled by administration of progestogens. Once the anemia is corrected, steroid hormone replacement can be withdrawn, with the expectation that cyclic events will be resumed without further difficulty.

UNDESCENDED TESTES

An undescended testis is one that fails to descend to its normal scrotal position by 1 year of age; if palpable, it cannot be brought manually into the upper part of the scrotum. Cryptorchid testes are located along the pathway of descent; ectopic testes are not. Undescended testes may be unilateral or bilateral; if unilateral, the right testis is more commonly affected.

Differentiation between an undescended testis and a retractile testis often is extremely difficult. By definition, retractile testes can be brought manually into the bottom of the scrotum. Examination of the patient while he is sitting with his legs crossed Indian style is frequently a useful maneuver. Numerous genetic disorders are associated with testicular malfunction or maldescent; hence special attention should be paid to the presence of other physical abnormalities.

Treatment of undescended testes often is vigorously debated despite the absence of clear-cut data. The optimal time for surgical intervention and the possible benefit of chorionic gonadotropin have not been determined by controlled prospective clinical studies. The reader is referred to the reviews by Myers and Kelalis[76] and Shapiro and Bodai[77] for further consideration of these questions.

Currently, our approach to these patients depends on their degree of involvement. Patients with unilateral or bilateral palpable but undescended testes are given a 6-week course of hGH 500 IU intramuscularly three times per week; numerous higher and lower dosage schedules have been proposed. In the prospective study by Sudmann[78] a shorter course of treatment caused descent of 31% of palpable testes. In cases of bilateral, undescended inguinal testes, serum testosterone should be measured after 1 week to demonstrate normal Leydig cell responsiveness.

hCG therapy almost surely does not cause the descent of nonpalpable (abdominal) testes. A 3-day course (2,000 IU/day intramuscularly) with measurement of serum testosterone on day 4 may be used to determine the presence of abdominal testes (see Appendix 9).[79] Although the risk of surgery may equal the risk of malignant degeneration of abdominal testes, we prefer to recommend an attempt at surgical correction before the patient starts school. If the testicles cannot be brought into a palpable location, they probably should be removed. Testicular prostheses should be offered, and replacement therapy with androgens started at about 12 years of age. Careful biopsies should be performed to assess testicular histology at the time of orchiopexy, and the family should be made aware that orchiopexy does not eliminate the increased risk of malignant degeneration. Other clinicians disagree with this approach and believe that bilateral abdominal testes are best left in situ for future endocrine function.[76, 77]

MICROPENIS

Occasionally boys are brought to the pediatrician or family physician because of the small size of the phallus. Usually the penis is truly within the normal range in size, although it may be embedded in suprapubic fat. In such instances reassurance, dietary restriction, and time are all that is necessary. In rare cases when the penis is truly hypoplastic the clinician must look for signs of hypopituitarism, Prader-Willi syndrome, or other dysmorphic disorders. Micropenis and hypoglycemia in a newborn boy are cardinal features of congenital hypopituitarism.[80] Short-term parenteral testosterone therapy (testosterone enanthate, 25 mg/mo intramuscularly for 3 to 4 months) may be beneficial, but should be prescribed only by experienced personnel.[81] Perhaps the best use of testosterone therapy is to preoperatively stimulate growth of the penis in patients with congenital hypospadias.[81]

APPENDIX 9

Dexamethasone Suppression Test

This test will determine the source of increased 17-KS excretion.

	Day 1	2	3	4	5	6
Treatment: Dexamethasone, 1.25 mg/m²/day in six divided doses, on days 3–6						
Serum DHEAS	X	X				X
Serum cortisol	X	X				X
Serum 17-OH-progesterone	X					X
or						
Urinary 17-KS	X	X			X	X
Urinary 17-OH corticosteroids	X	X				X
Urinary pregnanetriol	X					X

HCG Stimulation Test

This test will evaluate the steroidogenic capacity of undescended or structurally abnormal testes. According to Winter et al.,[79] the mean serum testosterone value for prepubertal boys on day 4 is 173 ± 27 ng/dL (SE: n = 8).

	Day 1	2	3	4
hCG, 2,000 IU/day IM	X	X	X	
Serum testosterone	X			X

REFERENCES

1. Cutler GB, et al: Pubertal growth: Physiology and pathophysiology, in *Recent Progress in Hormone Research*, vol. 42. Orlando, Fla, Academic Press, 1986.
2. Prader A: Biomedical and endocrinological aspects of normal growth and development, in Borms J, Hauspie R, Sand A, et al (eds): *Human Growth and Development — Proceedings From the Third International Congress on Auxology*, New York, Plenum Publishing Corp, 1984.
3. Marshall JC, Kelch RP: Gonadotropin-releasing hormone: Role of pulsatile secretion in the regulation of reproduction. *N Engl J Med* 1986; 315:1459.
4. Styne DM, Grumbach MM: Puberty in the male and female: Its physiology and disorders, in Yen SSC, Jaffe RB (eds): *Reproductive Endocrinology*. Philadelphia, WB Saunders Co, 1986, pp 313–384.
5. Grumbach MM: The neuroendocrinology of puberty, in Kreiger DT, Hughes JC (eds): *Neuroendocrinology*. Sunderland, Mass, Sinauer Associates, 1980.
6. Faiman C, Winter JSD: Sex differences in gonadotropin concentration in infancy. *Nature* 1971; 232:130.
7. August GP, Grumbach MM, Kaplan SL: Hormonal changes in puberty. III: Correlation of plasma testosterone, LH, FSH, testicular size, and bone age with male pubertal development. *J Clin Endocrinol Metab* 1972; 34:319.
8. Jenner MR, et al: Hormonal changes in puberty. IV: Plasma estradiol LH, and FSH in prepubertal children, pubertal females, and in precocious puberty, premature thelarche, hypogonadism and in a child with feminizing ovarian tumor. *J Clin Endocrinol Metab* 1972; 34:521.
9. Winter JSD, Faiman C: Pituitary-gonadal relationships in male children and adolescents. *Pediatr Res* 1972; 6:126.
10. Winter JSD, Faiman C: Pituitary-gonadal relations in female children and adolescents. *Pediatr Res* 1973; 7:948.
11. Winter JSD, Faiman C: The development of cyclic pituitary-gonadal function in adolescent females. *J Clin Endocrinol Metab* 1973; 37:714.
12. Kelch RP, Kaplan SL, Grumbach MM: Suppression of urinary and plasma follicle-stimulating hormone by exogenous estrogens in prepubertal and pubertal children. *J Clin Invest* 1973; 52:1122.
13. Conte FA et al: Correlation of luteinizing hormone-releasing factor-induced luteinizing hormone and follicle-stimulating hormone release from infancy to 19 years with the change in the pattern of gonadotropin secretion in agonadal patients: Relation to the restraint of puberty. *J Clin Endocrinol Metab* 1980; 50:163.

14. Lustig RH et al: Ontogeny of gonadotropin secretion in congenital anorchism: Sexual dismorphism versus syndrome of gonadal dysgenesis and diagnostic considerations. *J Urol* 1987; 138:587.

15. Jakacki RI et al: Pulsatile secretion of luteinizing hormone in children. *J Clin Endocrinol Metab* 1982; 55:453.

16. Zipf WB, et al: Suppressed responsiveness to gonadotropin-releasing hormone in girls with unsustained isosexual precocity. *J Pediatr* 1979; 95:38.

17. Hale PM et al: Increased LH pulse frequency during sleep in early pubertal boys: Effects of testosterone infusion. *J Clin Endocrinol Metab* 1988; 66:785.

18. Kulin HE: The maturation of ovulatory potential in man. *Horm Res* 1980; 12:46.

19. Boepple PA, et al: Use of a potent, long acting agonist of gonadotropin-releasing hormone in the treatment of precocious puberty. *Endocr Rev* 1986; 7:24.

20. Sauder SE, et al: The effects of opiate antagonism on gonadotropin secretion in children and in women with hypothalamic amenorrhea. *Pediatr Res* 1984; 18:321.

21. Reiter EO, et al: Secretion of the adrenal androgen, dehydroepiandrosterone sulfate, during normal infancy, childhood, adolescence, in sick infants, and in children with endocrinologic abnormalities. *J Pediatr* 1977; 90:766.

22. Yen SSC: Chronic anovulation caused by peripheral endocrine disorders, in Yen SSC, Jaffe RB (eds): *Reproductive Endocrinology*. Philadelphia, WB Saunders Co, 1986, pp 441–499.

23. Marshall WA, Tanner JM: Variations in pattern of pubertal changes in girls. *Arch Dis Child* 1969; 44:291.

24. Marshall WA, Tanner JM: Variations in the pattern of pubertal changes in boys. *Arch Dis Child* 1970; 45:13.

25. Frisch RE, Revelle R: Height and weight at menarche and a hypothesis of critical body weights and adolescent events. *Science* 1970; 169:397.

26. Kelch RP, Grumbach MM, Kaplan SL: in Saxena BB, Beling CG, Gandy HM (eds): *Gonadotropins*. New York, Wiley-Interscience, 1972, p 524.

27. Harlan WR, et al: Secondary sex characteristics of boys 12 to 17 years of age: The U.S. Health Examination Survey. *J Pediatr* 1979; 95:293.

28. Harlan WR, et al: Secondary sex characteristics of girls 12 to 17 years of age: The U.S. Health Examination Survey. *J Pediatr* 1980; 96:1074.

29. Tanner JM, Davies PW: Clinical longitudinal standards for height and height velocity for North American children. *J Pediatr* 1985; 107:317.

30. Link K, et al: The effect of androgens on the pulsatile release and the twenty-four-hour mean concentration of growth hormone in peripubertal males. *J Clin Endocrinol Metab* 1986; 62:159.

31. Beas F, et al: Familial male sexual precocity: Report of the eleventh kindred found, with observations on blood group linkage and urinary C19-steroid excretion. *J Clin Endocrinol Metab* 1962; 22:1095.

32. Van Wyk JJ, Grumbach MM: Syndrome of precocious menstruation and galactorrhea in juvenile hypothyroidism: An example of hormonal overlap in pituitary feedback. *J Pediatr* 1960; 57:416.

33. Penny R, et al: Correlation of serum follicular stimulating hormone (FSH) and luteinizing hormone (LH) as measured by radio-immunoassay in disorders of sexual development. *J Clin Invest* 1970; 49:1847.

34. Sigurjonsdottir TJ, Hayles AB: Precocious puberty, a report of 96 cases. *Am J Dis Child* 1968; 115:309.

35. Pescovitz OH, et al: The NIH experience in precocious puberty: Diagnostic subgroups and the response to short-term LHRH analogue therapy. *J Pediatr* 1986; 108:47.

36. Hopwood NJ, Kelch RP, Helder LJ: Familial precocious puberty affecting a brother and sister. *Am J Dis Child* 1981; 135:78.
37. Liu N, et al: Prevalence of electroencephalographic abnormalities in idiopathic precocious puberty and premature pubarche: Bearing on pathogenesis and neuroendocrine regulation of puberty. *J Clin Endocrinol Metab* 1965; 25:1296.
38. Hung W, et al: Computerized tomography in the evaluation of isosexual precocity. *Am J Dis Child* 1980; 134:25.
39. Lippe BM, Sample WF: Pelvic ultrasonography in pediatric and adolescent endocrine disorders. *J Pediatr* 1978; 92:987.
40. Danon M, et al: Cushing syndrome, sexual precocity and polyostotic fibrous dysplasia (Albright syndrome) in infancy. *J Pediatr* 1975; 87:917.
41. Huseman CA, et al: Sexual precocity in association with septo-optic dysplasia and hypothalamic hypopituitarism. *J Pediatr* 1978; 92:748.
42. Judge DM, et al: Hypothalamic hamartoma: A source of leuteinizing-hormone-releasing factor in precocious puberty. *N Engl J Med* 1977; 296:7.
43. Peters H, McNatty KP: *The Ovary*. Berkeley, University of California Press, 1980.
44. Potter EL: Th ovary in infancy and childhood, in Grady HG, Smith DE (eds): *The Ovary*. Baltimore, Williams & Wilkins, 1963.
45. Ross GT: Disorders of the ovary and female reproductive tract, in Wilson JD, Foster DW (eds): *Williams' Textbook of Endocrinology*, 7th ed Philadelphia, WB Saunders, 1985, p 206.
46. Eberlein VVR, et al: Ovarian tumors and cysts associated with sexual precocity. *J Peditar* 1960; 57:484.
47. Ein SH, Darte JMMM, Stephens CA: Cystic and solid ovarian tumors in children: A 44-year review. *J Pediatr Surg* 1970; 5:148.
48. Towne BH, et al: Ovarian cysts and tumors in infancy and childhood. *J Pediatr Surg* 1975; 10:311.
49. Root A, et al: Isosexual pseudoprecocity in a 6-year-old boy with a testicular interstitial cell adenoma. *J Pediatr* 1972; 80:264.
50. Rosenfield RL: Plasma 17 ketosteroids and 17 beta hydroxysteroids in girls with premature development of sexual hair. *J Pediatr* 1971; 79:260.
51. Rickman RA, et al: Adverse effects of large doses of medroxyprogesterone (MPA) in idiopathic isosexual precocity. *J Pediatr* 1971; 79:963.
52. Sadeghi-Nejad A, Kaplan SL, Grumbach MM: The effect of medroxyprogesterone acetate on adrenocortical function in children with precocious puberty. *J Pediatr* 1971; 78:616.
53. Sherins RJ, et al: Pituitary and testicular function studies: I. Experience with a new gonadal inhibitor 17 α-pregn-4-en-20-yno-(2,3-d) isoxazol-17-ol (Danazol). *J Clin Endocrinol Metab* 1971; 32:522.
54. Greenblatt RB, et al: Clinical studies with an antigonadotropin — Danazol. *Fertil Steril* 1971; 22:102.
55. Werder EA, et al: Treatment of precocious puberty with cyproterone acetate. *Pediatr Res* 1974; 8:248.
56. Teller WM, Murset G, Schellong G: Urinary C19 and C21 steroids patterns in isosexual precocious puberty during long-term treatment with gestagens. *Acta Paediatr Scand* 1969; 58:385.
57. Camacho AM, Williams DL, Montalvo JM: Alterations of testicular histology and chromosomes in patients with constitutional sexual precocity treated with medroxyprogesterone acetate. *J Clin Endocrinol Metab* 1972; 34:279.
58. Styne DM, et al: Treatment of true precocious puberty with a potent luteinizing hormone-releasing factor agonist: Effect on growth, sexual maturation, pelvic son-

ography, and the hypothalamic-pituitary-gonadal axis. *J Clin Endocrinol Metab* 1985; 61:142.

59. Luder AS, et al: Intranasal and subcutaneous treatment of central precocious puberty in both sexes with a long-acting analog of luteinizing hormone-releasing hormone. *J Clin Endocrinol Metab* 1984; 58:966.

60. Holland FJ, et al: Pharmacokinetic characteristics of the gonadotropin-releasing hormone analog D-Ser(TBU))-^{6}EA-^{10}luteinizing hormone-releasing hormone (Buserelin) after subcutaneous and intranasal administration in children with central precocious puberty. *J Clin Endocrinol Metab* 1986; 63:1065.

61. Holland FJ, et al: Ketoconazole in the management of precocious puberty not responsive to LHRH-analogue therapy. *N Engl J Med* 1985; 312:1023.

62. Holland FJ, Kirsch SE, Selby R: Gonadotropin-independent precocious puberty ("testotoxicosis"): Influence of maturational status on response to ketoconazole. *J Clin Endocrinol Metab* 1987; 64:328.

63. Kelch RP: Management of precocious puberty (editorial). *N Engl J Med* 1985; 312:1057.

64. Talbert LM, Sloan C: The effect of a low-dose oral contraceptive on serum testosterone levels in polycystic ovary disease. *Obstet Gynecol* 1979; 53:694.

65. Copeland KC, et al: Marihuana smoking and pubertal arrest. *J Pediatr* 1960; 96:1079.

66. Hopwood NJ: Pathogenesis and management of abnormal puberty, in Cohen MP, Foa PP(eds): *Special Topics in Endocrinology and Metabolism.* New York, Alan R Liss, 1986, p 175.

67. Van Dop C, et al: Isolated gonadotropin deficiency in boys: Clinical characteristics and growth. *J Pediatr* 1987; 111:684.

68. Kelch RP, et al: LH and FSH responsiveness to intravenous gonadotropin-releasing hormone (GnRH) in children with hypothalamic or pituitary disorders: Lack of effect of replacement therapy with human growth hormone. *J Clin Endocrinol Metab* 1976; 42:1104.

69. Kelch RP, et al: Diagnosis of gonadotropin deficiency in adolescents: Limited prognostic usefulness of a standard gonadotropin-releasing hormone (GnRH) tests in obese boys. *J Pediatr* 1980; 97:820.

70. Griffin JE, Wilson JD: Hereditary male psuedohermaphroditism. *Clin Obstet Gynecol* 1978; 5:457.

71. Griffin JE: Testicular feminization associated with a thermolabile androgen receptor in cultured human fibroblasts. *J Clin Invest* 1979; 64:1624.

72. Biglieri EG, Herron MA, Brust N: 17-hydroxylation deficiency in man. *J Clin Invest* 1966; 45:1946.

73. Kaplan JG, et al: Constitutional delay of growth and development: Effects of treatment with androgens. *J Pedtiar* 1973; 82:38.

74. Hopwood NJ, et al: The effect of synthetic androgens on the hypothalamic pituitary-gonadal axis in boys with constitutionally delayed growth. *J Pediatr* 1979; 94:657.

75. Santoro N, Filicori M, Crowley WF: Hypogonadotropic disorders in men and women: Diagnosis and therapy with pulsatile gonadotropin-releasing hormone. *Endocr Rev* 1986; 7:11.

76. Myers RP, Kelalis PP: Cryptorchidism reassessed: Is there an optimal time for surgical correction? *Mayo Clin Proc* 1973; 48:94.

77. Shapiro SR, Bodai BI: Current concepts of the undescended testis. *Surg Gynecol Obstet* 1978; 147:617.

78. Sudmann E: The undescended testis. *Acta Chir Scand* 1971; 137:815.

79. Winter JSD, Taraska S, Faiman C: The hormonal response to HCG stimulation in male children and adolescents. *J Clin Endocrinol Metab* 1972; 34:348.

80. Lovinger RD, et al: Congenital hypopituitarism associated with neonatal hypoglycemia and microphallus: Four cases secondary to hypothalamic hormone deficiencies. *J Pediatr* 1975; 87:1171.

81. Guthrie RD, Smith DW, Graham CB: Testosterone treatment for micropenis during early childhood. *J Pediatr* 1973; 83:247.

Obesity

One of the most frustrating problems in pediatrics is the overweight child. He or she is frequently referred to the endocrinologist because of suspicion of a hormonal disorder, or with a tentative diagnosis of Fröhlich's syndrome. However, the great majority of overweight patients seen in our clinic fall into no diagnostic category other than exogenous obesity, and children with a chief complaint of excessive weight almost never demonstrate an endocrine abnormality as the primary cause. The patients and their parents are frequently disappointed when told that the only justifiable treatment is caloric restriction. Unfortunately many dietary programs ultimately fail because the patient lacks sufficient motivation for this form of therapy.

NATURAL HISTORY

The incidence of obesity in children and adolescents in the United States has been estimated at 5% to 25%[1] (probably dependent on the definition used), and there is an increase with age. In one study the incidence in grades 4, 5, and 6 was 9.1% vs. 14.8% in grades 9, 10, and 11.[2]

It has been documented that mothers who are overweight prior to pregnancy and those who gain the most weight during gestation have infants with increased subcutaneous fat.[3] Kramer et al.[4] concluded that birth weight remained the best predictor of weight at 13 months. Dine et al.[5] noted a tendency for obese infants to remain overweight at age 5 years, although it was emphasized that "approximately 70% of the variance in weight and ponderosity indices" at this age could not be accounted for by similar measurements during the 1st year of life. Fisch et al.[6] reported that extremely obese infants (95th to 100th percentile) tended to remain overweight at age 4 to 7 years, and Zack et al.[7] concluded that

TABLE 10–1.
Conditions Associated With Obesity

Endocrine abnormalities
  Hypothyroidism
  Cushing's disease
Syndromes
  Fröhlich
  Laurence-Moon-Biedl
  Prader-Willi
Clinical associations
  Psychologic problems
  Inactivity
  Positive family history
Metabolic and hormonal associations
  ↑ "Caloric efficiencies"
  Hyperinsulinism
  ↓ Growth hormone response to stimuli
  ↑ Cortisol production rate
  ↑ Cell number secondary to overfeeding
  ↑ β-Endorphin

childhood fatness was the most predictive factor for adolescent fatness. Thus, although there are limitations to the concept that overweight infants become obese adolescents and adults, there appears to be a definite trend in this direction.[8] The rate of spontaneous remission declines with advancing age and, as expected, with increasing obesity.[1]

Obesity is associated with an increased incidence of diabetes mellitus and cardiovascular disorders (hypertension, cerebrovascular accidents), although a causal relationship is not always apparent.[9] Patients with extreme obesity may develop the Pickwickian syndrome: hypoxemia, cardiomegaly, cyanosis, and somnolence secondary to decreased pulmonary reserve.

ETIOLOGY

Multiple causes for obesity have been proposed, and it is probable that obesity in most patients is a result of a combination of circumstances. Factors that may be associated with excessive weight are listed in Table 10–1.

Genetic and Environmental Factors

The overweight child usually has a strong family history of obesity.[10] Our experience is consistent with earlier reports that at least one parent is overweight in over 50% of cases.[11] Also, it has been stated, "By age 17, the children of two obese parents are three times as fat as the children of two lean parents," as judged by triceps fatfold measurements.[12]

However, there is still controversy regarding the relative contributions of genetic vs. environmental factors. Garn et al.[13] reported similarities in skinfold measurements between children and their adoptive parents, and an ad hoc committee of the American Academy of Pediatrics has suggested that obesity within families is related closely to learned attitudes toward eating and exercise.[12] However, the data of Stunkard et al.[14] and of Biron et al.[15] indicate that weight patterns are explained primarily by heredity. Finally, Vuille and Mellbin have reported that, at age 10 years, excessive weight is intimately related to heredity and physical activity in girls, but to environment and appetite in boys.[16]

Psychological Factors

Bruch[17] has studied the psychological aspects of obesity in large groups of patients and found evidence of emotional disturbance in many. There seems little doubt that children who are depressed or otherwise disturbed often respond by overeating. However, it is not clear how frequently emotional problems are the primary cause of obesity, as obesity itself causes psychological difficulties.

A sociological study of families of obese adolescents revealed significant differences when compared with family groups in which children were of average weight.[18] The obese child appeared to be a scapegoat in the power struggle and rivalry among siblings. A warm relationship existed infrequently between the obese adolescent and his family. Parents tended to "go through the motions of seeking help for their obese youngsters without really becoming involved." Again, the precise relationship of these problems to the cause of obesity is not easily determined.

Hormonal and Metabolic Factors

Although children with Cushing's disease (see Chapter 7) and hypothyroidism (see Chapter 6) tend to become obese, these conditions are extremely rare in patients whose chief complaint is excessive weight. Several metabolic abnormalities are found in overweight patients but invariably prove to be a result rather than a cause of obesity, although they may make weight reduction more difficult (most such studies have been performed in adults); these include hyperinsulinism,[19, 20] increased cortisol production rate,[21, 22] and diminished growth hormone response to provocative stimuli[23] (which might contribute to the lag in free fatty acid release that can be demonstrated in overweight persons after prolonged fasting.)

A recent study suggests a possible direct role for increased plasma β-endorphin in the induction of overeating in obese children.[24] Various neurotransmitters also appear to be involved in the control of appetite.[25]

Physical Activity

Lack of exercise obviously favors excessive weight gain. Obese individuals usually are less active physically than their peers.[18] It has been found that television watching is correlated with and precedes adiposity.[26]

Caloric Efficiencies

Although many obese children simply eat more calories than is appropriate for their age and height, a history (presumably reliable) of a rather modest intake sometimes is obtained. Conversely, everyone is aware of individuals whose food consumption appears abundant but who do not gain excessive weight. Although differences in caloric efficiencies have not been found by oxygen consumption studies,[27] it seems probable that there are significant individual variations in the utilization of food, possibly related to some of the metabolic factors already described. Likewise, De Luise et al.[28] have provided evidence to suggest that energy efficiency is increased in obese adults. Therefore it must be emphasized to overweight children that their caloric intake may not be excessive for a nonobese sibling, but that it is too much for them.

Cell Number

In recent years there has been considerable interest in the study of the cell number in obese individuals. It has been shown that overfeeding during the first few months of life results in an increase in cell number.[29, 30] Reversal of this process apparently does not occur in patients who are subsequently able to lose weight.[31] It is possible that the permanent increase in cell number predisposes to the obese state and militates against successful weight reduction, but this hypothesis is unproved.

SYNDROMES ASSOCIATED WITH OBESITY

Fröhlich's Syndrome[32]

The original description of Fröhlich's syndrome appeared in 1901. The patient was a boy with obesity and sexual infantilism, who was subsequently found to have a brain tumor. Obesity presumably was caused by disturbed hypothalamic function, and the retarded sexual development by decreased secretion of gonadotropins.

Many patients are referred to an endocrinologist with a tentative diagnosis of Fröhlich's syndrome, but demonstrable intracranial tumors rarely are found in these circumstances. In many cases apparent sexual immaturity is a result of excessive fat, which obscures normal genitalia. Since obese children often are tall for their age,[33] genitalia commensurate with chronological age rather than height age may seem inappropriately small. On the other hand, the genitalia of some obese boys appear truly immature. Although no space-occupying lesion of the central nervous system (CNS) is present, it is possible that some functional or microscopic abnormality in the region of the hypothalamus may be conducive to excessive weight gain[34] and delayed maturation in these children. Although obesity may be etiologically related to CNS malfunction in some instances, cases consistent with the original description by Fröhlich are extremely rare.

Laurence-Moon-Beidl Syndrome[35-37]

This condition is characterized by obesity, hypogonadism, mental retardation, polydactyly, and retinitis pigmentosa. In addition, renal anomalies appear to be common. In one series,[37] all nine patients studied had abnormal intravenous pyelograms. There was a wide spectrum of renal lesions, including mesangial tissue proliferation, glomerular sclerosis, and cyst formation. Two had nephrogenic diabetes insipidus, and five had some degree of uremia.

The relationship of these various anomalies to one another is not clear but this syndrome is inherited on an autosomal recessive basis.

Prader-Willi Syndrome[38-41]

These children demonstrate hypotonia during infancy. Obesity and hypogenitalism are present, as in the syndromes of Fröhlich and of Laurence-Moon-Biedl. The hypogonadism is of the hypogonadotrophic variety, but at least one case of primary gonadal deficiency has been reported.[39] Additional features of the Prader-Willi syndrome are short stature, small hands and feet, glucose intolerance, and hypotonia during infancy. Abnormalities of chromosome 15 have been found in about half of all patients,[40] and a functional deficiency of pancreatic polypeptide has also been reported.[41]

Miscellaneous Syndromes

Three additional syndromes, all familial, characterized by excessive weight are (1) X-linked hypogonadism, gynecomastia, mental retardation, and short stature[42]; (2) mental retardation, short stature, contractures of the hands, and genital anomalies[43]; and (3) acanthosis nigricans, insulin resistance, and hyperandrogenemia.[44]

Diagnosis of these syndromes and others associated with obesity is academically rewarding but usually does not facilitate effective treatment.

DIAGNOSTIC EVALUATION

Important historical information includes the incidence of obesity in other family members, age at which excessive weight gain was first noted, and assessment of caloric intake and physical activity. The patient should be questioned for symptoms of hypothyroidism and Cushing's syndrome. For example, slow growth of hair and nails is suggestive of thyroid deficiency.

It is useful to evaluate the child's attitude toward his or her weight problem and to inquire who initiated the visit to the physician (e.g., patient, parent or school counselor). This information helps in determining whether the patient is sufficiently motivated to adhere to a weight control program.

Ideally, adiposity should be diagnosed and monitored on the basis of caliper measurements of skinfold thickness.[9] This technique may not be entirely reliable in the hands of an inexperienced operator. Obesity can be defined by a weight for height ratio greater than 120% of ideal.[1] However, from a practical viewpoint most obese children and adolescents who seek medical attention are sufficiently overweight, by clinical observation and by growth chart, that the problem is readily appreciated.

Physical examination may reveal evidence of the aforementioned congenital syndromes or of an endocrine disorder. It should be noted that children with exogenous obesity may have striae and the buffalo hump appearance of the upper back suggestive of Cushing's syndrome. However, the striae of patients with Cushing's syndrome usually are more deeply discolored, and the obesity is centripetal in distribution. Of considerable diagnostic importance is the fact that both hypothyroidism and excessive glucocorticoid production cause a decreased linear growth rate, whereas children with exogenous obesity frequently are tall for their age.[33]

If an obese child has maintained a growth rate above the 50th percentile for height and there is no historical or physical evidence for an endocrine abnormality, it may be justifiable to make a diagnosis of exogenous obesity in the absence of any laboratory studies. However, it has been our practice to obtain serum thyroxine and cortisol determinations in these patients, recognizing that a single random cortisol level usually cannot be relied on to rule out Cushing's syndrome with certainty. Although the yield is low, these two relatively simple procedures are useful psychologically in convincing the patient and his family that no endocrine abnormality exists.

If the serum cortisol concentration is elevated or the index of suspicion is high for other reasons, a dexamethasone suppression test may be necessary; the overnight test might eliminate the need for hospitalization (see Chapter 7). (Note that 24-hour urinary 17-hydroxysteroid excretion is often elevated in obese individuals because of the increased cortisol production rate; therefore this determination cannot always enable one to distinguish between Cushing's syndrome and simple obesity).

Although there is a higher incidence of carbohydrate intolerance among obese patients, we generally omit the glucose tolerance test from the routine outpatient evaluation unless there is a strong family history of diabetes mellitus.

A glycosylated hemoglobin determination can be obtained but may not be sufficiently sensitive to rule out non-insulin-dependent diabetes with certainty. Depressed plasma testosterone,[45] and increased conversion of androstenedione[46] and testosterone to estradiol[47] have been reported in adult men, with resultant gynecomastia in some cases.

TREATMENT

Endocrine disorders are treated as described in the other chapters. The various approaches to exogenous obesity are discussed in the sections that follow. Treatment programs are the same for patients with congenital syndromes such as Prader-Willi, but less success is to be expected.

Caloric Restriction

Caloric restriction is the most physiologic means of weight reduction. In children with mild obesity, the trend may be partially reversed by a few practical suggestions, such as a switch to low-calorie foods such as skimmed milk and diet soft drinks, elimination of excessive snacks of cookies and potato chips, and limiting bread and desserts at mealtimes. Likewise, this approach might be appropriate for children with mental retardation or those with normal intelligence who simply are not sufficiently motivated to adhere to a more specific dietary plan. The alternative is to prescribe a more formal diet. About 1,000 calories/day usually is suitable for most children over 5 years of age and, if followed reasonably well, should result in a loss of roughly 1 lb/wk. Diets of 1,200 to 1,500 calories sometimes are adequate for adolescents and may result in greater acceptance, but a dietary history is important in deciding the optimum intake. In any case, weight loss is invariably greater in the first month, and the rate decreases as a more normal weight is approached and motivation declines. A group of children at the University of Michigan who adhered to diets of 1,000 to 1,200 calories with varying degrees of compliance lost an average of approximately 3 lb during the first month, but only about 1 lb in the following 4 weeks.[48]

The course of children on dietary programs is frequently unsatisfactory. In a series of 45 obese children followed at our hospital, 21 were not treated with diet because of psychiatric problems and apparent lack of motivation. Of the 24 placed on caloric restriction, 16 failed to return to the clinic after the first two or three visits. Of the remaining 8, three were discharged with normal weight and 5 were progressing satisfactorily at the time the data were collected.[49] This rather depressing success rate also is reflected in other studies.[31, 50] Unfortunately, early failures tend to prejudice children against subsequent attempts at caloric restriction.

Dietary programs are probably more successful if combined with "behavior modification."[51] The basis of this approach is an attempt to disrupt situational stimuli to eating and to teach the patient to take responsibility for what he consumes. Unfortunately, comprehensive behavior modification programs require a considerable commitment of time and/or the assistance of qualified paramedical personnel (social worker, dietitian) and therefore may not be practical for the practicing physician. However, books that discuss the important elements of these plans (e.g., restricting food intake to a specific eating area) are available to the consumer for his/her self-education.[52] Also, a study has supported the feasibility and short-term effectiveness of a behavior modification program conducted through the schools.[53]

Programs such as Weight Watchers and TOPS (Take Off Pounds Sensibly) are available in many areas. These facilities provide good dietary instruction, and the "group therapy" concept has proved successful in many cases. Our patients are encouraged to investigate such programs, but children often feel uncomfortable at these meetings, which are attended primarily by adults. In some areas special programs designed for children and adolescents are available. Summer camps specifically for obese children also are recommended, but frequently these are expensive.

Dietary modifications initiated during the first year of life may have some preventive value. Pisacano et al. conducted a study in which a group of 80 infants in a private practice setting participated in a dietary program.[54] At age 3 years, the prevalence of overweight was significantly less than in a control group.

Psychological Help

Psychiatric counseling probably is of some benefit in childhood obesity in view of the positive correlation between excessive weight and emotional difficulties.[16] However, since multiple factors may contribute to obesity, this approach is by no means successful in all, or even in the majority of, patients. Furthermore, such treatment is not always possible because of the expense or because qualified psychologists or psychiatrists are not locally available. In practice, therefore, this approach is feasible for relatively few patients. A psychologically stable and supportive family, able to set appropriate limits, is an important determinant of the success of a weight-reduction program. A family-oriented approach is therefore recommended.[1]

It should be kept in mind that adverse psychological reactions may accompany weight loss[55] as well as weight gain.

Exercise

Physical activity is to be encouraged, but rarely does exercise alone result in satisfactory weight reduction. For example, 30 minutes of running uses about 300 calories and would be of limited benefit in a patient who has a daily intake of 3,000 calories. However, the data of Berkowitz et al.[56] indicate that "high physical activity reduces the risk of developing adiposity," and exercise is, at the least, a valuable adjunct to diet.[57]

Drugs

In the past, it was often tempting to prescribe anorectic agents in refractory cases or when substantial pressure was applied by the patient or parent. The effect of this form of therapy was invariably transient and left the child short of his or her ideal weight.[58] Because of the low benefit-risk ratio, these drugs can no longer be considered appropriate for the treatment of obesity in children and adolescents.

"Total" Starvation[59-61]

Experience with the use of very restricted diets of 200 to 500 calories/day has been gained primarily in adult patients, but obese adolescents also have participated in such programs.

Primary advantages of this approach are rapid weight loss, with attendant psychological benefit, and the development of ketosis, with decreased appetite. On the other hand, hospitalization is required to supervise adherence to the diet and to monitor the metabolic consequences, primarily hypoglycemia and hyperuricemia. In our experience low blood sugar may become a problem in adolescents after several days of a 200-calorie diet, requiring periodic increases to approximately 500 calories. Uric acid levels frequently rise above 10 mg/dL, at which time treatment with allopurinol is instituted.

Other undesirable side effects include postural hypotension, headaches, weakness, and transient nausea. If the diet does not contain adequate amounts of potassium, this should be provided as a supplement. Daily multivitamin tablets should be prescribed.

A weight loss of 0.5 lb/day or more can be expected on this program. However, prolonged hospitalization is necessary, and the expense may be prohibitive. Also, adolescents frequently become disruptive on the ward, and some fail to lose weight as a result of obtaining extra food from hospital canteens or from other patients. A comprehensive schedule of activities to reduce boredom is important in such a program. Finally, excessive weight gain may occur following discharge from the hospital unless intensive outpatient follow-up is available. The involvement of a psychiatrist both during and after hospitalization is beneficial, but not always feasible.

Figure 10–1 illustrates the case of a 15-year-old boy with exogenous obesity (321 lb) in addition to some psychological problems. He was hospitalized for weight reduction. A diet of 200 to 500 calories resulted in a loss of about 80 lb over a period of nearly 5 months. Diet was liberalized during subsequent admission to a psychiatric unit, but significant weight loss continued. A gain of about 20 lb occurred following discharge. When the patient was last seen, his weight was 203 lb, representing a net loss of 118 pounds over about 1 year.

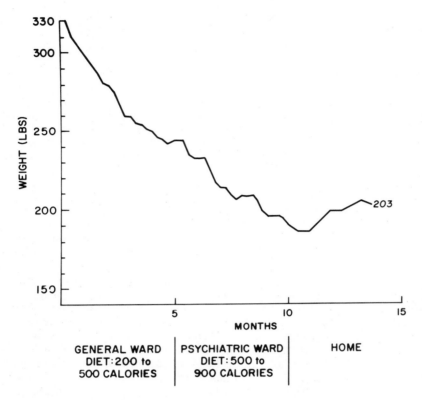

GENERAL WARD | PSYCHIATRIC WARD | HOME
DIET:200 to | DIET:500 to
500 CALORIES | 900 CALORIES

FIG 10–1.
Results of "total" starvation in a 15-year-old boy. Net weight loss was more than 100 lb. See text for discussion.

"Total" starvation was reasonably successful in this patient, but the expenditure of professional time and money was extraordinary. Therefore the use of severe caloric restriction in the adolescent age group should be limited to carefully selected patients. Younger children should not be considered candidates for this type of program, but a patient whose obesity is causing significant cardiorespiratory problems (Pickwickian syndrome) deserves hospitalization.

A less drastic alternative to "total" starvation has been suggested by Sidbury.[62] The patient is hospitalized for several days, fasts until ketosis occurs, then is discharged on a diet sufficient to maintain ketonuria (approximately 700 calories for an adolescent), which is monitored at home with reagent strips. The anorectic effect of ketosis is important to this program, and fasting should be resumed if ketones disappear from the urine.

Surgery[63-67]

Surgery should be reserved for carefully selected patients with morbid obesity who have proved refractory to more conservative measures. Jejunoileal bypass is no longer recommended because of significant long-term complications, such as nutritional cirrhosis and hepatic accumulation of fat. Gastric bypass or plication are now the procedures of choice. Bypass has been used in patients with Prader-Willi syndrome, although the results are typically less gratifying.

In summary, the causes of obesity are multiple but classic endocrine abnormalities rarely are important etiologic factors. Dietary programs frequently fail because of inadequate motivation. Other forms of treatment often are impractical or unphysiologic and therefore not appropriate in the majority of children. A reasonable approach would include modest caloric restriction and exercise, combined with a behavior modification program implemented in a supportive family environment.

Further discussion of childhood obesity, and additional bibliography, may be found in the excellent reviews by Weil[9] and by Dietz.[1]

REFERENCES

1. Dietz WH, Jr: Childhood obesity: Susceptibility, cause, and management. *J Pediatr* 1983; 103:676.
2. Huse DM, et al: The challenge of obesity in childhood: I. Incidence, prevalence, and staging. *Mayo Clin Proc* 1982; 57:279.
3. Udall JN, et al: Interaction of maternal and neonatal obesity. *Pediatrics* 1978; 62:17.
4. Kramer MS, et al: Infant determinants of childhood weight and adiposity. *J Pediatr* 1985; 107:104.
5. Dine MS, et al: Where do the heaviest children come from? A prospective study of white children from birth to 5 years of age. *Pediatrics* 1979; 63:1.
6. Fisch RO, et al: Obesity and leanness at birth and their relationship to body habitus in later childhood. *Pediatrics* 1975; 56:521.
7. Zack PM, et al: A longitudinal study of body fatness in childhood and adolescence. *J Pediatr* 1979; 95:126.
8. Lloyd JK, Wolff OH, Wheeler WS: Childhood obesity. *Br Med J* 1961; 2:145.
9. Weil WB, Jr: Current controversies in childhood obesity. *J Pediatr* 1976; 91:175.
10. Garn SM: The origins of obesity. *Am J Dis Child* 1976; 130:465.
11. Mayer J: Genetic, traumatic and environmental factors in the etiology of obesity. *Physiol Rev* 1953; 33:472.
12. Garn SM, Clark DC: Trends in fatness and the origins of obesity. *Pediatrics* 1976; 57:443.
13. Garn SM, Bailey SM, Higgins ITT: Fatness similarities in adopted pairs. *Am J Clin Nutr* 1976; 29:1067.
14. Stunkard AJ, et al: An adoption study of obesity. *N Engl J Med* 1986; 314:193.
15. Biron P, et al: Familial resemblance of body weight and weight/height in 374 homes with adopted children. *J Pediatr* 1977; 91:55.
16. Vuille J, Mellbin T: Obesity in 10-year-olds: an epidemiologic study. *Pediatrics* 1979; 64:564.

17. Bruch H: Obesity in childhood. Physiologic and psychologic aspects of the food intake of obese children. *Am J Dis Child* 1940; 59:739.
18. Hammar SL, et al: An interdisciplinary study of adolescent obesity. *J Pediatr* 1972; 80:373.
19. Martin MM, Martin ALA: Obesity, hyperinsulinism, and diabetes mellitus in childhood. *J Pediatr* 1973; 82:192.
20. Golay A, et al: Effect of obesity on ambient plasma glucose, free fatty acid, insulin, growth hormone, and glucagon concentrations. *J Clin Endocrinol Metab* 1986; 63:481.
21. Garces LY, et al: Cortisol secretion rate during fasting of obese adolescent subjects. *J Clin Endocrinol Metab* 1968; 28:1843.
22. O'Connell M, et al: Experimental obesity in man: III. Adrenocortical function. *J Clin Endocrinol Metab* 1973; 36:323.
23. Carnelutti M, del Guercio MJ, Chiumello G: Influence of growth hormone on the pathogenesis of obesity in children. *J Pediatr* 1970; 77:385.
24. Genazzani AR, et al: Hyperendorphinemia in obese children and adolescents. *J Clin Endocrinol Metab* 1986; 62:36.
25. Levine AS, Morley JE: Appetite control. Neuropeptides and the regulation of food intake. *Practical Gastroenterol* 1984; 8:19.
26. Dietz WH, Jr, Gortmaker SL: Do we fatten our children at the television set? Obesity and television viewing in children and adolescents. *Pediatrics* 1985; 75:807.
27. Iliff A, et al: Basal metabolic rate in obese children. *Pediatrics* 1949; 4:744.
28. De Luise M, Blackburn GL, Flier JS: Reduced activity of the red-cell sodium-potassium pump in human obesity. *N Engl J Med* 1980; 303:1017.
29. Knittle JL: Obesity in childhood: A problem in adipose tissue cellular development. *J Pediatr* 1972; 81:1048.
30. Knittle JL, et al: The growth of adipose tissue in children and adolescents: Cross-sectional and longitudinal studies of adipose cell number and size. *J Clin Invest* 1979; 63:239.
31. Ginsberg-Fellner F, Knittle JL: Weight reduction in young obese children: I. Effects on adipose tissue cellularity and metabolism. *Pediatr Res* 1981; 15:1381.
32. Bruch H: The Frohlich syndrome: Report of the original case. *Am J Dis Child* 1939; 58:1282.
33. Forbes GB: Nutrition and growth. *J Pediatr* 1977; 91:40.
34. Hirsch J: Hypothalamic control of appetite. *Hospital Practice*, Feb 1984, p 131.
35. Reinfrank RF, Nichols FL: Hypogonadotropic hypogonadism in the Laurence-Moon syndrome. *J Clin Endocrinol Metab* 1964; 24:48.
36. Bauman ML, Hogan GR: Laurence-Moon-Biedl syndrome. *Am J Dis Child* 1973; 126:119.
37. Hurley RM, et al: The renal lesion of the Laurence-Moon-Biedl syndrome. *J Pediatr* 1975; 87:206.
38. Hall BD, Smith DW: Prader-Willi syndrome. *J Pediatr* 1972; 81:286.
39. Seyler LE, Jr, et al: Hypergonadotropic-hypogonadism in the Prader-Labhart-Willi syndrome. *J Pediatr* 1979; 94:435.
40. Ledbetter DH, et al: Chromosome 15 abnormalities and the Prader-Willi syndrome: A follow-up report of 40 cases. *Am J Hum Genet* 1982; 34:278.
41. Zipf WB, et al: Pancreatic polypeptide responses to protein meal challenges in obese but otherwise normal children and obese children with Prader-Willi syndrome. *J Clin Endocrinol Metab* 1983; 57:1074.
42. Sotos JF, et al: X-linked hypogonadism, gynecomastia, mental retardation, short stature, and obesity — a new syndrome. *J Pediatr* 1979; 94:55.

43. Urban MD, et al: Familial syndrome of mental retardation, short stature, contractures of the hands, and genital anomalies. *J Pediatr* 1979; 94:52.
44. Richards GE, et al: Obesity, acanthosis nigricans, insulin resistance, and hyperandrogenemia: Pediatric perspective and natural history. *J Pediatr* 1985; 107:893.
45. Amatruda JM, et al: Depressed plasma testosterone and fractional binding of testosterone in obese males. *J Clin Endocrinol Metab* 1978; 47:268.
46. Kley HK, et al: Enhanced conversion of androstenedione to estrogens in obese males. *J Clin Endocrinol Metab* 1980; 51:1128.
47. Schneider G, et al: Increased estrogen production in obese men. *J Clin Endocrinol Metab* 1979; 48:633.
48. Bacon GE, Lowrey GH: A clinical trial of fenfluramine in obese children. *Curr Ther Res* 1967; 9:626.
49. Robertson AF, Lowrey GH: Overweight children. *Mich Med* 1964; 63:629.
50. Stunkard A, McLaren-Hune M: The results of treatment for obesity: A review of the literature and report of a series. *Arch Intern Med* 1959; 103:79.
51. Brightwell DR: Treating obesity with behavior modification. *Postgrad Med* 1974; 55:52.
52. Stuart RB, Davis B: *Slim Chance in a Fat World* (condensed ed) Champaign Ill, Research Press, 1972.
53. Botvin GJ, et al: Reducing adolescent obesity through a school health program. *J Pediatr* 1979; 95:1060.
54. Pisacano JC, et al: An attempt at prevention of obesity in infancy. *Pediatrics* 1978; 61:360.
55. Stunkard AJ, Rush J: A critical review of reports of untoward responses during weight reduction for obesity. *Ann Intern Med* 1974; 81:526.
56. Berkowitz RI, et al: Physical activity and adiposity: A longitudinal study from birth to childhood. *J Pediatr* 1985; 106:734.
57. Epstein LH, et al: Effect of diet and controlled exercise on weight loss in obese children. *J Pediatr* 1985; 107:358.
58. Lorbert J: Obesity in childhood: A controlled trial of anorectic drugs. *Arch Dis Child* 1966; 41:309.
59. Drenick EJ, et al: Prolonged starvation as treatment for severe obesity. *JAMA* 1964; 187:100.
60. Mayer J: Reducing by total fasting. *Postgrad Med* 1964; 35:279.
61. Drenick EJ, Smith R: Weight reduction by prolonged starvation: Practical management. *Postgrad Med* 1964; 36:A95.
62. Sidbury, JA: Personal communication.
63. Bray GA: Current status of intestinal bypass surgery in the treatment of obesity. *Diabetes* 1977; 26:1072.
64. Alden JF: Gastric and jejunoileal bypass. A comparison in the treatment of morbid obesity. *Arch Surg* 1977; 112:799.
65. Freeman JB, Burchett H: Failure rate with gastric partitioning for morbid obesity. *Am J Surg* 1983; 145:113.
66. Alpers DH: Surgical therapy for obesity. *N Engl J Med* 1983; 308:1026.
67. Soper RT, et al: Gastric bypass for morbid obesity in children and adolescents. *J Pediatr Surg* 1975; 10:51.

Abnormalities of Calcium and Phosphorus Homeostasis

Significant advances in our understanding of the hormonal control of calcium and phosphorous homeostasis have occurred in the last 2 decades. In many instances, these advances have led to a much better understanding of the pathophysiology of disorders associated with abnormal calcium or phosphorous metabolism, and to more rational and specific therapies.[1-6] The purposes of this chapter are to present a clinically useful review of the hormonal control of calcium and phosphorous homeostasis and to apply this knowledge in the diagnosis and management of common clinical disorders.

CALCIUM AND PHOSPHOROUS HOMEOSTASIS

The precise regulation of the serum concentration of ionized calcium reflects the important role of calcium ions in many biologic processes, including neuronal conduction, synaptic transmission, mitotic division, cardiac automaticity, muscle contraction, membrane function and permeability, blood coagulation, secretion of peptide hormones, and numerous enzymatic reactions. Serum calcium is narrowly regulated by the interactions of parathormone, vitamin D and its metabolites, calcitonin, direct response of bone (sluggish), serum proteins, and to a lesser extent by glucocorticoids, sex steroids, thyroid hormones, and growth hormone.

The average adult human body contains 1,000 to 1,200 g of calcium. The vast majority of the body's calcium (99%) is in the deep layers of bone in the form of hydroxyapatite crystals. Approximately 1 g is in the extracellular fluid, whereas the rapidly exchangeable pool approximates 5.0 g. The daily intake of calcium for an adult is 500 to 1,000 mg; intestinal secretions add another 600 mg to the intestinal contents. Intestinal absorption of calcium depends on the activated form of vitamin D (1,25-dihydroxyvitamin D₃),[1-6] net absorption averages 200 to 250 mg/day. Calcium excretion is primarily fecal; urinary calcium should be less than 200 mg/day (<4 mg/kg or <0.25 mg/mg creatinine in healthy children) despite a filtered load of approximately 10,000 mg/day. Renal tubules normally reabsorb more than 97% of the filtered calcium load. Small quantities of calcium are lost in sweat and other fluids. In adults bone accretion equals resorption (approximately 350 mg calcium exchange/day), whereas in the growing child accretion exceeds resorption (approximately 275 mg/day in infancy and up to 400 mg/day in the rapidly growing adolescent boy). Bone resorption or osteolysis is stimulated by parathyroid hormone, cortisol, thyroid hormones, and growth hormone, and is inhibited by calcitonin, estrogens, and androgens.

The total serum calcium averages 10 mg/dL (5 mEq/L or 2.5 mM), with a range between 8.8 and 10.7 mg/dL. There is only slight variability with age, attributable to differences in serum protein concentrations.

Calcium in serum occurs in three major forms: ionized (45%); protein bound, primarily to albumin (40%); and diffusable but complexed to such organic anions as sulfate, phosphate, lactate, and citrate (15%). The concentration of ionized calcium (mean, 4.5 mg/dL; range, 4.0 to 5.6 mg/dL) is the important, closely regulated variable. Measurements of ionized calcium are not routinely available, but new methodologies have allowed clinicians access to these determinations in specialized laboratories. Serum protein determinations may aid in the interpretation of total serum calcium values, but often the correlation between total protein and serum ionized calcium is poor. This seems to be especially true in the neonatal period,[7-10] when falsely high estimates of ionized calcium are commonly derived from the McLean-Hastings nomogram. Normally, 80% of protein-bound calcium is associated with albumin and 20% with globulins. A rough but useful guideline for the interpretation of total serum calcium values in hypoalbuminemic patients is to allow 0.8 mg/dL reduction from the normal range for every 1 g/dL reduction in serum albumin below normal (4.0 g/dL). *Venous blood sampling for calcium determinations should be performed quickly, because prolonged venous stasis results in the loss of protein-free fluid and increased serum protein and calcium concentrations.*

In contrast to serum calcium, serum inorganic phosphate is highly variable and depends on age, diet, and hormonal status. Indeed, the concentration of serum phosphate falls after every meal. The normal range for adults is 2.6 to 4.3 mg/dL, men having slightly lower values than women. Serum phosphate is high in growing children (5 to 6.5 mg/dL) and in conditions with increased bone resorption (thyrotoxicosis), decreased filtration (renal failure), increased tubular reabsorption (hypoparathyroidism), and high intake (Fleet's Phosphosoda). Decreased absorption (aluminum hydroxide gels) or intake as well as low tubular reabsorption of inorganic phosphate (TRP) (hyperparathyroidism, rickets, renal tubular disorders) lower serum phosphate concentrations. *Because of the significant variability of serum inorganic phosphate concentrations, determinations should be performed in the morning after an overnight fast whenever precise evaluation of calcium-phosphorous homeostasis is necessary.*

Milk, cheese, meat, and fish are rich sources of phosphorus. Phosphate is absorbed readily (approximately 70% of dietary intake). Absorption is increased by a low calcium intake, acids, vitamin D, parathormone, and growth hormone, and is decreased by high calcium diets, aluminum hydroxide gels, and severe impairment of calcium absorption. The principal route of excretion is renal. TRP depends on dietary load:

Phosphate Intake	TRP
Normal	80%–90%
Low	90%
High	75%

TRP is low in hyperparathyroidism (primary or secondary) and in many renal diseases, whereas it is high in hypoparathyroidism.

Parathyroid Hormone

Parathyroid hormone (PTH) is a polypeptide hormone whose secretion by the parathyroid glands is reciprocally related to changes in the concentration of serum ionized calcium. Initially, a preproparathyroid hormone is synthesized that has additional amino acids on each end of the final peptide chain. Proparathyroid hormone, the immediate precursor of PTH, has six additional amino acids on the amino end. PTH is secreted as an 84-amino acid, single-chain polypeptide. However, several different forms (presumably metabolites) appear in the circulation. The active portion of the molecule consists of the first 27 amino acids; fragments that do not contain this sequence, common in serum, are inactive regardless of length or composition. After binding to its receptor, intact PTH splits into an inactive C-terminal fragment and an active N-terminal fragment.

The multiplicity of circulating immunoreactive forms of PTH, with highly variable half-lives, marked differences in antisera specificity, and the previous lack of a universally accepted standard, have limited somewhat the usefulness of PTH immunoassays. The oldest and most widely available PTH assays measure circulating C-terminal fragments. In most instances, these assays have provided clinically useful results for the diagnosis of hyperparathyroidism. However, C-terminal assays cannot be relied on in patients with renal failure because C-terminal fragments are normally metabolized in the kidney. Assays specific for the N-terminus, the middle of the molecule, and assays that measure the intact hormone molecule are less widely available.

Assays specific for the intact hormone most accurately reflect the steady-state or integrated level of hormone secretion and appear to most reliably differentiate hyperparathyroidism from nonparathyroid causes of hypercalcemia. The midregion assays are variable and are not always specific for intact hormone. On the other hand, N-terminal assays are better for studies of acute changes in glandular secretion but have not proved very useful in clinical practice. In summary, when available, assays specific for the intact hormone provide the best clinical information. If not available, C-terminal assays should be used, but N-terminal assays are preferred in patients with renal failure.[11]

Clinicians must be aware of the specificity and limitations of PTH assays available to them. PTH assays, even though they may be directed at the same portion of the molecule, vary significantly among clinical laboratories, and each laboratory must establish its own range of normal. Assays from different laboratories cannot be compared directly.

Parathyroid hormone regulates calcium and phosphate homeostasis through its effects on three end organs: bones, renal tubule, and intestinal mucosa. It increases serum calcium mainly by stimulating bone breakdown; both bone mineral and matrix are released.[3, 11, 12] It also increases intestinal absorption and renal tubular reabsorption of calcium. The other major effect of PTH is to increase renal phosphate clearance (decrease TRP). In addition, PTH increases renal excretion of sodium, potassium, amino acids, and bicarbonate, and decreases the excretion of calcium, magnesium, and hydrogen. The action of PTH on the kidney is mediated by stimulation of adenylcyclase activity and subsequently, increased formation of cyclic adenosine monophosphate (cAMP). Indeed, almost all of the cAMP found in urine results from the action of parathormone on the renal tubule. Measurement of urinary cAMP in a carefully timed 1- to 2-hour urine collection is a very useful test for the diagnosis of hyperparathyroidism, but results should be expressed as a function of glomerular filtration rate.[11]

The renal effects of parathormone occur within minutes and the bone effects within hours, whereas the intestinal response is slow (days or weeks). Both the bone and intestinal effects of PTH are at least partially dependent on vitamin D. Some recent evidence has linked the effects of PTH and vitamin D metabolism even further. PTH seems to control the renal synthesis of 1,25-dihydroxyvitamin D_3 (biologically active form), which in turn acts directly as a feedback inhibitor of PTH secretion (Fig 11–1).

Vitamin D

Technically speaking, recent knowledge indicates that vitamin D is not a vitamin but a hormone (see Fig 11–1).[1-6] Once vitamin D enters the circulation, either through formation in skin (quantitatively the most important source) or by intestinal absorption of dietary sources, it is bound by an α_2-globulin known as vitamin D binding protein.

Vitamin D is not active as such until it undergoes a series of metabolic transformations, first in the liver and then in the kidney. It is well established that vitamin D undergoes hydroxylation at position 25 in the liver; this reaction occurs in both microsomes and mitochondria. The mitochondrial enzyme is not regulated by the vitamin D status of the individual, but the microsomal enzyme is partially controlled by previously formed vitamin D metabolites. This reaction is not regulated tightly, however. Although there is marked variability in the serum concentrations of 25-hydroxyvitamin D (25-OHD) that depend to a great degree on the amount of available substrate, the plasma concentration of 25-OHD is an accurate reflection of vitamin D reserves in humans. For example,

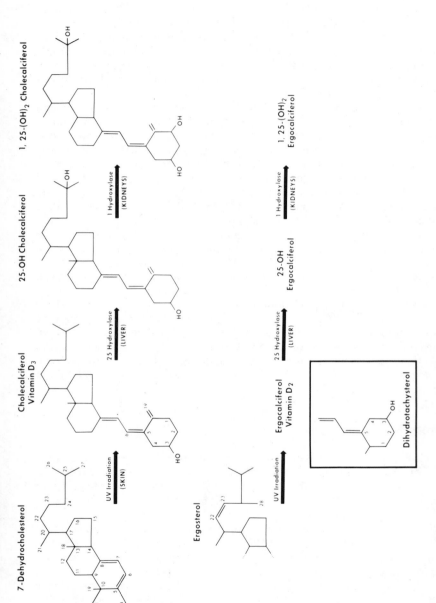

FIG 11–1.

Metabolism of vitamins D_2 and D_3: Vitamins D_2 and D_3 differ only in the structure of the side chain. Vitamin D_2 is found primarily in plants and is present in most commercial vitamin D preparations. Ultraviolet irradiation produces the same changes in *7-dehydrocholesterol* and *ergosterol*. Dietary sources of vitamin D are required when clothing, housing, smog, and a harsh climate prevent adequate exposure to sunlight. The inset illustrates the lower (A) ring of *dihydrotachysterol*. Note that rotation of the A ring has made *dihydrotachysterol* structurally similar to 1-

very high, but not toxic, concentrations of 25-OHD have been found in life-guards. Furthermore, administration of pharmacologic amounts of vitamin D_2 or D_3 (e.g., 2 or 3 mg/day; 80 to 120,000 U/day) results in 25-OHD concentrations 10-fold greater than normal. In contrast to vitamin D_2 and vitamin D_3, which have no appreciable direct biologic activity, 25-OHD is moderately active and can induce hypercalcemia and its associated toxicity. This explains the potential toxicity of vitamin D_2 or D_3 in patients who cannot further metabolize (activate) vitamin D via additional hydroxylation at the 1 position. To complicate matters further, most vitamin D_2 and D_3 is not metabolized, but is stored in adipose tissue and plasma and remains for months as available substrate for 25 hydroxylation. The biologic half-life of 25-OHD in patients treated with pharmacologic amounts of D_2 is approximately 3 weeks.[13, 14] These factors explain the potentially prolonged toxicity of vitamin D_2 (or D_3).

Although 25-OHD is active at high concentrations, it is not the physiologically active form. 25-OHD is metabolized further by the kidneys to 1,25-dihydroxyvitamin D (1,25(OH)$_2$D). 1,25(OH)$_2$D seems to be the principal metabolically active form of the hormone, and is remarkably potent, effective at dosages between 0.25 and 1.0 μg/day. The 1-hydroxylation step is stimulated by PTH, hypocalcemia, and hypophosphatemia. Growth hormone production and estrogens also increase 1,25(OH)$_2$D formation. The biologic half-life of 1,25(OH)$_2$D is short. Indeed, recent reports suggest that twice-per-day dosage schedules may be necessary for optimum replacement therapy. Other metabolites of 25(OH)$_2$D, also formed by the kidneys, are 24,25-dihydroxyvitamin D (24,25(OH)$_2$D) and 1,24,25-trihydroxyvitamin D (1,24,25(OH)$_3$D). 24,25(OH)$_2$D formation and serum concentrations are reciprocally related to 1,25(OH)$_2$-D; for example, normal or increased serum concentrations of calcium and phophorus increase 24 hydroxylase in both the kidney and intestine. The precise role(s) and significance of these metabolites is not agreed upon, but it seems likely that they may represent initial steps in the degradation of vitamin D.

The major action of vitamin D (1,25(OH)$_2$D) is to stimulate intestinal absorption of calcium. It also stimulates the mobilization of calcium from bone, a process that requires the presence of parathormone. Vitamin D may improve renal tubular reabsorption of calcium, but this must be a minor effect. Vitamin D also increases serum phosphate by stimulating intestinal absorption, renal tubular reabsorption, and release of phosphate from bone.

The discovery of active metabolites of vitamin D has led to a better understanding of the effectiveness, or ineffectiveness, of various forms of vitamin D therapy and to the development of new, useful analogues. For example, it is now clear why conventional therapy with vitamin D_2 is relatively ineffective in severe renal disease, whereas dihydrotachysterol (structurally similar to 1-hydroxyvitamin D) is more effective. Animal and clinical studies have confirmed that 1α-hydroxyvitamin D_3 and 1,25(OH)$_2$D$_3$ are equally effective in the absence of functioning kidneys.[2] When 1,25(OH)$_2$D became available for clinical use several years ago, it was unclear whether it would provide significant therapeutic advantages over dihydrotachysterol and vitamin D_2. Recent studies clearly indicate that it is the preferred form of vitamin D therapy in several conditions, for example, renal osteodystrophy and X-linked hypophosphatemic rickets.[3, 15, 16]

Tables 11–1 and 11–2 list the normal serum concentrations of vitamin D metabolites in infants and children and the clinically available vitamin D preparations.[8, 14, 17, 18]

Calcitonin

Calcitonin is a single-chain, 32-amino acid polypeptide secreted by the calcitonin-producing cells (C cells, parafollicular cells) of the thyroid gland. Despite a great deal of knowledge about its embryology, synthesis, and biochemical effects, the importance of calcitonin in calcium homeostasis is uncertain.[19] For example, thyroidectomized patients who have normal parathyroid gland function have no appreciable abnormality in calcium homeostasis. The principal stimulus for calcitonin secretion is an increased concentration of ionized calcium. However, oral intake of calcium stimulates calcitonin secretion without appreciable increases in serum calcium. The latter effect appears to be mediated by the secretion of gastrointestinal hormones; glucagon and pentagastrin are important stimuli for calcitonin secretion.

The major site of calcitonin activity is on bone, where it inhibits resorption and lowers serum calcium. Calcitonin also decreases renal tubular reabsorption of phosphate. Thus calcitonin and parathormone both act to lower serum phosphate, but have opposing actions on serum calcium. In addition, calcitonin affects the gastrointestinal tract: it delays gastric emptying and increases the secretion of water, sodium, and chloride. Whether these effects, which are demonstrable after pharmacologic administration of calcitonin, have physiologic significance is unknown. At present, synthetic salmon calcitonin has been useful in the treatment of Paget's disease,[19, 20] and calcitonin measurements (especially during calcium infusion tests or after pentagastrin stimulation) have been useful in detecting occult medullary carcinoma of the thyroid in affected families.[19]

TABLE 11–1.
Vitamin D Metabolite Concentrations in Infants and Children (Mean ± SD)

	25-OHD (ng/mL)	24,25(OH)$_2$D (ng/mL)	1,25(OH)$_2$D (pg/mL)
Infants (<18 mo)*			
Winter	45 ± 18	3.8 ± 1.6	72 ± 25
Summer	61 ± 16	4.6 ± 1.6	53 ± 16
Children (18 mo to 19 yr)†			
Winter	23 ± 7.4‡	2.3 ± 1.1‡	38 ± 9.8
Summer	36 ± 9.5‡	3.8 ± 1.3‡	40 ± 15

* Formula fed infants. (Data from Lichtenstein P, et al: Calcium-regulating hormones and minerals from birth to 18 months of age: A cross-sectional study. 1. Effects of sex, race, age, season, and diet on Vitamin D status. *Pediatrics* 1986; 77:883.)
† Data for children not receiving vitamin supplements. (Data from Taylor AF, Norman ME: Vitamin D metabolite levels in normal children. *Pediatr Res* 1984; 18:886.)
‡ Specifically measured as 25(OH)D$_3$ and 24,25(OH)$_2$D$_3$.

TABLE 11–2.
Clinically Available Vitamin D Preparations*

	Vitamin D_3 (Cholecalciferol)	Vitamin D_2 (Ergocalciferol)	Dihydrotachysterol (DHT)	Calcifediol (25-Hydroxycholecalciferol)	Calcitriol (1,25-Dihydroxycholecalciferol)
Physiologic dose (µg/day)	10	10	20	5	0.5
Pharmacologic dose† (µg/day)	...	1,250–5,000	100–1,000	20–100	0.25–1.0
Onset of maximal effect (days)	30	30	15	15	3
Available forms	Tablets: 10 and 25µg‡	Drops: 200 µg/mL‡ Capsules: 625, 1,250 µg Tablets: 1,250 µg IM: 12,500 µg/mL	Tablets: 125, 200, 400 µg Capsules: 125 µg Liquid: 200 µg/5mL; 200, 250 µg/mL	Capsules: 20, 50 µg	Capsules: 0.25, 0.5 µg

* 1.0 µg of vitamin D_2 has an activity of 40 IU.
† Dosage range for treating hypoparathyroidism, osteomalacia due to malabsorption or vitamin D resistance, and renal osteodystrophy in older children and adults.
‡ Available without prescription.

Synthetic salmon calcitonin rather than human calcitonin is used because of its greater and more prolonged activity.

HYPOCALCEMIA, HYPOPHOSPHATEMIA, AND RICKETS

Tables 11–3 and 11–4 are useful outlines of the causes of hypocalcemia and hypophosphatemia in childhood. The most common symptom of hypocalcemia is tetany, or tetanic equivalents resulting from a low plasma ionized calcium. Muscle weakness; fatigue; numbness and tingling of the hands, lips, and feet; muscle cramps; and frank carpopedal spasm are common complaints. Laryngeal stridor or generalized seizures may follow. Patients also may have psychological problems, such as emotional lability, anxiety, depression, delirium, delusions, and psychotic behavior. Chronic hypocalcemia results in irreversible brain damage and mental retardation.

Alkalosis must be considered in the differential diagnosis of tetany. A history of severe anxiety (hyperventilation syndrome), vomiting, or alkali ingestion is suggestive. Typically patients have normal total serum calcium and phosphate concentrations, normal urinary calcium excretion, and an alkaline plasma and urine at the time of the attack. Emotional stress is the most common cause and usually is seen in adolescents. Alkalosis results in a lowering of the serum ionized calcium by increasing protein binding of calcium. This effect alone, however, is not sufficient to explain alkalotic tetany.

Hypocalcemia secondary to renal insufficiency rarely results in tetany, because of the associated acidosis. Bicarbonate therapy, however, may unmask this tendency.

Phosphorus is a major intracellular anion instrumental in innumerable metabolic and enzymatic reactions.[24] Although total body phosphorous content is regulated closely, serum phosphorous concentrations vary widely and are age-dependent. By convention, serum phosphate concentrations are expressed in terms of the concentration (in milligrams per deciliter) of elemental phophorus.

Hypophosphatemia may be secondary to decreased intake, increased renal losses, or transcellular ionic shifts. Common causes of hypophosphatemia that are not listed in Table 11–4 include total parenteral nutrition without phosphorus; diabetic ketoacidosis; and in adults, alcoholism and phosphate-binding antacids. Clinical manifestations of hypophosphatemia are not usually apparent until serum phosphorus falls below 2.0 mg/dL. Neuromuscular manifestations include weakness, malaise, anorexia, bone pain, and joint stiffness. If the serum phosphorous falls below 1.0 mg/dL, anisocoria, ballismus, hyporeflexia, paresthesias, convulsions, and subsequently coma and death may occur. Hypophosphatemia also causes erythrocyte, leukocyte, and platelet dysfunction; decreased tissue respiration in the liver; and skeletal abnormalities such as rickets, large joint arthralgias, inflammatory arthritis, and pathologic fractures.

Rickets, a defect in endochondral bone formation that leads to inadequate or delayed mineralization of osteoid, develops whenever there is significant

TABLE 11–3.
Hypocalcemic Disorders of Childhood

Parathyroid hormone abnormalities
  Hypoparathyroidism
    Congenital
      DiGeorge's syndrome
      Retinoic acid embryopathy
      X-linked recessive form
    Transient neonatal
      Idiopathic
      Secondary to maternal hypoparathyroidism
    Later onset
      Familial
      Idiopathic
      Candidal endocrinopathy syndrome
      Infiltration with iron, tumor, or lymphocytes
      Postsurgical
  Pseudohypoparathyroidism: several phenotypic forms
  Hypomagnesemia
    Imparied gut absorption
    Excessive renal wasting
    Prolonged diarrhea
Vitamin D abnormalities
  Dietary deficiency
  Reduced sunlight exposure
  Malabsorption syndromes
  Hepatocellular disorders that impair absorption and 25-OHD
    synthesis and enterohepatic circulation
  Vitamin D dependency or resistance
    1-Hydroxylase deficiency
      Autosomal recessive forms
      Severe renal disease
    End organ unresponsiveness to calcitriol (often associated with
      alopecia)
    Augmented metabolism of 25-OHD to inactive polar metabolites
      by drugs such as phenobarbital, phenytoin, ethanol
Miscellaneous conditions[21]
  Hypoproteinemia
  Alkalosis
  Hyperphosphatemia
    Postrauma (e.g., rhabdomyolysis)
    Postchemotherapy (e.g., tumor lysis syndrome)
  Massive transfusions
  Hypernatremia, hypokalemia
  Sepsis
  Pancreatitis
  Toxic shock syndrome
  Fat embolism
  Caffey-Kenny-Linarelli syndrome[22]

calcium or phosphate deficiency or acid accumulation.[3] Except in premature infants, nutritional vitamin D deficiency rickets is relatively rare today because of the mandatory fortification of milk (400 IU/qt). However, urban black breast-fed infants, infants of malnourished mothers, and infants excessively clothed and restricted to some vegetarian diets because of social or religious beliefs are at increased risk for the development of rickets.[25] Usually the first radiographic sign of rickets is widening of the growth plate. Currently, severe renal disease with phosphate retention is the most common cause of rickets and secondary hyperparathyroidism (renal osteodystrophy)[1]; other causes include vitamin D dependency, X-linked hypophosphatemia, Fanconi syndrome, and renal tubular disorders.

Neonatal Tetany

Neonatal hypocalcemia usually is defined as a total serum calcium concentration less than 8 mg/dL some time during the first 4 weeks of life. Serum phosphate concentrations may be normal but usually are increased, especially in the "classic" form. The incidence of neonatal hypocalcemia depends on duration of gestation, ease of delivery, and maternal condition. Hypocalcemia is uncommon in healthy full-term infants (approximately 1%), but may occur in 50% or more of premature or severely stressed newborn infants.[8, 9, 26] Boys are affected more often than girls.

Two forms of neonatal hypocalcemia are now well recognized: an early ("first-day") hypocalcemia and the classic or late form. Early hypocalcemia occurs during the first 24 to 48 hours of life in infants who have had an abnormal, stressful birth. Prematurity and the presence of maternal diabetes also are predisposing factors. The classic form of neonatal hypocalcemia (neonatal tetany) usually occurs between the fifth and tenth days of life. Again, prematurity is a predisposing factor, but a high dietary intake of phosphorus seems to be more important.

The cause of neonatal hypocalcemia no doubt is multifactorial. Hypercalcemia in cord blood, functional hypoparathyroidism, hypercalcitonemia, decreased ability to excrete a phosphate load, and decreased responsiveness to

TABLE 11–4.
Hypophosphatemic Disorders of Childhood

Primary hypophosphatemic rickets (X-linked dominant)
Hereditary hypophosphatemic rickets with hypercalciuria[23]
Oncogenous rickets with phosphaturia ("tumoral rickets")[3]
Bone or soft-tissue mesenchymal tumors
Polyostotic fibrous dysplasia
Neurofibromatosis
Complex proximal tubulopathy
Fanconi syndrome
Idiopathic
Numerous secondary causes: Wilson's disease, hereditary fructose intolerance; galactosemia
Secondary to increased parathormone secretion
Primary hyperparathyrodism (associated with hypercalcemia)
Vitamin D deficiency
Vitamin D dependence or resistance

parathormone have been demonstrated in neonates.[26, 27] Further, decreased concentrations of 25-OHD have been found in plasma samples from socioeconomically deprived mothers and their hypocalcemic infants.[28]

Early hypocalcemia may result from functional hypoparathyroidism (secondary to fetal hypercalcemia) combined with increasing phosphate release into the circulation because of hypoxia. Hyperphosphatemia secondary to a low dietary calcium-phosphorus ratio, renal immaturity, and functional hypoparathyroidism probably account for the classic form. Vitamin D deficiency and increased circulating levels of calcitonin also may be important in neonatal hypocalcemia. The use of artificial formulas similar in composition to breast milk has decreased the incidence of classic neonatal tetany.

Most of the signs and symptoms of neonatal tetany are the result of increased neuromuscular excitability. Irritability, twitching, unilateral or bilateral clonic or tonic seizures, and vomiting are common. Laryngospasm, edema, gastrointestinal bleeding, and cyanosis frequently occur. Chvostek and peroneal signs are not helpful, as they are frequently seen in normal newborn infants. Severe intracranial disease (e.g., hemorrhage, anoxia, meningitis) may mask or mimic hypocalcemia. Hypocalcemic infants without CNS damage, however, usually appear well between convulsive episodes. It should be obvious that calcium, phosphate, and total protein concentrations must be monitored closely in sick neonates. Hypocalcemia causes prolongation of electrical systole and hence prolongation of the QT interval. An article by Colletti et al. emphasizes the usefulness of electrocardiographic findings in neonatal hypocalcemia.[29] A corrected Q-oT interval (the interval from the origin of the Q wave to the origin of the T wave, corrected for heart rate by the formula $Q - oT_c = \left(\dfrac{Q - oT}{\sqrt{R - R}}\right) \geq 0.19$ seconds in premature infants and ≥ 0.20 seconds in full-term infants suggests the presence of hypocalcemia. The QT interval, however, is not always prolonged in hypocalcemia. Hypokalemia may also cause prolongation of the QT interval, and hypomagnesemia causes more marked prolongation in the hypocalcemic state. However, as recently reported, treatment of hypocalcemia in very low birth weight (VLBW) infants did not affect cardiac function.[30]

Acute treatment of neonatal tetany consists of intravenous administration of calcium salts. Calcium gluconate is given intravenously as a 10% solution, no faster than 1 mL/min. During the infusion the infant's heartbeat must be monitored electrocardiographically or by an assistant. The infusion should be stopped as soon as the symptoms have abated or at the first sign of bradycardia. Usually 1 to 3 mL calcium gluconate terminates seizures. Care must be taken to avoid subcutaneous or intramuscular administration of calcium salts, because severe tissue necrosis will be produced. Calcium infusion should be given with extreme caution in hypokalemic infants and infants receiving digitalis preparations. Several (3 to 4) intravenous doses of calcium gluconate may be necessary over the first 24 hours to control symptoms: 1 to 2 mL/kg body weight may be given every 6 or 8 hours.

After the acute symptoms have been controlled, a soluble calcium salt should be added to the infant's formula to achieve a calcium-phosphorus ratio of approximately 4:1. This can be achieved by adding 4 g of calcium gluconate (9% calcium by weight) or 3 g of calcium lactate powder (13% calcium by weight) to 1 L of a commercially available low-phosphate formula (e.g., Similac PM 60/40 or SMA-S-26). This provides an excess of calcium, which causes precipitation of dietary phosphate in the intestinal lumen as insoluble $Ca_3(PO_4)_2$. Calcium gluconate is commercially available as a syrup (Syrup of NeoCalglucon) that provides 115 mg calcium per teaspoon. Because of its convenience, calcium gluconate syrup is used most frequently, but some infants develop diarrhea because of the large amount of sugar. Calcium lactate powder is easily dissolved in milk, but the required amount must be weighed and packaged by a pharmacist. Calcium lactate tablets are unsatisfactory because of their poor solubility, even after they have been crushed. Some clinicians recommend calcium chloride (1.5 g/ day in three to four doses) because of its acidifying effect and better absorption; however, calcium chloride is irritating to the gastrointestinal tract and is seldom, if ever, necessary. Treatment with supplemental calcium salts usually is required for at least 7 to 10 days. When the serum calcium has reached normal levels, the calcium supplement may be tapered gradually; if the serum calcium level remains normal, treatment may be discontinued after a total duration of 2 to 3 weeks. In severe cases aluminum hydroxide gel may be helpful. PTH and vitamin D are seldom indicated in the treatment of neonatal tetany.

In severe or persistent cases of neonatal tetany, especially in infants who fail to respond to calcium salt supplementation alone, maternal hyperparathyroidism,[31] congenital absence of the parathyroid glands with or without thymic dysplasia (DiGeorge's syndrome),[32] X-linked neonatal hypoparathyroidism,[33] and Caffey-Kenny-Linarelli syndrome[22] must be considered. All of these are rare conditions.

Hypoparathyroidism

The differential diagnosis of hypoparathyroidism depends on the age of the child. Transient neonatal hypoparathyroidism and the syndromes of congenital absence of the parathyroid glands occur early in life. Idiopathic hypoparathyroidism usually becomes obvious between the ages of 5 and 15 years. This condition frequently is accompanied by cutaneous moniliasis[34] secondary to a defect(s) in the delayed-type immune system. Idiopathic hypoparathyroidism may be familial, in which case it is often associated with Addison's disease and sometimes with diabetes mellitus, pernicious anemia, or thyroiditis. Hypoparathyroidism may also develop after accidental removal or destruction of the glands during thyroidectomy. Pseudohypoparathyroidism usually is distinguished by characteristic physical findings and positive family history.

In addition to the signs and symptoms of hypocalcemia, patients with hypoparathyroidism may have increased intracranial pressure, hyperreflexia, choreiform movements, visual and auditory problems, metastatic calcification (conjunctiva, sclera, lens, basal ganglia), and diarrhea due to hyperexcitability of the gastrointestinal tract. Magnesium deficiency also may occur in these patients, and necessitates replacement therapy before eucalcemia can be restored.

Primary malabsorption syndromes may produce hypocalcemia and hyperphosphatemia and may be difficult to differentiate.[35] Vitamin D therapy, however, does not cure the gastrointestinal symptoms of primary malabsorption syndrome.

Ectodermal problems also are a prominent feature of all types of hypoparathyroidism. These include dry, puffy, yellowish skin; brittle, transversely ridged nails; and alopecia. Idiopathic hypoparathyroidism also is associated with dental abnormalities such as enamel hypoplasia, transverse ridging, delayed eruption, and caries and with longitudinally rigged, cracked nails with transverse whitish patches. Cutaneous moniliasis may be severe and may precede hypocalcemia; these cases usually are familial. On the other hand, adrenal insufficiency usually develops after hypoparathyroidism.

Hypocalcemia, inappropriately low serum PTH concentrations, hyperphosphatemia, and normal alkaline phosphatase levels are classic laboratory findings in hypoparathyroidism.

Except for the low PTH values, similar laboratory findings are seen in pseudohypoparathyroidism type 1. However, round facies, short stature, typical brachydactyly, mental dullness, and a positive family history strongly support this diagnosis. Subcutaneous calcifications are common; moniliasis is not seen in this syndrome. Hypoparathyroidism is inherited and affects girls approximately twice as often as boys. In view of the reported instances of male-male transmission, an autosomal dominant gene with variable penetrance appears to be the cause of pseudohypoparathyroidism type 1. Hyperplastic parathyroid glands, high concentrations of serum immunoreactive PTH, and renal unresponsiveness to PTH are the hallmarks of this condition.[36] However, there is a spectrum of involvement; for example, some patients have all of the physical features of the condition but are eucalcemic. Furthermore, both hypocalcemic and eucalcemic patients with physical findings of pseudohypoparathyroidism may be present in the same kindred. The awkward term *pseudo-psuedohypoparathyroidism* has been used to describe such eucalcemic patients. Another term, *type 2 pseudohypoparathyroidism*, should be limited to describing patients who respond to PTH with a prompt increase in urinary cAMP but have no phosphaturic response. Patients with type 2 disease have hypocalcemia, hyperphosphatemia, and high PTH concentrations, but do not have distinguishing anatomic features.[37] Finally, patients who have renal resistance to PTH but normal bone responsiveness have also been reported (pseudohypohyperparathyroidism); these patients have had osteitis fibrosa, presumably the result of excess PTH secretion.[38]

Several tests have been designed to determine PTH responsiveness: increased phosphate excretion (Ellsworth-Howard test), increased urinary cAMP, and appropriate serum changes in calcium and phosphorus. These tests are somewhat difficult to perform and usually are not required. When the precise diagnosis is in doubt, responsiveness to PTH may be determined by administering synthetic human PTH-(1-34) (Parathar) intravenously (3 U/kg over 10 minutes up to a maximum dose of 200 U) and measuring urinary cAMP and phosphate excretion for 1 to 2 hours before and after injection.[39]

The therapeutic goal in all forms of hypoparathyroidism should be maintenance of eucalcemia *without complications* of hypocalcemia (e.g., seizures, CNS damage, cataracts, alopecia, dystrophic nails) or hypercalcemia (e.g., renal stones, nephrocalcinosis, renal failure). The disorder in children is more difficult to manage than in adults (probably because of greater calcium needs for growth), and therapy is more difficult in idiopathic hypoparathyroidism than in pseudohypoparathyroidism. (For a detailed discussion of therapeutic problems, interested readers are referred to references 1, 14, 16, and 40.)

Mild or partial hypoparathyroidism, as may occur after subtotal thyroidectomy, may be managed sometimes by administration of calcium salts alone. However, at least 4 to 5 g of calcium is required per day in the older child. Because this would mean more than 30 g of calcium lactate per day, calcium carbonate, which is 40% calcium by weight is usually recommended. Calcium carbonate produces mild alkalosis that may slightly worsen hypocalcemic symptoms during the first few days of treatment. However, as the serum calcium increases, symptoms disappear despite persistence of a mild metabolic alkalosis. When patients are maintained on calcium salts alone, special care must be taken to avoid complications of hypocalcemia; careful ophthalmologic evaluation is necessary to detect the presence of early lenticular opacities, which would necessitate more intensive treatment.

Patients with severe or complete hypoparathyroidism require treatment with pharmacologic amounts of vitamin D_2, dihydrotachysterol, or calcitriol. Calcium salts (1 to 2 g of elemental calcium/day) usually are required early in therapy but may be discontinued later. When possible, patients should be maintained on vitamin D alone to avoid the complications of marked hypercalciuria. Furthermore, calcium therapy is not accepted well by many children because of the large amounts necessary. In the absence of PTH, which increases tubular reabsorption of calcium, hypercalciuria may develop even when the serum calcium concentration is slightly low or in the low normal range. *This obviously emphasizes the need for quantitative serum and urinary calcium determinations to monitor therapy.*

Treatment of patients with hypoparathyroidism must be individualized and should be supervised by physicians with experience in this area. Our goal is to maintain serum calcium between 8.5 and 10 mg/dL and the urinary calcium below 3 mg/kg/day or 0.25 mg/mg creatinine. The maintenance dose of vitamin D_2 may vary between 0.025 and 0.05 mg/kg/day (1,000 to 2,000 IU/kg/day). Most patients do well with an average dose of 50,000 IU/day or its equivalent (see Table 11–2). Initial treatment should be approximately 5,000 IU/kg/day until the serum calcium level begins to increase. As reliable dosage forms became available, we preferred to treat our patients with dihydrotachysterol because of its more rapid action and shorter half-life. Dihydrotachysterol, on a weight basis, is two to four times as potent as vitamin D_2; the usual maintenance dosage is between 0.01 and 0.02 mg/kg/day. *Close follow-up is mandatory.* Initially, serum calcium and phosphorus levels should be checked twice a week until the patient is eucalcemic. Subsequently monthly checks usually suffice, and when a satisfactory regimen has been established, patients should be evaluated three or four times per year.

Patients and their families should be advised to report the first signs of hypercalcemia: nocturia, polyuria, polydipsia, anorexia, and constipation. A note of caution is necessary about possible difficulties encountered when therapy is changed from vitamin D_2 to shorter acting analogues such as dihydrotachysterol or $1,25(OH)_2D_3$. Metabolites of vitamin D_2 may persist for as long as 12 months after discontinuation, and thus the maintenance dosage of the new compound may not be established quickly.[41]

Hypoparathyroidism with associated endocrine diseases, especially Addison's disease, is difficult to manage and patients should be under the care of an endocrinologist. Likewise, patients with moniliasis and hypoparathyroidism require the combined expertise of an immunologist and an endocrinologist.

Vitamin D Deficiency Rickets

Occasional "simple" rickets is seen in premature infants, patients with severe malabsorption, and severely deprived children. The earliest symptoms are apathy and muscular weakness. Irritability, delayed closure of the fontanelle, abdominal distention, and prominence of the costochondral junctions are later signs; bowing of the lower extremities appears after significant weight bearing. Widening and irregularity of the epiphyseal plates, cupped metaphyses, fractures, and bowing are seen roentgenographically.

There are three stages in the development of vitamin D deficiency in infancy. In the first stage serum calcium is low, but serum phosphate and PTH are normal and aminoaciduria is absent. Within several days stage 2 develops, in which serum calcium returns to normal but PTH increases, phosphate decreases, and aminoaciduria develops. Most cases are diagnosed in stage 3, when there are hypocalcemia, hypophosphatemia, aminoaciduria, and increased PTH and alkaline phosphatase levels. The reason for the failure of PTH to rise promptly in stage 1 is unclear but may be secondary to the negative feedback effects of the small amounts of residual vitamin D. PTH certainly seems to be the cause of the mild acidosis and aminoaciduria.

Mild, simple rickets may be treated nicely with daily administration of 1,000 to 2,000 IU of vitamin D_2 for several months until healing occurs. Serum phosphorus usually returns to normal within 1 week, and radiographic improvement occurs in 2 weeks. When healing is completed, a dietary intake of 400 IU/day prevents recurrence. Much larger doses of vitamin D_2 may be used when therapeutic compliance is uncertain or when more rapid improvement is desirable. Furthermore, large dosages eliminate the possibility of an initial hypocalcemic effect secondary to the more prompt rise in serum inorganic phosphate. A 3-week course of 12,000 to 16,000 IU/day of vitamin D_2 produces unquestionable biochemical and radiographic improvement in uncomplicated vitamin D deficiency rickets. After this course, vitamin D intake may be reduced to a prophylactic dose of 400 IU/day. Finally, massive dosage, or stosstherapy, may also be given: 600,000 IU of vitamin D_2 given in 1 day (six doses of 100,000 IU given orally at 2-hour intervals). If this approach is chosen, concentrated preparations of vitamin D_2 must be given (50,000 IU capsules), because administration of the commonly available propylene glycol solution of D_2 (Drisdol, 8,000 IU/mL) would cause intoxication.

Vitamin D Dependency

There are at least three forms of vitamin D dependency: an autosomal recessive form due to a deficiency of 1-hydroxylase[3, 42, 43]; an autosomal recessive form due to end organ resistance to $1,25(OH)_2D_3$[44]; and an anticonvulsant-induced form.[45, 46] Serum calcium is low; phosphorous may be normal or low.

The inherited form of vitamin D dependency type I (often called pseudo-deficiency rickets) is most rare. Typical signs and symptoms of rickets appear during infancy. However, as the name implies, these patients do not respond to the usual replacement doses of vitamin D. Indeed, they usually require approximately 100 times the usual daily requirement of vitamin D_2. Recent studies indicate that these patients have a defect in the formation of $1,25(OH)_2D_3$ from 25-OHD, an autosomal recessive disorder; physiologic doses of $1,25(OH)_2D_3$ (0.25 to 1.0 μg) have been effective. These uncommon patients have been maintained on 40,000 to 80,000 IU of D_2/day, with close observation, but safer and more rational therapy is $1,25(OH)_2D_3$.[3]

Shortly after the discovery of the importance of $1,25(OH)_2D_3$ and development of specific assays for its measurement in serum, several familial instances of probable end organ resistance were reported; the inheritance pattern is autosomal recessive, but the gene locus is unknown.[44] Patients have had severe rickets, secondary hyperparathyroidism, and increased concentrations of $1,25(OH)_2D_3$; the majority have also had alopecia. Vitamin D dependency type 2 has been used to describe the disorder in these patients; however, it seems likely that further classification will evolve as we learn more about the cellular actions of vitamin D. Treatment of this rare disorder consists of huge doses of calcitriol and calcium supplementation.[3, 47]

Vitamin D dependency also may be induced by prolonged treatment with anticonvulsants such as phenytoin and phenobarbital. In these instances the greater requirements of vitamin D are the result of an increased rate of metabolism and excretion of the hormone, as well as inhibition of calcium transport by the intestinal mucosa. Treatment with 800 to 2,000 IU/day of vitamin D_2 usually corrects the rickets, but some patients have needed 10,000 to 50,000 IU/day.[46]

X-Linked Hypophosphatemia

X-linked hypophosphatemia, frequently termed vitamin D-resistant rickets, is an inherited defect of phosphate transport present in both the kidneys and intestine[3]; it is the most common form of hypophosphatemic rickets. Serum calcium often is normal, and PTH is mildly increased or normal.[48] Recent studies indicate the serum concentrations of $1,25(OH)_2D_3$ are low or normal, despite marked hypophosphatemia, a potent stimulus for 1-hydroxylation. These findings have reopened discussions about the pathogenesis and treatment of this disorder.[3, 49, 50] The condition becomes apparent early in infancy because of growth failure, rickets, and severe hypophosphatemia. Because of X linkage, boys are more severely affected than girls.

Treatment of X-linked hypophosphatemia has consisted of oral phosphate (1 to 4 g of elemental phosphorus/day) and sufficient vitamin D_2 (1,000 to 2,000 IU/kg/day), dihydrotachysterol (0.01 to 0.02 mg/kg/day), or preferably calcitriol (35 ng/kg/day) to prevent hypocalcemia[3, 50–55] and produce healing of the rickets. Recent studies suggest that $1,25(OH)_2D_3$ gives the best results. Growth acceleration and further healing of rickets were noted when patients were given up to 4 µg/day of $1,25(OH)_2D_3$ along with phosphate supplementation.[54, 55] Massive doses of vitamin D_2 alone, as previously used, have been detrimental (hypercalcemia, nephrocalcinosis) in some patients[56] and will not restore serum phosphate to normal. Despite the advantages of phosphate therapy, patient acceptance often is poor because of dosage frequency (five to six times per day) and the unpleasant taste of neutral phosphate solutions. Phosphate therapy can be accomplished by administering Joulies' solution,* which provides 30 mg of inorganic phosphorus/mL, or Neutra-Phos-K, which provides 250 mg inorganic phosphorus per 75 mL. The latter is preferred because it has a more pleasant taste and lacks sodium. As always when vitamin D is given in pharmacologic amounts, close observation of serum calcium concentration and urinary calcium excretion is mandatory; we recommend keeping the urinary calcium-creatinine ratio below 0.2. With careful therapy most, if not all, of the skeletal deformities can be prevented. However, after the adolescent growth spurt has been completed, surgical correction of residual bowing is recommended to lessen the likelihood of the development of severe osteoarthritis later in life.

Rickets also occurs in many renal tubular disorders, for example, Fanconi's syndrome, cystinosis, Lowe's syndrome, and renal tubular acidosis. Treatment must be individualized and supervised by an experienced physician. Oral phosphate, modest doses of vitamin D_2, and oral alkali (e.g., Shohl's solution, a solution of sodium citrate and citric acid; Polycitra, a flavored solution of sodium and potassium citrate) are the principal forms of therapy.

Juvenile Idiopathic Osteoporosis

Idiopathic osteoporosis is a disease of the elderly. Rarely, however, it occurs in young adults, adolescents, and even children.[57–59] The juvenile form of the disease occurs most often between the ages of 8 and 12 years. Severe pain and compression fractures of the spine are common findings. The diagnosis should only be reached by exclusion. Malnutrition, malabsorption syndromes, anorexia nervosa, chronic immobilization, chronic illnesses (e.g., collagen diseases), hyperparathyroidism, Cushing's disease, and hyperthyroidism must be considered and ruled out.

---

* Joulies' solution: diabasic sodium phosphate, 136 g/vol; phosphoric acid (National Formulary, 85%), 58.8 g/vol; distilled water to 1,000 mL.

Numerous forms of treatment including vitamin D, calcium, androgens, estrogens, fluoride, phosphate salts, and calcitonin have been reported, but a definite effect on remineralization has not been clearly demonstrated. Because symptoms usually subside spontaneously in these patients, conservative therapy with modest doses of vitamin D_2 (1,000 to 5,000 IU/day), supplemental calcium (1 g/day), supplemental oral phosphate (1 to 2 g elemental phosphorus/day), analgesics as needed, and gradually increased activity would seem wise.

Magnesium Deficiency

Despite the important intracellular role of the magnesium ion, disorders of magnesium metabolism are uncommon. Primary intestinal malabsorption of magnesium has been reported.[60] However, magnesium deficiency is more likely to be secondary to malabsorption syndromes, protein-calorie malnutrition, hypercalcemia from any cause, renal tubular acidosis, diuretic therapy, hyperaldosteronism, chronic alcoholism, or renal tubular dysfunction secondary to treatment with aminoglycoside antibiotics such as gentamicin. Hyperexcitability and frank tetany are the presenting features.

The role of magnesium in PTH action and regulation is complex. Magnesium deficiency, however, impairs parathyroid gland responsiveness to hypocalcemia.[61-63] This may explain the necessity of magnesium replacement in some patients with hypocalcemic tetany. Magnesium deficiency should be suspected in any patient with "refractory hypocalcemia" or tetany.

In the case of documented hypomagnesemia (Mg <1.3 mEq/L in the neonatal period or <1.6 mEq/L later) therapy with Mg_2SO_4, 0.2 mL/kg/day of a 50% solution, may be given intramuscularly. Magnesium depletion may be corrected by daily oral administration of 1 to 4 mEq/kg of Mg chloride or citrate salt.

Metabolic Bone Disease of Prematurity

During the past 10 years, metabolic bone disease has become a widely recognized problem in VLBW premature infants (<1,500 g) who now usually survive in modern neonatal intensive care units. The bone disease is usually subclinical, but elevated alkaline phosphatase concentration, decreased bone mineralization, and even fractures are common findings. Because many factors contribute to the occurrence and severity of this disorder, the term "metabolic bone disease of prematurity" has gained acceptance and is preferred over rickets or osteopenia. The principal cause of this disorder has been recognized as failure of earlier conventional therapy to meet the significant demands for calcium and phosphorus imposed by the rapidly growing VLBW infant. Other factors, especially long-term therapy with furosemide and immaturity of the vitamin D metabolic system also contribute significantly.

The best therapy of metabolic bone disease of prematurity is prevention through phosphorus and calcium supplementation of enteral or parenteral feedings.[64] Vitamin D_2, 400 IU/day, appears to be sufficient to prevent vitamin D deficiency in mineral-sufficient enterally fed VLBW infants, but many investigators have recommended 800 to 1,000 IU/day; 100 to 200 IU/day of vitamin D has been recommended for parenterally fed infants. Finally, the minimal clinically effective dose of furosemide should be used to lessen urinary calcium losses and nephrocalcinosis.

HYPERCALCEMIA

In contrast to hypocalcemia, hypercalcemic disorders are rare in children. For all practical purposes, the differential diagnosis of hypercalcemia is limited to primary hyperparathyroidism, familial hypocalciuric hypercalcemia, idiopathic infantile hypercalcemia, immobilization hypercalcemia, and vitamin D intoxication. Malignancies with or without osseous metastases, multiple myeloma, sarcoidosis, and the milk-alkali syndrome are common causes in adults but are unusual in children. Severe leukemic infiltration of bone may, however, produce hypercalcemia. Addison's disease, hyperthyroidism, hypothyroidism, vitamin A intoxication, subcutaneous necrosis, and hypophosphatasia also are rare causes of hypercalcemia.

The progression of symptoms of hypercalcemia is as follows:

1. Asymptomatic
2. General malaise, fatigue, psychoneurotic complaints, weight loss, pruritus
3. Renal colic, polyuria, polydipsia
4. Constipation, epigastric pain, anorexia, nausea, vomiting
5. Lethargy, muscular weakness, confusion, psychosis, stupor, coma

Hypercalcemic crisis (serum calcium usually >15 mg/100 mL) is characterized by fever, stupor, coma, hypertension, profound dehydration, bradycardia, seizures, and if not controlled promptly, death. These symptoms may be explained by the effects of excess calcium: decreased membrane excitability, decreased membrane permeability and subsequent tremendous renal losses of water and solute, and vascular constriction. Acidosis also may accompany hypercalcemia, especially if it is secondary to hyperparathyroidism.

Emergency treatment of severe hypercalcemia should consist of vigorous intravenous hydration and maintenance of massive sodium diuresis along with elimination of vitamin D intake and a low calcium diet. Furosemide (1 mg/kg intravenously every 6 to 8 hours) or ethacrynic acid is useful, but *thiazide diuretics are contraindicated* because of their hypercalcemic potential. Infusions of sodium sulfate or sodium citrate may be superior to saline solution. Pharmacologic doses of glucocorticoids (e.g., prednisone, 2 mg/kg/day) oppose the actions of vitamin D, but their effect on serum calcium takes several days. Oral phosphate (1 to 3 g of inorganic phosphate/day in four divided doses) promotes deposition of calcium in bone (and possibly soft tissues). Potassium and magnesium concentrations must be followed closely and appropriate replacement therapy given.

Synthetic salmon calcitonin (Calcimar) may be given intravenously or intramuscularly (5 to 8 MRC units/kg every 6 to 12 hours) to correct the hypercalcemia until the glucocorticoids become effective. Mithramycin, an antitumor, cytotoxic antibiotic, has also been used successfully in patients with metastatic disease (25 μg/kg as an intravenous bolus).[65] Its effect is rapid (within several hours) and lasts up to 48 hours.

Primary Hyperparathyroidism

Recurrent episodes of abdominal pain and pancreatitis may be common findings in children with parathyroid adenomas.[66] However, the use of more frequent laboratory screening studies has led to the recognition of many cases of asymptomatic hypercalcemia, especially in adults.[67, 68] Diagnosis of primary hyperparathyroidism should not be difficult: hypercalcemia, hypophosphatemia, increased alkaline phosphatase, increased immunoreactive PTH compared with a simultaneous calcium determination, subperiosteal bone resorption (especially phalangeal),[69] and hyperchloremia are typical findings. The cause of primary hyperparathyroidism (adenoma or hyperplasia) is unknown.[70] Virtually all infants with primary hyperparathyroidism have parathyroid hyperplasia, whereas affected children usually have a parathyroid adenoma.[71] Both autosomal recessive and autosomal dominant transmission have been documented in families with children who have parathyroid hyperplasia.[6] Primary hyperparathyroidism may be part of both multiple endocrine adenomatosis (MEA) type I (pituitary, parathyroid, pancreas, and less commonly, thyroid and adrenal adenomas) and MEA type II (medullary carcinoma of thyroid, pheochromocytomas, and hyperparathyroidism). The preferred treatment of primary hyperparathyroidism is surgical removal of involved parathyroid tissue by an experienced surgeon.[72, 73] However, the prognosis in untreated, asymptomatic primary hyperparathyroidism is unknown and thus the indications for surgery are unclear.[71] When all four parathyroid glands are hyperplastic, total parathyroidectomy may be necessary. Autotransplantation of part of one gland to within the muscles of the forearm has been recommended in such cases.[6] This may allow close monitoring of the function of the transplanted tissue and easy removal if hypercalcemia recurs.

Familial Hypocalciuric Hypercalcemia

Familial hypocalciuric hypercalcemia is an uncommon autosomal dominant disorder of the regulation of divalent cations.[74–76] Serum calcium concentrations in this disorder are similar to those in patients with symptomatic primary hyperparathyroidism. Nonetheless, these patients are asymptomatic throughout life. Serum magnesium values are also increased, and this is the only known cause of hypercalcemia not associated with hypomagnesemia. Serum PTH concentrations are usually normal, but some investigators have reported modest increases in PTH in a few patients. A positive family history and lack of hypercalciuria assist greatly with the differentiation from primary hyperparathyroidism. This disorder has been associated with both neonatal hyperparathyroidism and hypoparathyroidism in infants of affected mothers: neonatal hypoparathyroidism is usually transient, but severe neonatal primary hyperparathyroidism resulting from diffuse hyperplasia has required total parathyroidectomy.[75, 76]

Idiopathic Infantile Hypercalcemia

Infantile hypercalcemia (Williams syndrome or Lightwood's syndrome) is a rare disorder of unknown cause. The severe form of this syndrome is characterized by failure to thrive; symptomatic, often severe hypercalcemia without hypophosphatemia; elfin facies; mental retardation; strabismus; dense mineralization of bone; and cardiovascular anomalies, usually supravalvular aortic stenosis.[77, 78] Nephrocalcinosis and renal failure may develop. Less severely affected infants may merely show (between 3 and 8 months) failure to thrive; hypercalcemia may have abated spontaneously by that time, and the diagnosis can only be suspected.

The cause of this syndrome is unclear. Vitamin D intoxication, increased maternal or fetal sensitivity to vitamin D, abnormal metabolism of vitamin D, impaired secretion of calcitonin, or hyperfunction of the placental calcium transport mechanism have been proposed as important factors. Treatment should be aimed at rapid normalization of serum calcium to prevent further CNS damage. Calcium-free formulas, temporary elimination of vitamin D, avoidance of sunlight, and pharmacologic doses of glucocorticoids may be necessary initially. Differential diagnosis seldom is a problem; however, infantile primary hyperparathyroidism secondary to parathyroid hyperplasia must be considered. The natural history and detailed features of Williams syndrome are summarized well by Morris et al.[78]

Immobilization Hypercalcemia

Disuse atrophy of bone, soft-tissue ossification, hypercalciuria, and urinary calculi are relatively common complications of chronic immobilization. Hypercalcemia, however, is rare.[79, 80] Most of the reported cases were in adolescent boys with a fractured femur or multiple fractures. For example, a 13-year-old boy was referred to us in severe hypercalcemic crisis. He had been immobilized for 6 weeks because of a severely fractured right femur. During his hospitalization he had been given vitamin D_2 and calcium supplements and was urged to drink 2 quarts of milk a day — all inappropriate and dangerous.

Differentiating between immobilization hypercalcemia and primary hyperparathyroidism with a pathologic fracture might be difficult. However, radiographic evidence of hyperparathyroidism, increased PTH concentrations, hyperchloremia, increased alkaline phosphatase level, and marked hypophosphatemia would be expected in primary hyperparathyroidism.

Prevention is the best treatment of immobilization hypercalcemia. Low calcium intake, increased fluid intake, active and passive exercises, and prompt mobilization should suffice. Treatment of hypercalcemia was outlined above.

Vitamin D Intoxication

Hypercalcemia, normal or increased serum phosphate or alkaline phosphatase levels, and a history of intake of pharmacologic doses of vitamin D_2 (50,000 to 100,000 IU/day) are typical of vitamin D intoxication. Many of these patients have received inappropriate treatment. For example, a recent patient of ours was given prolonged treatment with vitamin D_2 for what really was "physiologic bowing" of the lower extremities. Treatment should consist of a low-calcium diet, increased fluid intake, and steroids; however, the long biologic half-life (several weeks) of vitamin D_2 makes treatment difficult. Usually glucocorticoids can be tapered after 2 weeks of treatment.

REFERENCES

1. Audran M, Kumar R: The physiology and pathophysiology of Vitamin D. *Mayo Clin Proc* 1985; 60:851.
2. Brommage R, DeLuca HF: Evidence that 1,25-dihydroxyvitamin D_3 is the physiologically active metabolite of vitamin D_3. *Endocr Rev* 1985; 6:491.
3. Chesney RW: Metabolic bone diseases. *Pediatr Rev* 1984; 5:227.
4. Norman AW, Roth J, Orci L: The vitamin D endocrine system: Steroid metabolism, hormone receptors, and biological response (calcium binding proteins). *Endocr Rev* 1982; 3:331.
5. Harrison HE: Vitamin D, the parathyroid and the kidney. *Johns Hopkins Med J* 1979; 144:180.
6. Harrison HE, Harrison HC: *Disorders of Calcium and Phosphate Metabolism in Childhood and Adolescence*. Philadelphia, WB Saunders Co, 1979.
7. Burritt MF, Pierides AM, Offord KP: Comparative studies of total and ionized serum calcium values in normal subjects and patients with renal disorders. *Mayo Clin Proc* 1980; 55:606.
8. Lichtenstein P, et al: Calcium-regulating hormones and minerals from birth to 18 months of age: A cross-sectional study. I. Effects of sex, race, age, season and diet on vitamin D status. *Pediatrics* 1986; 77:883.
9. Specker BL, et al: Calcium-regulating hormones and minerals from birth to 18 months of age: A cross-sectional study: II. Effects of sex, race, age, season, and diet on serum minerals, parathyroid hormone, and calcitonin. *Pediatrics* 1986; 77:891.
10. Venkataraman PS, et al: Pathogenesis of early neonatal hypocalcemia: Studies of serum calcitonin, gastrin, and plasma glucagon. *J Pediatr* 1987; 110:599.
11. Levine MM, Kleeman CR: Hypercalcemia: Pathophysiology and treatment. *Hosp Practice* July 15, 1987, p 93.
12. Rasmussen H, et al: Hormonal control of skeletal and mineral homeostasis. *Am J Med* 1974; 56:751.
13. Lund BJ, et al: Vitamin D metabolism in hypoparathyroidism. *J Clin Endocrinol Metab* 1980; 51:606.

14. Kumar R, Riggs BL: Vitamin D in the therapy of disorders of calcium and phosphorus metabolism. *Mayo Clin Proc* 1981; 56:327.

15. Chesney RW, et al: Long-term influence of calcitriol (1,25-dihydroxyvitamin D) and supplemental phosphate in X-linked hypophosphatemic rickets. *Pediatrics* 1983; 71:559.

16. Chan JCM, et al: Calcium and phosphate metabolism in children with idiopathic hypoparathyroidism or psuedohypoparathyroidism: Effect of 1,25 dihydroxyvitamin D₃. *J Pediatr* 1985; 106:421.

17. Chesney RW, et al: Serum 1,25-dihydroxyvitamin D levels in normal children and in vitamin D disorders. *Am J Dis Child* 1980; 134:135.

18. Taylor AF, Norman ME: Vitamin D metabolite levels in normal children. *Pediatr Res* 1984; 18:886.

19. Austin LA, Heath III H: Calcitonin physiology and pathophysiology. *New Engl J Med* 1981; 304:269.

20. Deftos LJ, First BP: Calcitonin as a drug. *Ann Int Med* 1981; 95:192.

21. Zaloga GP, Chernow B: Hypocalcemia in critical illness. *JAMA* 1986; 256:1924.

22. Frech RS, McAlister WH: Medullary stenosis of the tubular bones associated with hypocalcemia, convulsions and short stature. *Radiology* 1968; 91:457.

23. Tieder M, et al: "Idiopathic" hypercalciuria and hereditary hypophosphatemic rickets. Two phenotypical expressions of a common genetic defect. *N Engl J Med* 1987; 316:125.

24. Gertner JM: Phosphorus metabolism and its disorders in childhood. *Pediatr Ann* 1987; 16:957.

25. Rudolf M, Arulanantham K, Greenstein RM: Unsuspected nutritional rickets. *Pediatrics* 1980; 66:72.

26. Tsang RC, et al: Possible pathogenetic factors in neonatal hypocalcemia of prematurity. *J Pediatr* 1973; 82:432.

27. Kruse K, Kustermann W: Evidence for transient peripheral resistance to parathyroid hormone in premature infants. *Acta Paediatr Scand* 1987; 76:115.

28. Rosen JF, et al: 25-Hydroxyvitamin D. *Am J Dis Child* 1974; 127:220.

29. Colletti RB, et al: Detection of hypocalcemia in susceptible neonates: The Q-oTce interval. *N Engl J Med* 1974; 290:931.

30. Venkataraman PS, et al: Effect of hypocalcemia on cardiac function in very-low-birth-weight preterm neonates: Studies of blood ionized calcium, echocardiography, and cardiac effect of intravenous calcium therapy. *Pediatrics* 1985; 76:543.

31. Ertel NH, Reiss JS, Spergel G: Hypomagnesemia in neonatal tetany associated with maternal hyperparathyroidism. *N Engl J Med* 1969; 280:260.

32. DiGeorge AM: Congenital absence of the thymus and its immunological consequences: Concurrence with congenital hypoparathyroidism. *Birth Defects* 1968:4:116.

33. Peden VH: True idiopathic hypoparathyroidism as a sex-linked recessive trait. *Am J Hum Genet* 1960; 12:323.

34. Blizzard RM, Gibbs JH: Candidiasis: Studies pertaining to its association with endocrinopathies and pernicious anemia. *Pediatrics* 1968; 42:231.

35. Carson RJ, Schubert WK, Partin JC: Idiopathic hypoparathyroidism, magnesium deficiency, and steatorrhea. *(Abstract) J Pediatr* 1973; 83:150.

36. Lee JB, et al: Familial pseudohypoparathyroidism. *N Engl J Med* 1968; 279:1179.

37. Drezner M, Neelon F, Lebovitz HE: Pseudohypoparathyroidism Type II. A possible defect in the reception of the cyclic AMP signal. *N Engl J Med* 1973; 289:1056.

38. Singleton EB, Tent CT: Pseudohypoparathyroidism with bone changes simulating hyperparathyroidism. *Radiology* 1962; 78:388.

39. Mallette LE, et al: Synthetic human parathyroid hormone-(1-34) for the study of pseudohypoparathyroidism. *J Clin Endocrinol Metab* 1988; 67:964.

40. Avioli LV: The therapeutic approach to hypoparathyroidism. *Am J Med* 1974; 57:34.

41. Aksnes L, Aarskog D: Vitamin D metabolites in serum from hypoparathyroid patients treated with vitamin D_2 and 1 α-hydroxyvitamin D_3. *J Clin Endocrinol Metab* 1980; 51:823.

42. Suster P, Paala JV: Pseudo vitamin D-deficiency rickets. *J Pediatr* 1970; 76:937.

43. Arnaud C, et al: Vitamin D deficiency: An inherited postnatal syndrome with secondary hyperparathyroidism. *Pediatrics* 1970; 46:871.

44. Tsuchiya Y, et al: An unusual form of vitamin D-dependent rickets in a child: Alopecia and marked end-organ hyposensitivity to biologically active vitamin D. *J Clin Endocrinol Metab* 1980; 51:685.

45. Lifshitz F, MacLaren NK: Vitamin D-dependent rickets in institutionalized, mentally retarded children receiving long-term anticonvulsant therapy. I: A survey of 288 patients. *J Pediatr* 1973; 83:612.

46. Hunt PA, et al: Bone disease induced by anticonvulsant therapy and treatment with calcitriol (1,25-dihydroxyvitamin D_3). *Am J Dis Child* 1986; 140:715.

47. Takeda E, et al: 1α-hydroxyvitamin D_3 treatment of three patients with 1,25-dihydroxyvitamin D-receptor-defect rickets and alopecia. *Pediatrics* 1987; 80:97.

48. Lewy JE, et al: Serum parathyroid hormone in hypophosphatemic vitamin D-resistant rickets. *J Pediatr* 1972; 81:294.

49. Hirschman GH, DeLuca HF, Chan JCM: Hypophosphatemic vitamin D-resistant rickets: Metabolic balance studies in a child receiving 1,25-dihydroxy-vitamin D_3, phosphate, and ascorbic acid. *Pediatrics* 1978; 61:451.

50. Chesny RW, et al: Supranormal 25-hydroxyvitamin D and subnormal 1,25-dihydroxyvitamin D: Their role in X-linked hypophosphatemic rickets. *Am J Dis Child* 1980; 134:140.

51. McEnery RT, Luerman FNS, West CD: Acceleration of growth with combined vitamin D-phosphate therapy of hypophosphatemic resistant rickets. *J Pediatr* 1972; 80:763.

52. Glorieux FH, et al: Use of phosphate and vitamin D to prevent dwarfism and rickets in X-linked hypophosphatemia. *N Engl J Med* 1972; 287:481.

53. Scriver CR: Familial hypophosphatemia. The dilemma of treatment. *N Engl J Med* 1973; 289:531.

54. Chan CM, Lovinger RD, Mamunes P: Renal hypophosphatemic rickets: Growth acceleration after long-term treatment with 1,25-dihydroxyvitamin D_3. *Pediatrics* 1980; 66:445.

55. Lovinger RD: Rickets. *Pediatrics* 1980; 66:359.

56. Stickler GB, Jowsey J, Bianco AJ: Possible detrimental effect of large doses of vitamin D in familial hypophosphatemic vitamin D-resistant rickets. *Pediatrics* 1971; 79:68.

57. Dent CE, Friedman M: Idiopathic juvenile osteoporosis. *Q J Med* 1965; 34:177.

58. McRae WM, Sweet EM: Diagnosis of osteoporosis in childhood. *Br J Radiol* 1965; 40:104.

59. Gooding CA, Ball JH: Idiopathic juvenile osteoporosis. *Radiology* 1969; 93:1349.

60. Paunier L, et al: Primary hypomagnesemia with secondary hypocalcemia in an infant. *Pediatrics* 1968; 41:385.

61. Suh SM, Csina A, Fraser D: Pathogenesis of hypocalcemia in magnesium depletion: Normal end organ responsiveness to parathyroid hormone. *J Clin Invest* 1971; 50:2668.

62. Suh SM, et al: Pathogenesis of hypocalcemia in primary hypomagnesemia: Normal end organ responsiveness to parathyroid hormone, impaired parathyroid gland function. *J Clin Invest* 1973; 52:153.

63. Levine BS, Coburn JW: Magnesium, the mimic/antagonist of calcium. *N Engl J Med* 1984; 310:1253.

64. Carey DE, Rowe JC: Metabolic bone disease in premature infants. *Pediatr Ann* 1987; 16:947.

65. Elias EG, Reynoso G, Mittelman A: Control of hypercalcemia with mithramycin. *Ann Surg* 1972; 175:431.

66. Daum F, Rosen JF, Boley SJ: Parathyroid adenoma, parathyroid crisis, and acute pancreatitis in an adolescent. *J Pediatr* 1973; 83:275.

67. Avioli LV: Primary hyperparathyroidism: Recognition and management. *Hosp Prac* September 30, 1987, p 69.

68. Marx SJ: New insights into primary hyperparathyroidism. *Hosp Prac* March, 1984, p 55.

69. Genant HK, et al: Primary hyperparathyroidism. *Radiology* 1973; 109:513.

70. Reiss E, Canterbury JM: Spectrum of hyperparathyroidism. *Am J Med* 1974; 56:794.

71. Allen DB, Friedman AL, Hendricks SA: Asymptomatic primary hyperparathyroidism in children. Newer methods of preoperative diagnosis. *Am J Dis Child* 1986; 140:819.

72. Purnell DC, et al: Treatment of primary hyperparathyroidism. *Am J Med* 1974; 56:800.

73. Mannix H: Primary hyperparathyroidism in children. *Am J Surg* 1975; 129:528.

74. Marx SJ, et al: Familial hypocalciuric hypercalcemia. The relation to primary parathyroid hyperplasia. *N Engl J Med* 1982; 307:416.

75. Marx SJ, et al: An association between neonatal severe primary hyperparathyroidism and familial hypocalciuric hypercalcemia in three kindreds. *N Engl J Med* 1982; 306:257.

76. Page LA, Haddow JE: Self-limited neonatal hyperparathyroidism in familial hypocalciuric hypercalcemia. *J Pediatr* 1987; 111:261.

77. Wiltse HE, et al: Infantile hypercalcemia syndrome in twins. *N Engl J Med* 1966; 275:1157.

78. Morris CA, et al: Natural history of Williams syndrome: Physical characteristics. *J Pediatr* 1988; 113:318.

79. Lawrence GD, et al: Immobilization hypercalcemia. *J Bone Joint Surg [Am]* 1973; 55:87.

80. Stewart AF, et al: Calcium homeostasis in immobilization: An example of resorptive hypercalciuria. *N Engl J Med* 1982; 306:1136.

12

Diabetes Insipidus and Inappropriate Antidiuretic Hormone Secretion

DIABETES INSIPIDUS

In a healthy individual, urine volume is controlled by vasopressin (antidiuretic hormone, ADH), a relatively simple octapeptide that is easily synthesized. It is produced primarily in the supraoptic nuclei of the hypothalamus, but is transported by way of axons to the posterior pituitary (neurohypophysis), where it is stored. It is released in response to decreased extracellular fluid and increased plasma osmolality, the latter being most important.[1] The net effect of vasopressin is to retain fluid. This is achieved by altering the permeability of the distal renal tubule, which results in reabsorption of the relatively hypotonic fluid in this portion of the nephron. The effect is mediated through increased production of cyclic adenosine monophosphate (cAMP); administration of this nucleotide will mimic some of the actions of vasopressin.

True diabetes insipidus (DI, central or neurogenic) is a result of a deficiency of vasopressin, but similar clinical findings may be caused by insensitivity of the renal tubule to the action of ADH (nephrogenic DI) or compulsive water drinking (psychogenic DI).

264

Diabetes Insipidus Due to Vasopressin Deficiency

Vasopressin-deficient DI may occur at any age. A frequent cause is a tumor of the central nervous system (CNS); often a craniopharyngioma.[2, 3] In these patients evidence of anterior pituitary dysfunction sometimes is present. In addition, DI may follow surgical procedures for removal of tumors in the hypothalamic-pituitary area. Less frequently, DI is due to histiocytosis X, head trauma,[4] or congenital malformations of the CNS. Rarely, DI occurs in children with meningitis,[5, 6] encephalitis, or leukemia.[7] Transient DI in the newborn period has been reported in association with listeriosis, disseminated intravascular coagulation,[8] and intraventricular hemorrhage.[9] In a significant number of patients, DI is idiopathic, indicating that no cause can be demonstrated by available diagnostic techniques. Undetected tumors may be present in some of these patients. Anterior pituitary abnormalities may also occur in association with idiopathic DI. In one series, six of 17 patients followed up to 26 years eventually developed growth hormone deficiency.[10]

Vasopressin-deficient DI usually occurs sporadically, but rare familial cases have been reported.[11, 12] Two modes of inheritance have been postulated: autosomal dominant and sex-linked.[13]

The signs of vasopressin deficiency, polyuria and polydipsia, often occur abruptly. Patients frequently show a preference for ice water. Urine is colorless. Children with idiopathic DI have no other complaints. Headache, vomiting, and visual disturbance suggest the presence of a CNS tumor. Congenital CNS malformations causing DI sometimes are associated with blindness, aplasia of the olfactory tracts, midline facial defects, and/or varying degrees of pituitary dysfunction (septo-optic dysplasia).

The laboratory investigation and treatment of DI will be discussed later.

Nephrogenic Diabetes Insipidus

Nephrogenic DI is a congenital condition in which a concentration defect may be manifested in the first few weeks of life, although the problem may escape detection until the patient has been toilet trained. The mode of inheritance is controversial; there is evidence for X-linked transmission[13, 14] with variable defects in heterozygote females,[14] but autosomal dominance with incomplete penetrance in girls has been proposed.[15, 16] The disease is a result of renal unresponsiveness to vasopressin. It has been shown that urinary cAMP in these patients fails to rise in response to ADH stimulation.[17] However, in a subsequent study, administration of cAMP to children with nephrogenic DI did not cause an antidiuretic effect, suggesting that the defect is located beyond this step.[18]

Patients with nephrogenic DI who retain modest concentrating ability may have a reduced glomerular filtration rate rather than partial responsiveness to ADH.[19] There have been reports of transient nephrogenic DI during administration of demeclocycline (Declomycin)[20] and following transplacental lithium intoxication.[21]

As in ADH-deficient DI, polyuria and polydipsia are the cardinal features of nephrogenic DI. However, because of the occurrence of this condition in infancy, secondary signs of water loss are more prominent. These include irritability, fevers without apparent infection, and failure to thrive. There often is a preference for water instead of milk. The infants are prone to episodes of hypertonic dehydration, with possible convulsions, brain damage, and death. Vasopressin insensitivity usually is an isolated defect initially, but renal insufficiency may occur in later childhood, presumably secondary to previous episodes of dehydration.

Psychogenic Diabetes Insipidus

Psychogenic DI appears to be less common in children as a cause of polyuria than either ADH-deficient or nephrogenic DI. It may occur at any age during childhood, but is rare in infancy. Onset is typically more gradual than in the other forms of DI, and the preference for ice water over other liquids is not a feature of this condition.

Diagnosis

Some form of DI is suspected in any child with polyuria (excretion >30 mL/kg/day) and polydipsia who excretes a dilute urine (<250 mOsm/kg). Serum sodium and osmolality may be increased. The differential diagnosis includes hypercalcemia and other renal tubular disorders. Hypernatremia may occur in the presence of adequate ADH reserve, as a result of an abnormal thirst mechanism and impaired osmotic regulation of ADH release[22, 23] ("essential" hypernatremia), with or without structural abnormalities.[24, 25] Instances of diabetes mellitus and DI in the same patient have been reported.[26]

Onset of polyuria (without glucosuria) in infancy and a positive family history is consistent with nephrogenic DI. Rapid onset during childhood suggests ADH deficiency. Gradual appearance of symptoms favors compulsive water drinking.

Initially, a water deprivation test should be performed (this and other tests for DI are described in the appendix to this chapter). In children with ADH-deficient or nephrogenic DI, urinary specific gravity usually remains below 1.005 and osmolality less than 150 mOsm/kg. There also should be evidence of increased serum tonicity: sodium greater than 150 mEq/L or osmolality greater than 290 mOsm/kg. (In fact, random serum osmolalities may be of predictive value, tending to be low in psychogenic DI and high in the other two types.) Failure of urinary output to decrease appreciably and an associated weight loss approaching 5% during the deprivation test also are consistent with nephrogenic or ADH-deficient DI. The test should be terminated if weight loss exceeds 5%.

Healthy individuals and compulsive water drinkers should achieve a urinary specific gravity of at least 1.010, and often higher, during the deprivation test. Urinary output should decrease, and significant weight loss does not occur. The ratio of urine:plasma osmolality will be at least 2.[27]

In a few cases the deprivation test results in an intermediate response that is difficult to interpret. This may occur in partial ADH-deficient[28] or nephrogenic DI. Likewise, children with primary polydipsia of long standing may fail to respond fully. A test to differentiate partial from complete ADH deficiency involves water deprivation followed by administration of ADH.[28, 29] The reader is referred to the reports of Miller et al. for details.[28, 29]

Patients who fail to respond normally to water deprivation should be given a diagnostic trial of aqueous vasopressin (Pitressin). Children with nephrogenic DI respond minimally or not at all, whereas those with ADH deficiency should be able to concentrate their urine to a specific gravity of at least 1.010 and usually greater. If the response to vasopressin is marginal, the test should be repeated with a double dose (see Appendix 12). As an alternative to aqueous vasopressin, intranasal DDAVP (a synthetic vasopressin analogue, 1-deamino-8-D-arginine vasopressin; desmopressin) can be substituted; Hendricks et al. recommend that it be used at the conclusion of the water deprivation test[30] (see Appendix 12).

Sensitive assays for vasopressin have been developed and tested under various conditions[31]; these are useful adjuncts, but are not totally reliable for the diagnosis of DI when used alone.

In children with ADH-deficient DI, careful funduscopic, neurologic, and visual field examination (if age permits), in addition to computed tomographic brain scans or magnetic resonance imaging, are essential to rule out a brain tumor. Close follow-up is important.

Treatment

A major advance in recent years has been the availability of DDAVP.[32-34] This preparation is administered intranasally and requires that the patient (or parent) blow the solution into the nose through a plastic tube. Two doses per day are often sufficient, but response varies. Side effects (usually headache) are infrequent. Suggested dose is 5 to 30 μg (0.05 to 0.3 mL) daily for children 3 months to 12 years of age. Older children and adults may require up to 40 μg (0.4 mL) daily; average adult dose is 10 μg (0.1 mL) twice a day.

This product has largely replaced the painful intramuscular injections of vasopressin tannate in oil or the 8-lysine vasopressin nasal spray[35, 36] (duration of action 3 to 6 hours) as the treatment of choice for central DI. Chlorpropamide (usually 150 to 400 mg/day in three doses) has been used successfully in patients with partial DI,[37-40] but significant hypoglycemia can occur[41]; those with associated anterior pituitary deficiency are at increased risk because of the lack of counterregulatory hormones.

Treatment of nephrogenic DI is not satisfactory. A low-sodium diet usually reduces urine volume to some degree. A trial of a thiazide derivative also is justified as an adjunct to sodium restriction. These drugs have a paradoxical antidiuretic action, which appears to be related to contraction of body fluid volume.[42] The suggested dose is 1 g/m²/day in three divided doses for chlorothiazide, and one-tenth this amount for hydrochlorothiazide. The thiazides are much less efficient than vasopressin in children with ADH-deficient DI.

A concise summary of ADH regulation and the therapy of DI has been written by Moses.[43]

SYNDROME OF INAPPROPRIATE ANTIDIURETIC HORMONE SECRETION

The syndrome of inappropriate antidiuretic hormone secretion (SIADH) was described by Schwartz et al. in 1957[44] and later by Barrter and Schwartz.[45] It is characterized by a concentrated urine associated with a hypotonic serum. In adults it sometimes occurs as a result of bronchogenic carcinoma; the tumor itself appears to secrete an antidiuretic substance. In infants and children, possible causes include a number of conditions involving the CNS: encephalitis, meningitis,[46] brain abscess or hemorrhage, hypoplastic corpus callosum,[47] and head trauma. Occasionally it is associated with abnormalities outside the CNS, such as pneumonia, cystic fibrosis,[48] or atelectasis,[49] but the etiologic relationship is not clear. Transient SIADH of several days' duration often follows DI after removal of midbrain tumors. In fact, most cases of SIADH in the pediatric age group are of limited duration if the primary illness is temporary.

Diagnosis

The diagnosis of SIADH is suspected in children with hyponatremia, hypochloremia, and persistent natriuresis in the absence of volume depletion. Serum osmolality is low. Urinary specific gravity usually is inappropriately high and the osmolality of the urine often exceeds that of the serum. However, it has been emphasized that a urine osmolality of only 100 mOsm/kg or more is compatible with SIADH when hyponatremia is present.[50] Serum potassium concentration typically is normal, but occasionally is low.

The aforementioned studies are generally adequate for presumptive diagnosis, although normal renal and adrenal function must be established. Hypoadrenalism is unlikely unless serum potassium is elevated. However, a serum cortisol determination and/or measurement of 24-hour urinary 17-hydroxysteroid excretion provide confirmatory information. If reasonable doubt still exists, further investigation of the hypothalamic-pituitary-adrenal axis is indicated (see Chapter 7).

Direct vasopressin measurements have not proved totally reliable in the diagnosis and usually serve only to confirm the clinical impression.[50] However, in a child with SIADH, Skowsky and Fisher[51] demonstrated a serum vasopressin concentration that was only minimally elevated but not suppressible by water loading. This case report is recommended for further discussion of SIADH and additional bibliography.

Treatment

The hyponatremia of SIADH generally responds poorly to infusion of saline or administration of mineralocorticoids. The simplest therapy is carefully monitored water restriction, which is the initial treatment of choice. There has also been some interest in the use of lithium carbonate,[52, 53] which blocks the action of ADH at the renal collecting tubules, in the management of recurrent SIADH. Likewise, it has been suggested that demeclocycline, which acts in a similar manner, may be superior to lithium.[54] The review of ADH excess by Friedman and Segar[55] is recommended for additional reading.

APPENDIX 12

Water Deprivation Test

After a 24-hour period of adequate hydration and stable weight, fluids are restricted for 7 hours. Urinary specific gravity and volume and body weight are measured hourly. Serum sodium and urine and serum osmolality are measured before and after the test. Hematocrit and blood urea nitrogen (BUN) also may be obtained at these times but are not critical. *Subjects must be carefully observed to assure that fluids are not ingested during the test.*

Interpretation

Specific gravity remains below 1.005 in patients with ADH-deficient or nephrogenic DI. Urine osmolality remains below 150 mOsm/kg, and there should be no significant reduction of urine volume. A weight loss up to 5% usually occurs. At the end of the test, a serum osmolality > 290 mOsm/kg, Na > 150 mEq/L, and a rise of BUN and hematocrit provide evidence that the patient did not receive water.

In healthy children and those with psychogenic DI, urinary specific gravity rises to at least 1.010 and usually greater. The urinary:plasma osmolality ratio exceeds 2. Urine volume decreases significantly, and there should be no appreciable weight loss. (See text for discussion of intermediate responses.)

Precautions

The test should be started in the morning to avoid the possibility of significant dehydration occurring unobserved during the night. The test should be terminated if weight loss approaches 5%.

The report of Frasier et al.[56] contains further details and discussion of the response to water deprivation.

Vasopressin Test

The test is preceded by a 24-hour control period during which intake, output, and urinary specific gravity are measured while the patient receives fluids ad lib. The bladder is then emptied and *aqueous* vasopressin is administered, 0.3 mL/m² subcutaneously. (Note that aqueous vasopressin contains 20 U/mL, whereas vasopressin tannate in oil contains 5 U/mL.) Intake is monitored, and urinary output and specific gravity are determined every 30 to 60 minutes. A response should occur in 4 to 6 hours. If there is no effect after 6 hours, the test is repeated using 0.6 mL/m².

Interpretation

Patients with ADH-deficient DI concentrate their urine (to 1.010 and usually greater) and also demonstrate a reduction of urine volume and decreased fluid intake. Patients with nephrogenic DI have no significant change in intake, urine volume, or specific gravity. Constant intake associated with decreased output and increased specific gravity suggests psychogenic DI.

Precautions

Temporary water intoxication is a possible, but infrequent, complication of vasopressin administration in patients with a positive response. This is particularly true of compulsive water drinkers if they continue to drink excessively as urine flow decreases; however, this test presumably would not be performed in these children, since they should have responded normally to water deprivation.

DDAVP Test

DDAVP (10 μg in infants and 20 μg in children) is administered intranasally, preferably at the termination of the water deprivation test. Urine is then monitored hourly for specific gravity for 4 hours. If specific gravity reaches 1.014 during this period, the test can be terminated. Otherwise, urine (U) and serum (S) osmolalities are obtained after 4 hours: a U/S ratio >1.5 or final urine osmolality ≥ 450 mOsm is considered a positive response. The reader is referred to the original report for a more detailed discussion of the method and interpretation of this test.[30]

•   •   •

Additional useful information on the diagnosis of DI can be found in the 1985 article by Robertson.[57]

REFERENCES

1. Robertson GL, Athar S: The interaction of blood osmolality and blood volume in regulating plasma vasopressin in man. *J Clin Endocrinol Metab* 1976; 42:613.
2. Thomas WC: Diabetes insipidus. *J Clin Endocrinol Metab* 1957; 17:565.
3. Blotner H: Primary or idiopathic diabetes insipidus, a system disease. *Metabolism* 1958; 7:191.
4. Paxson CL, Jr, Brown DR: Post-traumatic anterior hypopituitarism. *Pediatrics* 1976; 57:893.
5. Pai K, et al: Hypothalamic-pituitary dysfunction following group B beta hemolytic streptococcal meningitis in a neonate. *J Pediatr* 1976; 88:289.
6. Lam A, et al: Transient diabetes insipidus as a complication of haemophilus meningitis. *Pediatrics* 1978; 61:785.

7. Bergman GE, et al: Diabetes insipidus as a presenting manifestation of acute myelogenous leukemia. *J Pediatr* 1976; 88:355.

8. Fenton LJ, Kleinman LI: Transient diabetes insipidus in a newborn infant. *J Pediatr* 1974; 85:79.

9. Adams JM, et al: Central diabetes insipidus following intraventricular hemorrhage. *J Pediatr* 1976; 88:292.

10. Czernichow P, et al: Diabetes insipidus in children. III: Anterior pituitary dysfunction in idiopathic types. *J Pediatr* 1985; 106:41.

11. Forssman H: Two different mutations of the X-chromosome causing diabetes insipidus. *Am J Hum Genet* 1955; 7:21.

12. Martin F I R: Familial diabetes insipidus. *Q J Med* 1959; 28:573.

13. Forssman H: On hereditary diabetes insipidus. With special reference to a sex-linked form. *Acta Med Scand* 1945; 159(suppl):1.

14. Carter C, Simpkiss M: The "carrier state" in nephrogenic diabetes insipidus. *Lancet* 1956; 2:1069.

15. Cannon JF: Diabetes insipidus: Clinical and experimental studies with consideration of genetic relationships. *Arch Intern Med* 1955; 96:215.

16. Robinson MC, Kaplan SA: Inheritance of vasopressin resistant ("Nephrogenic") diabetes insipidus. *Am J Dis Child* 1960; 99:164.

17. Fichman MP, Brooker G: Deficient renal cyclic adenosine 3'-5' monophosphate production in nephrogenic diabetes insipidus. *J Clin Endocrinol Metab* 1972; 35:35.

18. Proesmans W, et al: The effect of exogenous 3'-5'-adenosine monophosphate on urinary output in children with vasopressin-resistant diabetes insipidus. *Pediatr Res* 1975; 9:509.

19. McConnell RF, Jr, et al: The mechanism of urinary concentration in nephrogenic diabetes insipidus. *Pediatr Res* 1977; 11:33.

20. London AL, et al: Nephrogenic diabetes insipidus due to demethylchlortetracycline hydrochloride in a child. *Pediatrics* 1978; 61:91.

21. Mizrahi EM, et al: Nephrogenic diabetes insipidus in transplacental lithium intoxication. *J Pediatr* 1979; 94:493.

22. Conley SB, et al: Recurrent hypernatremia: a proposed mechanism in a patient with absence of thirst and abnormal excretion of water. *J Pediatr* 1976; 89:898.

23. DeRubertis FR, et al: "Essential" hypernatremia. *Arch Intern Med* 1974; 134:889.

24. Schaff-Blass E, Robertson GL, Rosenfield RL: Chronic hypernatremia from a congenital defect in osmoregulation of thirst and vasopressin. *J Pediatr* 1983; 102:703.

25. Hayek A, Peake GT: Hypothalamic adipsia without demonstrable structural lesion. *Pediatrics* 1982; 70:275.

26. Gossain VV, et al: Co-existent diabetes mellitus and diabetes insipidus, a familial disease. *J Clin Endocrinol Metab* 1975; 41:1020.

27. Utiger R: Therapeutic grand rounds: Diabetes insipidus. *JAMA* 1969; 207:1699.

28. Miller M, et al: Recognition of partial defects in antidiuretic hormone secretion. *Ann Intern Med* 1970; 73:721.

29. Miller M, Moses AM: Mechanism of chlorpropamide action in diabetes insipidus. *J Clin Endocrinol Metab* 1970; 30:488.

30. Hendricks SA, et al: Differential diagnosis of diabetes insipidus: Use of DDAVP to terminate the 7-hour water deprivation test. *J Pediatr* 1981; 98:244.

31. Robertson GL, et al: Development and clinical application of a new method for the radioimmunoassay of arginine vasopressin in human plasma. *J Clin Invest* 1973; 52:2340.

32. Lee W-NP, et al: Vasopressin analog DDAVP in the treatment of diabetes insipidus. *Am J Dis Child* 1976; 130:166.

33. Seif SM, et al: DDAVP (1-desamino-8-D-arginine-vasopressin) treatment of central diabetes insipidus — mechanism of prolonged antidiuresis. *J Clin Endocrinol Metab* 1978; 46:381.
34. Cobb WE, et al: Neurogenic diabetes insipidus: management with dDAVP (1-desamino-8-D arginine vasopressin). *Ann Intern Med* 1978; 88:183.
35. Moses AM: Synthetic lysine vasopressin nasal spray in the treatment of diabetes insipidus. *Clin Pharmacol Ther* 1964; 5:422.
36. Dingman JF, Hauger-Klevene JH: Treatment of diabetes insipidus: Synthetic lysine vasopressin nasal solution. *J Clin Endocrinol Metab* 1964; 24:550.
37. Vallet HL, et al: Chlorpropamide treatment of diabetes insipidus in children. *Pediatrics* 1970; 45:246.
38. Ehrlich RM, Kooh SW: The use of chlorpropamide in diabetes insipidus in children. *Pediatrics* 1970; 45:236.
39. Webster B, Bain J: Antidiuretic effect and complications of chlorpropamide therapy in diabetes insipidus. *J Clin Endocrinol Metab* 1970; 30:215.
40. Ettinger B, Forsham PH: Mechanism of chlorpropamide antidiuresis in diabetes insipidus. *J Clin Endocrinol Metab* 1970; 31:552.
41. Kuhns LR, et al: Chlorpropamide-induced hypoglycemia in a child with diabetes insipidus. *JAMA* 1969; 210:907.
42. Ramos G, et al: Mechanism of the antidiuretic effect of saluretic drugs. Studies in patients with diabetes insipidus. *Clin Pharmacol Ther* 1967; 8:557.
43. Moses A: Diabetes insipidus and ADH regulation. *Hosp Pract* July 1977, p 37.
44. Schwartz WB, et al: A syndrome of renal sodium loss and hyponatremia probably resulting from inappropriate secretion of antidiuretic hormone. *Am J Med* 1957; 23:529.
45. Barrter FC, Schwartz WB: The syndrome of inappropriate secretion of antidiuretic hormone. *Am J Med* 1972; 42:790.
46. Kaplan SL, Feigin RD: The syndrome of inappropriate secretion of antidiuretic hormone in children with bacterial meningitis. *J Pediatr* 1978; 92:758.
47. Fyhrquist F, et al: Inappropriate secretion of antidiuretic hormone, hypertension, and hypoplastic corpus callosum. *J Clin Endocrinol Metab* 1977; 45:691.
48. Cohen LF, et al: The syndrome of inappropriate antidiuretic hormone secretion as the cause of hyponatremia in cystic fibrosis. *J Pediatr* 1977; 90:574.
49. Paxson CL, et al: Syndrome of inappropriate antidiuretic hormone secretion in neonates with pneumothorax or atelectasis. *J Pediatr* 1977; 91:459.
50. Zerbe RL: Inappropriate antidiuretic hormone secretion. *Hosp Med* January 1984 p 241.
51. Skowsky WR, Fisher DA: Intermittent, idiopathic, inappropriate vasopressin secretion in a child. *J Pediatr* 1973; 83:62.
52. White MG, Fetner CD: Treatment of the syndrome of inappropriate secretion of antidiuretic hormone with lithium carbonate. *N Engl J Med* 1975; 292:390.
53. Baker RS, et al: Treatment of recurrent syndrome of inappropriate secretion of antidiuretic hormone with lithium. *J Pediatr* 1977; 90:480.
54. Forrest JN, Jr, et al: Superiority of demeclocycline over lithium in the treatment of chronic syndrome of inappropriate secretion of antidiuretic hormone. *N Engl J Med* 1978; 298:173.
55. Friedman AL, Segar WE: Antidiuretic hormone excess. *J Pediatr* 1979; 94:521.
56. Frasier SD, et al: A water deprivation test for the diagnosis of diabetes insipidus in children. *Am J Dis Child* 1967; 114:157.
57. Robertson GL: Diagnosis of diabetes insipidus. *Front Horm Res* 1985; 13:176.

Index